Serono Symposia USA
Norwell, Massachusetts

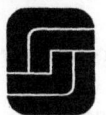

Springer Science+Business Media, LLC

PROCEEDINGS IN THE SERONO SYMPOSIA USA SERIES

Continued after Index

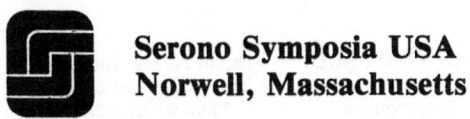

Serono Symposia USA
Norwell, Massachusetts

Thomas R. Ziegler   Glenn F. Pierce
David N. Herndon

Editors

Growth Factors and Wound Healing

Basic Science and Potential Clinical Applications

With 61 Figures

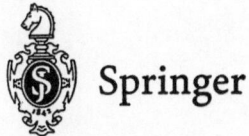

Springer

Thomas R. Ziegler, M.D.
Department of Medicine
Emory University
  School of Medicine
Atlanta, GA 30322
USA

Glenn F. Pierce, Ph.D., M.D.
Department of
  Preclinical Development
PRIZM Pharmaceuticals
San Diego, CA 92121
USA

David N. Herndon, M.D.
The University of Texas
  Medical Branch
Shriners Burns Institute
Galveston, TX 77550
USA

Proceedings of the International Symposium on Growth Factors and Wound Healing: Basic Science and Potential Clinical Applications, sponsored by Serono Symposia USA, Inc., held September 28 to October 1, 1995, in Boston, Massachusetts.

For information on previous volumes, contact Serono Symposia USA, Inc.

Library of Congress Cataloging-in-Publication Data

Growth factors and wound healing: basic science and potential
  clinical applications/Thomas R. Ziegler, Glenn F. Pierce, David N.
  Herndon, editors.
       p. cm.
     "Proceedings of the International Symposium on Growth Factors and
  Wound Healing: Basic Science and Potential Clinical Applications,
  sponsored by Serono Symposia USA, Inc., held September 28 to October
  1, 1995, in Boston, Massachusetts"—T.p. verso.
     Includes indexes.
     ISBN 978-1-4612-7321-9   ISBN 978-1-4612-1876-0 (eBook)
     DOI 10.1007/978-1-4612-1876-0
     1. Wound healing—Congresses.   2. Growth factors—Congresses.
  I. Ziegler, Thomas R. (Thomas Ralph), 1955-   . II. Pierce, Glenn
  F.
     [DNLM: 1. Wound Healing—physiology—congresses.   2. Wounds and
  Injuries—therapy—congresses.   3. Growth Substances—physiology—
  congresses.   4. Growth Substances—therapeutic use—congresses.
  WO 185 G884 1997]
  RD94.G76 1997
  617.1'4—DC21   97-9561

Printed on acid-free paper.

Production coordinated by Chernow Editorial Services, Inc., and managed by Francine McNeill; manufacturing supervised by Johanna Tschebull.
Typeset by TechType, Inc., Ramsey, NJ.

9 8 7 6 5 4 3 2 1

ISBN 978-1-4612-7321-9

INTERNATIONAL SYMPOSIUM ON GROWTH FACTORS AND WOUND HEALING: BASIC SCIENCE AND POTENTIAL CLINICAL APPLICATIONS

Scientific Committee

Thomas R. Ziegler, M.D., Chair
Emory University School of Medicine
Atlanta, Georgia

Glenn F. Pierce, Ph.D., M.D., Co-Chair
PRIZM Pharmaceuticals
San Diego, California

David N. Herndon, M.D., Co-Chair
The University of Texas Medical Branch
Shriners Burns Institute
Galveston, Texas

Organizing Secretary

Leslie Nies
Serono Symposia USA, Inc.
100 Longwater Circle
Norwell, Massachusetts

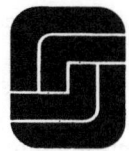

Preface

The biology of wound healing and tissue repair are increasingly being defined. At the same time, the availability of recombinant peptide growth factors for clinical investigation has prompted numerous trials of growth factor administration as adjunctive therapy to enhance the rate and quality of acute and chronic wound repair. New basic science information on growth factor function and regulation obtained in the research laboratory is actively being applied in animal studies and in clinical research settings. In addition to studies of surface wounds, an increasing number of investigations on growth factor administration have focused on healing and repair in nondermal tissues such as the intestinal tract and other organs.

While the amount of new information on the molecular biology of growth factor expression, signaling, and function has been exponential in recent years, results of many clinical trials on growth factor administration in wound healing have been disappointing. This may be due, in part, to the heterogeneity of clinical wounds and the patients who harbor them, less than adequate standardization of care in experimental and control groups, issues related to drug dosing, and inadequate control for important issues relevant to healing such as nutrient intake and underlying nutritional status. Nonetheless, several clinical trials of recombinant growth factor administration in human wound healing have been positive and numerous additional trials are in progress. In addition, growth factors are being investigated as adjunctive anabolic therapy in settings as diverse as short bowel syndrome, severe catabolic illness, and wasting syndromes.

This book contains the proceedings from the International Symposium on Growth Factors and Wound Healing: Basic Science and Potential Clinical Applications, held September 28 to October 1, 1995, in Boston, Massachusetts. The meeting drew a large and diverse group of individuals from the basic and clinical research community, as well as a number of industry representatives, from around the world. The symposium was convened to provide an overview of basic science studies, animal experiments, and clinical trials defining the potential clinical applications of recombinant growth factors in wound healing and tissue repair. The meeting was designed to include presentations covering pure basic science aspects of growth factor biology, including molecular mechanisms of action, interactions and tissue-specific effects, and the results of recent clinical trials on growth factor administration in wound healing and catabolic states. The symposium also included several presentations on the role of nutritional status, specific nutrients, and the interactions of nutrients with growth factors in healing, topics that have been little covered in previous wound healing symposia. Several interesting posters highlighting new work were also presented by the symposium participants.

This volume begins with an overview of general concepts relevant to wound healing. Wound healing biology and angiogenesis are discussed, as is regulation of important peptides such as fibroblast growth factor and the growth hormone/insulin-like growth factor (GH/IGF) axis. New information on the use of cultured skin cells and other novel products for wound closure is also covered. This information provides a basis for subsequent sections on the role of nutrients in wound healing responses and endogenous growth factors in wound healing. The discussions on nutrient–growth factor interactions support the concept that both underlying nutritional status and exogenous administration of specific nutrients such as zinc, vitamin A, arginine, and glutamine are important for optimal tissue repair under certain conditions. The section on endogenous growth factors highlights the important molecular biology of growth factor expression and signaling in wound healing.

Because of the great number of studies now published on clinical applications of GH and IGF-I therapy in catabolic states and tissue healing, a section is devoted to covering important clinical trials and animal studies using these agents. Specific presentations were made on GH therapy in burn injury, GH effects in experimental colonic healing and repair, use of GH in the postoperative setting and other catabolic states, and the modulation of IGF-I therapy with IGF binding protein-3. The final section focuses on potential clinical applications of other peptide growth factors, including keratinocyte growth factor (KGF), hepatocyte growth factor (HGF), and vascular endothelial growth factor (VEGF). The presentations include state-of-the-art information on KGF, HGF, and VEGF molecular biology, and the relevance of these factors in cell function and healing of specific tissues, such as the gut, wounds, and optic tissue. The final chapter, from the Food and Drug Administration, discusses important governmental regulatory concerns for wound healing biologics.

The editors thank the attendees and poster presenters for their outstanding contributions to the symposium and for the lively and informative discussions. We are particularly grateful for the help of Leslie Nies and her outstanding staff for their assistance with the organization of the meeting and the publication of these proceedings. We are also thankful for the provision of travel funds to young investigators and for the staff's help and patience throughout the editorial process of this book. Finally, we thank the contributors to this volume and hope that its publication will spur research in the area of growth factors and wound healing biology.

THOMAS R. ZIEGLER
GLENN F. PIERCE
DAVID N. HERNDON

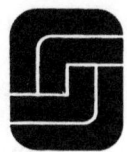

Contents

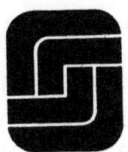

Contributors

DAVID H. ADAMS, Liver Labs, Clinical Teaching Block, Queen Elizabeth Hospital, Edgbaston, Birmingham, UK.

STEVEN ADAMS, Celtrix Pharmaceuticals, Santa Clara, California, USA.

JORGE E. ALBINA, Department of Surgery, Brown University and Rhode Island Hospital, Providence, Rhode Island, USA.

WES J. ARLEIN, Department of Surgery, University of Minnesota, Minneapolis, Minnesota, USA.

SHARON LEA AUKERMAN, PRIZM Pharmaceuticals, San Diego, California, USA.

ANDREW BAIRD, PRIZM Pharmaceuticals, San Diego, California, USA.

ADRIAN BARBUL, Department of Surgery, Sinai Hospital of Baltimore and the Johns Hopkins Medical Institutions, Baltimore, Maryland, USA.

ROBERT E. BARROW, Shriners Hospitals for Crippled Children, Burns Institute, Galveston, Texas, USA.

DONALD P. BOTTARO, Laboratory of Cellular and Molecular Biology, National Cancer Institute, National Institutes of Health, Bethesda, Maryland, USA.

FRANK BURSLEM, Pfizer Limited, Sandwich, Kent, UK.

MICHAEL D. CALDWELL, Department of Surgery and Biochemistry, University of Minnesota, Minneapolis, Minnesota, USA.

ANDREW M.-L. CHAN, Ruttenberg Cancer Center, Mount Sinai School of Medicine, New York, New York, USA.

HENRIK CHRISTENSEN, Surgical Department L, Aarhus University Hospital, and Department of Connective Tissue Biology, University of Aarhus, Aarhus, Denmark.

VITTORIA CIOCE, Laboratory of Biochemical Genetics, National Heart, Lung and Blood Institute, National Institutes of Health, Bethesda, Maryland, USA.

I. KELMAN COHEN, Division of Plastic and Reconstructive Surgery, Medical College of Virginia, Richmond, Virginia, USA.

PATRICIA A. D'AMORE, Laboratory for Surgical Research, Children's Hospital, Boston, Massachusetts, USA.

NAPOLEONE FERRARA, Department of Cardiovascular Research, Genentech, Inc., South San Francisco, California, USA.

JOHN L. GALLOWAY, Department of Surgery, Emory University School of Medicine, and Nutrition and Metabolic Support Service, Emory University Hospital, Atlanta, Georgia, USA.

JANE S. GIBSON, Orlando Regional Health Science Center, Orlando, Florida, USA.

DANIEL P. GRIFFITH, Nutrition and Metabolic Support Service, Emory University Hospital, Atlanta, Georgia, USA.

JOSÉ ANTONIO GUERRERO, University Department of Surgery, San Cecilio University Hospital, Granada, Spain.

JOHN F. HANSBROUGH, Department of Surgery, University of California, San Diego Medical Center, San Diego, California, USA.

DAVID N. HERNDON, The University of Texas Medical Branch, and Shriners Hospitals for Crippled Children, Burns Institute, Galveston, Texas, USA.

ARVIND Y. KRISHNA, Department of Medicine, Division of Endocrinology and Metabolism, Emory University School of Medicine, Atlanta, Georgia, USA.

CHRISTOPHER A. MAACK, Onyz Pharmaceuticals, Richmond, California, USA.

SHAWN P. MACAULEY, Department of Oral Biology, University of Florida, Gainesville, Florida, USA.

BRUCE A. MAST, Institute for Wound Research, Department of Surgery, Division of Plastic and Reconstructive Surgery, University of Florida, Gainesville, Florida, USA.

LYLE L. MOLDAWER, Institute for Wound Research, Department of Surgery, University of Florida, Gainesville, Florida, USA.

JEROME A. MOORE, Celtrix Pharmaceuticals, Santa Clara, California, USA.

DAVID M. ORNITZ, Department of Molecular Biology and Pharmacology, Washington University School of Medicine, St. Louis, Missouri, USA.

LAWRENCE S. PHILLIPS, Department of Medicine, Division of Endocrinology and Metabolism, Emory University School of Medicine, Atlanta, Georgia, USA.

GLENN F. PIERCE, PRIZM Pharmaceuticals, San Diego, California, USA.

EDGAR J. PIERRE, Shriners Hospitals for Crippled Children, Burns Institute, Galveston, Texas, USA.

ALAN B. PUCKETT, Nutrition and Metabolic Support Service, Emory University Hospital, Atlanta, Georgia, USA.

HANS OLIVER RENNEKAMPFF, Department of Surgery, University of California, San Diego Medical Center, San Diego, California, USA.

STEPHANIE ROHOVSKY, Laboratory for Surgical Research, Children's Hospital, Boston, Massachusetts, USA.

J. KEITH ROSE, Shriners Hospitals for Crippled Children, Burns Institute, Galveston, Texas, USA.

DAVID M. ROSEN, Celtrix Pharmaceuticals, Santa Clara, California, USA.

JEFFREY S. RUBIN, Laboratory of Cellular and Molecular Biology, National Cancer Institute, National Institutes of Health, Bethesda, Maryland, USA.

ESTRELLA RUIZ-REQUENA, University Department of Biochemistry, San Cecilio University Hospital, Granada, Spain.

MICHAEL R. SCHÄFFER, Department of Surgery, Chirurgische Klinik, Eberhard-Karls-Universität Tübingen, Tübingen, Germany.

GREGORY S. SCHULTZ, Institute for Wound Research, Department of Obstetrics and Gynecology, University of Florida, Gainesville, Florida, USA.

ANDREAS SOMMER, Celtrix Pharmaceuticals, Santa Clara, California, USA.

MICHAEL C. STACEY, Department of Surgery, Fremantle Hospital, Fremantle, Western Australia.

KARINA N. STOKES, Shriners Hospitals for Crippled Children, Burns Institute, Galveston, Texas, USA.

KURT STROMBERG, Center for Biologics Evaluation and Research, Food and Drug Administration, Bethesda, Maryland, USA.

ROY W. TARNUZZER, Institute for Wound Research, Department of Obstetrics and Gynecology, University of Florida, Gainesville, Florida, USA.

NAOMI TRENGROVE, Department of Surgery, Fremantle Hospital, Fremantle, Western Australia.

ANDERS E. ULLAND, Department of Surgery, University of Minnesota, Minneapolis, Minnesota, USA.

RAFAEL VARA-THORBECK, University Department of Surgery, San Cecilio University Hospital, Granada, Spain.

GABRIEL WAKSMAN, Department of Biochemistry, Washington University School of Medicine, St. Louis, Missouri, USA.

THOMAS R. ZIEGLER, Department of Medicine, Emory University School of Medicine, and Nutrition and Metabolic Support Service, Emory University Hospital, Atlanta, Georgia, USA.

Part I

General Concepts

1

An Overview of Wound Healing Biology

I. Kelman Cohen

This introductory chapter on growth factors and wound healing presents a brief summary of the biologic principles of wound healing and relates this information to the current status of growth factors in the modulation and control of tissue repair. I will add a few of my own philosophical observations as to the rather flamboyant, disjointed history of cytokines, wound healing, and industry during the past decade. Although I may be somewhat critical of the past, I will try to predict some of the exciting clinical advances with the use of cytokines we may expect in future decades.

For centuries, man has described new and better ways to promote healing of wounds. However, no one lotion, potion, or medication has ever been demonstrated to be superior to any other. Over the past decade, there has been a wave of excitement about the idea that cytokines will enhance the healing of chronic wounds. Although chronic wounds represent only a small segment of the potential for cytokines in the process of tissue repair, it is the chronic wound that has received the major focus of industrial research support. Industry reasoned that since chronic wounds represented a major health problem, development of drugs to heal these wounds would be very profitable. Many pharmaceutical companies jumped into clinical growth factor studies for the healing of chronic wounds without careful planning. Millions of dollars were wasted! Rather than careful preplanning ("Ready, aim, fire!") investigators and industry said, "Fire, ready, aim!" Rather than focus on the biology of the chronic wound environment, they rushed to dump cytokines into the "black box" of the open chronic wound. As one looks back at the disappointing results over the past decade, it is not surprising that industry is now somewhat gun-shy about putting money into this controversial area. However, most current clinical studies in this area have been designed well, and perhaps some efficacious results will now be found. My view is that efficacy of any cytokine will be limited until one understands and controls the basic biology of the chronic wound itself; the "black box" must be illuminated. The chapters in this book demonstrate

3

some of the ongoing efforts to do just this—define the biology of the chronic wound.

I have always been surprised that applied cytokine wound healing research has focused so much attention on the chronic wound. There are so many variables in any clinical study of chronic wound healing that results are always difficult to interpret and end points rather vague. This book touches on liver, gut, and the immune response, with some discussion of hard tissue healing (bone and cartilage). I believe that this latter area will be the most productive and lucrative areas for industry to support with research dollars.

Biology and Definitions of the Normal Healing Process

A basic understanding of tissue repair is required for an appreciation of the chapters in this book. A basic foundation of information on tissue repair can be found elsewhere (1-4).

Any type of tissue injury may result in regeneration, normal repair by scar formation, deficient healing, or excessive healing with overabundant matrix deposition. Mechanisms of repair include epitheliazation, contraction, and matrix deposition (mainly collagen). The nature of the tissue injury dictates the quantity of each repair mechanism necessary for healing. For example, a skin wound that is primarily closed heals mainly by matrix deposition from the suture coapted margins of tissue. The new collagen deposition at the margin of closure provides strength and integrity. Partial-thickness wounds heal by epitheliazation, while full-thickness open wounds heal mainly by contraction (with some epithelialization) as the wound margins are drawn together (1).

Wounds may also be divided into those that heal normally after injury, where there is an orderly and timely reparative process that results in sustained restoration of anatomical and functional integrity, and chronic wounds, which are the result of an underlying problem (3). Chronic wounds fail to proceed through an orderly and timely process to produce anatomical and function integrity, or they proceed through the repair process without establishing a sustained anatomical and functional result (3).

Normal healing is a finely orchestrated and overlapping sequence of events: coagulation, inflammation, fibroplasia, and remodeling (2). Cytokines are the messengers that mediate all the events of the healing process from the moment of injury until the final repair of the tissue. The cytokines from the coagulation process and throughout the inflammatory process [platelet-derived growth factor (PDGF), transforming growth factor-β (TGF-β), epidermal growth factor (EGF), basic fibroblast growth factor (bFGF) and many others] are major factors in repair (4). The role of these and other cytokines will become apparent as this book progresses. It is amazing to me how the role of inflammatory cytokines in the repair process was overlooked for so long. Equally amazing is that Cohnheim and Virchow predicted the presence of these messengers a century ago.

Growth factors, or cytokines, the subject of this book are a family of peptides that act on cells in a hormone-like fashion to regulate cell activity. They attach to specific cell membrane receptors and direct the cells intercellular activity. They can function in endocrine, paracrine autocrine, and intracrine fashion. They regulate cell migration, proliferation, matrix synthesis, and remodeling. These peptides gained the attention of tissue repair biologists and clinicians, leading to the hypothesis that the proper application of growth factors in wounds, sutures, and dressings, or growth factors systemically administered may promote the healing of chronic ulcers and accelerate the development of strength in the normal repair of acute wounds of skin, bone, tendon, and gut.

Among the most popular factors studied have been (a) TGF-β, which increases collagen accumulation by increasing collagen synthesis and decreasing collagen deposition and suppressing epithelial mitosis (5); (b) PDGF, which enhances collagen metabolism and is associated with the migration of fibroblasts and macrophages, and enhances chemotaxis, angiogenesis, and fibroblast proliferation (6, 7); (c) EGF, which increases both epitheliazation and fibroblast proliferation and angiogenesis (8, 9); and (d) bFGF, which is angiogenic, enhances epitheliazation and collagen deposition, and binds to a variety of heparin (10, 11).

There are several types of chronic wounds, each of which has a unique pathogenesis and responds in a specific fashion to different therapies. These include venous stasis ulcer, diabetic ulcers, vascular ulcers, pressures ulcers, drug-compromised wounds, and wounds resulting from malnutrition, radiation, and trauma (2).

Connective tissue matrix is "turning over" constantly, but under normal, healthy conditions the rate is slow. The rate of matrix metabolism is increased during the repair process. Matrix is composed mainly of collagen but also contains elastin, fibronectin, and various glycosoaminoglycans of which hyaluronic acid seems to be most important. Collagen is the most abundant protein in the body and a major component of skin, bone, tendon, and all supporting structures. Collagen is unique among proteins because it undergoes significant modification after initial synthesis and after being secreted from the cell where it is cross-linked, attaining the strength of steel on a per weight basis. There are several genetically distinct types of collagen that vary according to tissue source and age, and these collagens can be altered by various disease states. Collagen is normally degraded by a very specific enzyme, collagenase, which splits the collagen molecule at a specific amino acid site into three-quarter and one-quarter pieces.

Contraction is the process wherein wound edges are drawn together by inward movement of surrounding tissue. In contrast, a contracture is the pathologic result of excessive contraction. Briefly, this process appears to be performed by specialized fibroblasts that contain smooth muscle actin and have been termed *myofibroblasts*. The extracellular matrix is also thought to regulate the process of contraction. TGF-β also seems to stimulate contraction.

Clinically, several local and systemic factors can alter the healing process. These include tissue hypoxia, denervation, hematoma, infection, irradiation, mechanical forces, and dressing materials. Several general factors may be important as well, including age, drugs, infections, and malnutrition (12). Little is known as to how these conditions alter cytokine production and response.

Clinical Challenges

There are many areas in which cytokine therapy or inhibition of specific cytokines may be very important in tissue repair. In conditions of excessive scar formation, such as keloid, hypertrophic scar, and hepatic fibrosis, agents that block TGF-β receptor sites may have significant clinical usefulness. TGF-β enhances collagen deposition by increasing synthesis and inhibiting degradation, thereby leading to a net deposition of collagen, which is the end result in all the aforementioned disease process. If one could prevent TGF-β from stimulating particular cells, then these conditions may be controlled. Perhaps these agents and their antagonists could also help to prevent the formation of contractures. EGF and other epithelial stimulating growth factors should be helpful to the healing of partial thickness injuries. Although we have published work that EGF did not promote donor site healing in normal adult volunteers (1), it may very well be that various proteases in the wound site destroy the EGF before it has time to increase epithelial cell mitosis and migration.

References

1. Cohen IK, Diegelmann RF, Crossland MC. Wound healing and wound care. In: Schwartz SI, ed. Principles of surgery, 6th ed. New York: McGraw-Hill, 1994.
2. Cohen IK, Diegelmann RF, Lindblad WJ, eds. Wound healing: biochemical and clinical aspects. Philadelphia: W.B. Saunders, 1992.
3. Lazarus GS, Cooper DM, Knighton DR, Margolis DJ, Pecoraro RE, Rodeheaver G, et al. Definitions and guidelines for assessment of wounds and evaluation of healing. Arch Dermatol 1994;130:489–93.
4. McGee G, Davidson JM, Buckley A, et al. Recombinant basic fibroblast growth factor accelerates wound healing. J Surg Res 1988;45:145–53.
5. Roberts A. Transforming growth factor-β: activity and efficacy in animal models of wound healing. Wound Repair Regen 1995;3:408–18.
6. Mustoe TA, Pierce GF, Morishima C, et al. Growth factor-induced acceleration of tissue repair through direct and inductive activities in a rabbit dermal ulcer model. J Clin Invest 1991;87:694–703.

7. Lepisto J, Laato M, Miinikoski J, et al. Effects of homodimeric isoforms of platelet-derived growth factor (PDGF-AA and PDGF-BB) on wound healing in rat. J Surg Res 1992;53:596–601.
8. Franklin JD, Lynch JB. Effects of topical applications of epidermal growth factor on wound healing. Plast Reconstr Surg 1979;64:766–70.
9. Buckley A, Davidson JM, Kamerath CD, et al. Sustained release of epidermal growth factor accelerates wound repair. Proc Natl Acad Sci USA 1985; 82:7340–4.
10. Tsuboi R, Rifkin DB. Recombinant basic fibroblast growth factor stimulates wound healing in healing-impair db/db mice. J Exp Med 1990;172:245–51.
11. Kinsnorth AN, Vowles R, Nash JRG. Epidermal growth factor increases tensile strength in intestinal wounds in pigs. Br J Surg 1990;77:409–12.
12. Lawrence WT. Clinical management of nonhealing wounds. Wound healing: biochem clin aspects 1992;34–35.

2

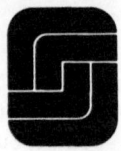

Growth Factors and Angiogenesis in Wound Healing

Stephanie Rohovsky and Patricia A. D'Amore

Several detailed reviews exist for this topic (1–3) and the mechanics of wound healing itself are mentioned in this chapter by way of introduction to regulators of angiogenesis and tissue repair.

Inflammation

Inflammation in wound healing can be divided into four major events: coagulation, fibrinolysis, neutrophil invasion, and macrophage recruitment. At the time of injury, the coagulation cascade is initiated, and clot formation ensues. Thrombin, which is activated by clotting, catalyzes the degradation of fibrinogen to fibrin, which binds to platelet surface receptors (for review see 4). Platelet adhesion to clot thus forms a thrombus. At the same time, platelets from injured blood vessels bind to surrounding collagen fibers (3). A platelet shape change ensues, leading to degranulation, which releases fibrinogen, fibronectin, von Willebrand factor, and thrombospondin. All of these factors promote additional platelet aggregation and thrombus formation (4). The thrombus then functions as a provisional matrix, not only for hemostasis, but also for subsequent cellular migration (5, 6).

Neutrophils migrate to the site of injury in response to signals from products of the coagulation cascade, activated complement products, and fibrin degradation products. Neutrophils clear wound bacteria by phagocytosis and intracellular lysis, and they debride the injured extracellular matrix through protease-mediated degradation (7). Macrophages, recruited from both circulating monocytes and resident tissue macrophages (8), are thought to be the main cell type responsible for the degradation of extracellular matrix. They debride a healing wound and phagocytose unused neutrophils at the site of injury (9). Macrophages release many substances, including reactive oxygen intermediates, prostaglandins, cytokines, growth factors [platelet-derived growth factor (PDGF), basic fibroblast growth factor (bFGF), transforming growth factor-β (TGF-β)], and chemoattractants for peripheral monocytes (for review see 11).

Tissue Formation

Approximately 12 hours after wounding, epithelial migration begins from the wound edges and proceeds inward (10). The dissolution of basement membrane at the site of injury allows the dermal-epidermal junction to loosen, facilitating epithelial cell migration (11) over a matrix of fibrin, fibronectin, and collagen (6, 8). Epithelial cells can also traverse desiccated tissue via activation of collagenases and plasminogen activators (12, 13).

After a few days, fibroblasts migrate from surrounding tissue matrix to the wound in response to growth factors and other chemotactic agents (8). During migration, they retract several intracellular organelles, form cytoplasmic actin condensations, and undergo a phenotypic change (14). They adopt the retractile properties and actin filaments characteristic of myofibroblasts, and they have been shown to contract in response to smooth muscle cell stimuli (15). Myofibroblasts, the most numerous cells in granulation tissue, are thought to be responsible for the wound contraction that occurs 4 days after injury. The signals for contraction have not yet been clearly defined, but they are hypothesized to be transmitted through intercellular channels that then trigger myofibroblast contractility (16). Contraction promotes orientation of a previously random matrix. As a wound matures, more collagen is deposited, cross-linked, and organized (for review see 17).

Angiogenesis begins at the same time as fibroblast migration and continues until the healing process is complete (18). It is thought that endothelial cells (ECs) in venules adjacent to wounded tissue initiate angiogenesis by projecting pseudopods across damaged basement membranes. Additionally, ECs are induced to produce matrix-degrading enzymes in response to various growth factors (17). In this way, endothelial cells traverse the perivascular space and form capillary sprouts (18, 19). After a hollow tube is formed, cell division occurs, and the sprouts go on to form capillary plexuses. Recruitment of smooth muscle cells and extracellular matrix allows formation of arterioles. The number of new vessels in experimental wounds has been shown to be highest at days 5 to 6 (20). New vessels function to regulate nutrient and cellular access to the provisional matrix. The mechanism of injury also impacts angiogenesis; the amount of debris and necrosis differ in crush injury, incisions, infarction, and ischemia (21).

Tissue Remodeling

Tissue remodeling is an ongoing process that continues after a wound has visibly healed the components of granulation tissue; components dynamically change (for review see 1), collagen becomes organized, the fibers become thicker, and cross-linking increases. The resulting scar eventually becomes acellular.

Regulators of Angiogenesis in Tissue Repair

A variety of factors have been postulated to contribute to the wound healing process (Table 2.1). Below we review the best studied of these as they relate to their role in angiogenesis.

Basic Fibroblast Growth Factor

Basic fibroblast growth factor (bFGF) is a member of a family of heparin-binding growth factors that has been implicated as an important mediator in wound healing. It exists as a single polypeptide in different molecular weight forms ranging from 18 to 25 kd, with the largest forms

TABLE 2.1. A partial listing of action of angiogenic factors in vivo and in vitro.

Factors	In vitro actions	In vivo actions in wound healing models
bFGF	Tube formation in 3D collagen gel (29)	Angiogenic response in rabbit ear after treatment with bFGF (36)
	Angiogenic in rat aortic explant (22)	Increased wound tensile strength, wound maturation, and organization (22)
	Shortened wound healing in organ culture (30)	Increased neovascularization in hairless mouse ear (37)
PDGF-BB	Mitogenic for brain capillary EC (57)	30% accelerated wound healing in rabbit ear (61)
	Increased capillary number, myofibroblasts and collagen in microvessel coculture (60)	Increased tissue repair in skin graft model (e.g., increased fibornectin, proliferating cells, fibroblasts, collagen, neovessels, and glycosaminoglycans (65)
	Angiogenic in rat aortic ring (59)	
TGF-b	Alters matrix accumulation by EC (81)	Enhances wound healing (117)
	Monocyte chemoattractant (80)	
	Inhibits EC proliferation (76)	
VEGF	Mitogenic for vascular EC (84)	Angiogenic in vivo (94, 95)
	Induces monocyte migration and activation (126)	Increases vascular permeability (126)

Relevant references in parentheses.

resulting from the use of an alternative upstream translation initiation site (for review see 23). Macrophages, smooth muscle cells, vascular ECs, fibroblasts, and some malignant tumor cells have all been shown by immunohistochemistry to contain bFGF (22, 23). bFGF is a cell-associated protein that has been localized to the cytoplasm and extracellular matrix (24–26). It does not have a secretion signal peptide (27), and its mechanism of release has not been clearly elucidated. bFGF can be released from heparan sulfate binding sites on the cell surface and in the matrix, or by proteinase degradation of the extracellular matrix (for review see 23). Researchers have shown that it can be released from cytosolic storage sites through plasma membrane disruptions (22, 24, 28), as well as through an uncharacterized mechanism of exocytosis independent of the endoplasmic reticulum–Golgi pathway (25). The cellular membrane damage theory has been invoked to explain elevated serum bFGF levels in some pathologic conditions (28).

Basic fibroblast growth factor has been shown to be angiogenic in vitro in a number of studies. ECs, in a three-dimensional collagen gel model, have been shown to form tubes in response to bFGF (29). In an in vitro rat aorta ring model, addition of bFGF increased both the length and number of microvessels sprouting from the explants (22); a 40% reduction in angiogenesis occurred after neutralizing bFGF antibodies were added. In a human cornea organ culture wound healing model, addition of bFGF shortened the wound healing time and increased corneal endothelial cell migration at the wound site (30). Finally, bFGF stimulated epidermal outgrowth in an in vitro epithelial explant model of wound healing (31).

Basic fibroblast growth factor has been shown to be angiogenic in vivo in both the chorioallantoic membrane (32, 33) and the corneal pocket assay as well (32). bFGF increased DNA synthesis in a dose-dependent manner in an in vivo rat sponge model (34). Continuous dosing in this model resulted in an amplified angiogenic response with an increased number of fibroblasts and blood vessels. Interestingly, a decrease in collagen content at 7 days was also noted, leading the authors to hypothesize that bFGF may have some collagenolytic activity. Degradation of collagen is a key event in clearing debris and allowing new cells to infiltrate during the tissue formation stage of wound healing. In another in vivo study, introduction of bFGF neutralizing antibodies led to decreased DNA synthesis, granulation tissue, and number of blood vessels as compared to control (35).

The effects of bFGF on tissue repair were demonstrated in three in vivo models. An angiogenic response was elicited in a rabbit ear wound healing model after treatment with bFGF, with increased numbers of ECs and neovessels compared with control (36). Tissue repair was accelerated by 4 days (30%) in the first 10 days, and an elevated wound collagenolytic rate was noted as well. Linear deposition of granulation tissue occurred in bFGF-treated wounds, and, by day 14, bFGF wounds contained twofold more new tissue than controls. A threefold increase in glycosaminoglycans and fibronectin was also present after 21 days. An absence of collagen at day 21 prompted study of the possibility of ongoing collagenolytic activity. A 50% increase in collagen degradation in the surrounding dermis was seen in the bFGF-treated wounds. This is consistent with other observations and lends credence to the role of bFGF in collagen breakdown. In support of this possibility, bFGF has been shown to lead to increased collagenase production by vascular ECs (17). In a second in vivo model, addition of bFGF not only increased wound tensile strength over controls but stimulated better wound maturation and organization (22). In a hairless mouse ischemic ear model, subcutaneous injections of bFGF resulted in increased neovascularization (37). The wound surface area in this model was markedly reduced at both 7 and 10 days as compared with controls.

Also, bFGF has been implicated in a number of experimental injury models that attempt to approximate human disease states. In a rat carotid balloon injury model, administration of bFGF caused a twofold increase in intimal thickening (38). This effect was blocked up to 80% by administration of anti-bFGF antibodies (39). Consistent with this observation, administration of anti-bFGF antibody at the time of carotid injury was found to lead to an 80% reduction in smooth muscle cells (40). In this carotid balloon model, the smooth muscle cell replication rate was increased by 50% (41). It was thus postulated that the bFGF synthesized by smooth muscle cells is released by arterial injury, stimulating the neighboring migration and replication of neighboring smooth muscle cells. bFGF has also been detected at the site of muscle damage in a rat myocyte crush injury/regeneration model (42). bFGF expression has been noted to change in an optic nerve injury model (43), at the site of focal brain injury (44), and in a cardiac myocyte injury model (45). Finally, an acid-stabilized form of bFGF has been shown to accelerate duodenal ulcer healing in a rat model (46); a ninefold increase in angiogenesis at the ulcer site was noted in the bFGF-treated ulcers.

In addition, bFGF has been implicated in a number of human disease states. Elevated levels of bFGF have been measured in the urine of some cancer patients (47), the cerebral spinal fluid of patients with brain tumors (48), and in the sera of patients with severe lower extremity atherosclerosis (49) and Duchenne's muscular dystrophy (33). Although the mechanism of bFGF release remains unknown, a unifying hypothesis in all of these cases is that bFGF may be either an effect of, or a reaction to, injury and thus aid in the healing process. bFGF has therefore earned the nickname of a "wound hormone." To support this title, future studies will have to demonstrate a causal role of bFGF in wound healing in vivo. The wound healing process would have to be reversed or altered by addition of a bFGF-neutralizing substance to prove that bFGF is necessary for effective wound healing.

Platelet-Derived Growth Factor

Platelet-derived growth factor (PDGF) is a dimeric glycoprotein with a molecular weight of 30,000, composed of A and B chains, that exists as both a heterodimer and a homodimer (for review see 50). PDGF is undetectable in normal human plasma and has a very short half-life in vivo (<2 minutes) (51). The activity of PDGF is thus thought to result from local (i.e., paracrine) effects rather than circulating effects. PDGF has demonstrated mitogenic and chemotactic activity, primarily in mesenchymal target cells. Many cells express receptors for PDGF, including some microvascular ECs (52), dermal fibroblasts, and vascular smooth muscle cells (SMCs) (reviewed in 50). Platelets (53), macrophages (54), ECs (55), and vascular SMCs (56) have all been shown to secrete PDGF. PDGF is a chemoattractant for neutrophils (57), monocytes (57), fibroblasts (58), SMCs (59), and macrophages (60). It is also a more potent vasoconstrictor than angiotensin II (61). The chemotactic activity coupled with evidence for a role in angiogenesis makes PDGF an important candidate as a wound healing growth factor.

Also, PDGF has been shown to be angiogenic both in vitro and in vivo. The PDGF-BB has been shown to be mitogenic for rat brain capillary ECs in culture (62), but not for adrenal capillary ECs (63). PDGF-AA and PDGF-BB both stimulated angiogenesis in vitro in a rat aortic ring model (64). PDGF-BB induced capillary tube formation fourfold over control in an in vitro microvessel fragment-myofibroblast coculture system (65). An increased amount of collagen synthesis by these myofibroblasts facilitated capillary network formation in vitro. The effect of PDGF-BB on capillary tube formation in culture could be reduced up to 47% by addition of anti–PDGF-BB antibodies (66). An increase in DNA synthesis by these cultured tube-forming ECs was noted, as was an increase in PDGF receptor mRNA. Finally, PDGF-BB has been shown to be angiogenic on the chick chorioallantoic membrane (CAM) (62). PDGF activity and the resulting increase in vessel density on the CAM was blocked by anti-PDGF antibodies.

The demonstration of PDGF as an angiogenic factor has led to intense study of its activity in wound healing. PDGF was shown to stimulate myofibroblast proliferation in vitro as well as to increase production of collagen type I (65). PDGF also increased wound fibroblast proliferation in vitro (67). This, coupled with the potent vasoconstrictor activity of PDGF, makes it an interesting possibility in the mediation of wound healing, as myofibroblast contraction and collagen synthesis are both well-characterized events in the wound healing process. PDGF-BB accelerated wound healing in a rabbit ear model by up to 30% over control after 10 days (66). An increased amount of glycosaminoglycans, specifically hyaluronic acid and proteoglycan sulfates, was noted in PDGF-stimulated wounds. Increased amounts of fibronectin deposition and provisional wound matrix were also noted. Initially, a lower amount of collagen was found in the PDGF-treated wounds, but by 21 days postwounding, the amount of collagen in the scar tissue was greater than control. PDGF was also shown to improve corneal wound strength in a rabbit model of corneal laceration and keratoplasty (68). Histologic examination of these wounds showed an increase in the number of fibroblasts as well as levels of collagen (types III and IV) in the PDGF-treated eyes. In addition, injured retinal pigment epithelial cells in culture increased the expression of PDGF-BB and PDGF-β receptors (69). In an in vivo skin graft neotissue model, PDGF was also shown to accelerate normal tissue repair (70). An increased amount of fibronectin, proliferating cells, fibroblasts, glycosaminoglycans, collagen, and new vessels were measured compared with control. Finally, increased levels of PDGF-BB have been detected in healing wounds in normal but not diabetic rats (71).

Clinical trials have been conducted examining PDGF-BB as an adjunct to wound healing. Using a randomized, prospective, double-blind, placebo-controlled study, Steed and Group (72) showed PDGF to stimulate healing in lower extremity diabetic neurotrophic ulcers. Forty-eight percent of the patients randomized to the PDGF-BB–treated group achieved complete wound healing compared with 25% of the control group. In another human study examining pressure ulcers, PDGF-BB was shown to increase fibroblast proliferation and new vessel formation in biopsy specimens (73). Accelerated wound healing was also noted. Normal skin and granulation tissue both contain PDGF-β receptors, hence the rationale for treating wounds with PDGF-BB. Interestingly, wounds treated with PDGF-BB showed markedly increased levels of PDGF-AA (74). Studies like these prompt further investigation into the efficacy of the PDGF family as wound healing agents.

Transforming Growth Factor-Beta (TGF-β)

Transforming growth factor-β_1 is the prototypic member of a large family of polypeptide growth regulators (for review see 75). It is a 25-kd homodimer originally isolated from a variety of sources including platelets. The functions of TGF-β are varied; it can stimulate or inhibit cell proliferation, depending on the cell type. Many of its actions are suspected to be mediated by the alterations that it induces in the nature and accumulation of extracellular matrix components.

Also, TGF-β has been widely implicated in the wound healing process, primarily because of its ability to induce connective tissue accumulation. TGF-β has been demonstrated to mediate fibrosis in a variety of conditions including glomerulonephritis (76). Use of TGF-β null mice should provide an excellent system in which to examine the contribution of the various TGF-β isoforms to the healing process. Unfortunately, these studies have been hampered by the fact that the homozygous null mice die at an early age as a result of diffuse inflammation (77). Therefore, most of the null mice studied are born to TGF-β heterozygotes and maternal transfer of TGF-β to the embryos has been demonstrated (78). This topic is outside of the scope of this chapter and the reader is referred to a number of comprehensive reviews regarding the role of TGF-β in connective tissue formation (79, 80).

The role of TGF-β in controlling microvascular growth is complex. TGF-β has been shown to be a potent inhibitor of capillary EC growth in vitro (81). Further, we (82) and others (83) have demonstrated, using coculture models, that contact between ECs and mural cells (pericytes in the microvasculature or smooth muscle cells in larger vessels) leads to the activation of latent TGF-β, which in turn inhibits EC proliferation. On the other hand, a bolus administration of TGF-β to an in vivo assay leads to angiogenesis (84). Although these observations are, at first glance, contradictory, there are several potential explanations. First, TGF-β has been shown to be a potent chemoattractant for monocytes (85), which via the release of a variety of peptide growth factors induce angiogenesis. Thus, TGF-β has been said to be an "indirect" angiogenic factor. Second, it is likely that there are significant differences between the bolus administration of high levels of TGF-β and the local delivery of low levels. The differences are both as the level of dose and as "mode of delivery." Locally high levels may be equivalent to what occurs in early wound healing when high concentrations of TGF-β are generated by release of platelet granules. At this stage TGF-β may have many effects including monocyte recruitment. Monocytes then release their granule constituents including the potent angiogenic factors bFGF and vascular endothelial growth factor (VEGF).

Other aspects of TGF-β action may occur later in the wound healing, process once significant angiogenesis has taken place. Once the early capillary tubes have formed, pericyte precursors are recruited. We speculate that once the pericyte makes contact with the endothelium, TGF-β is activated locally and acts to inhibit endothelial proliferation and induce the formation of a basement membrane, leading to a quiescent, differential capillary. Although some have called this phenomenon "anti-angiogenic," it seems more likely that under these conditions the TGF-β is acting to stabilize growing vessels, thus limiting continued remodeling (86).

Vascular Endothelial Growth Factor (VEGF)/Vascular Permeability Factor (VPF)

VEGF/VPF is a 34- to 42-kd homodimeric glycoprotein (for more complete review, see 87). The primary target of VEGF/VPF is a vascular endothelium that possesses two high-affinity tyrosine kinase receptors called flt-1 and flk-1 (or in humans KDR). VPF was first purified from tumor cells on the basis of its ability to cause hyperpermeability in a guinea pig skin model (88). Subsequently, two other groups purified a material from normal pituitary follicular cells that was a specific mitogen for vascular endothelium in vitro (89, 90).

VPF, the permeability inducing factor, and VEGF, the endothelial cell mitogen, have been conclusively demonstrated to be encoded by the same gene. The single gene leads to at least three splice variants: VEGF$_{189}$,

$VEGF_{165}$, and $VEGF_{121}$. The three vary in their affinity for heparin, with $VEGF_{121}$ displaying a minimal heparin affinity, $VEGF_{189}$ a strong heparin affinity, and $VEGF_{165}$ an intermediate heparin binding. Considering the relevance of heparin affinity in the biology of growth factor molecules (91-93), it is possible that this characteristic will eventually be shown to reflect some in vivo functional differences. Studies in which the VEGF gene (94, 95) or one of its receptors, flt-1 (96), has been deleted by targeted disruption and has been shown to lead to early embryonic lethality with phenotypes suggest a critical role for VEGF in the process of vasculogenesis. Early studies of the expression patterns of VEGF in tumors revealed elevated expression in cells bordering necrotic areas of tumors (97). These observations, in turn, lead to the suggestion that VEGF might be regulated by low local oxygen tensions, that is, hypoxia. A number of subsequent studies have shown this to be true and have begun to investigate the molecular basis of the hypoxic regulation of VEGF (97, 98). The angiogenic capacity of VEGF/VPF has been shown in a variety of in vivo experimental models (99, 100). Subsequently, a number of labs have demonstrated reduced tumor growth in vitro using neutralizing VEGF reagents (101, 102) as well as in models of ocular angiogenesis (103, 104).

The ability of VEGF to be regulated by hypoxia and the knowledge that the wound is a particularly low oxygen environment suggest a role for VEGF in wound healing. In addition, VEGF has a number of other characteristics that would be particularly consistent with the role in wound healing. In addition to its angiogenic capacity, VEGF has been shown to alter local protease production including plasminogen activator (105) and interstitial collagenase (106). In addition, VEGF has been shown to induce monocyte migration and activation (107) events critical to the successful wound healing response. VEGF has been shown to be expressed by macrophages in healing and to be dramatically increased in the keratocytes at the ages of healing wounds (108). Consistent with this, the VEGF receptor flt-1 has been shown to be upregulated in blood vessels at the wound edge (109). Finally, a defect in VEGF regulation during wound healing has been documented in diabetic db/db mice that show characteristic delay in wound repair (110). Definitive studies in which VEGF expression is experimentally blocked and delays in wound repair are documented have not been yet reported, yet the indirect evidence strongly suggests an important role for VEGF/VPF in the normal wound repair process.

Cytokines

The term *cytokine* was initially used to encompass a wide variety of substances, including growth factors, interleukins, and interferons. The definition of these low molecular weight polypeptides and glycoproteins was instituted before many of their specific actions and molecular biologic characteristics were characterized (for reviews see 23, 111, 112). Cytokines were thought to be released from leukocytes in response to specific stimuli and to act upon tumor cells (tumor necrosis factor) or the leukocytes themselves (interleukins). However, additional study has revealed the release of cytokines by and their action on a variety of cells in addition to leukocytes. As a group, cytokines generally exhibit more autocrine and paracrine than endocrine effects (112). Cytokines work in conjunction with one another, and their net effect is a result of the balance of synergistic and antagonistic actions of hormones and other soluble receptors. The integrated action of the many cytokines represent a way to introduce fine tuning and flexibility into the complicated process of wound healing.

Macrophages are a major source of most cytokines, and they have been shown to release a variety of substances, including interleukin-1 (IL-1), tumor necrosis factor-α (TNF-α), PDGF, and TGF-β (for review see 11). As noted above, macrophages play a critical role in wound healing and debridement.

Interleukins in Angiogenesis

Many of the interleukins have been studied in terms of their angiogenic effects. IL-1, which is released from both macrophages and epithelial cells, has been shown to stimulate angiogenesis in a rat sponge model (113). This activity was abolished by addition of IL-1 receptor blockers. IL-1 has been shown to stimulate macrophage synthesis of other cytokines as well (112). Interleukin-8 (IL-8) stimulated angiogenesis in vivo, and its activity was blocked by IL-8 antisera (113). IL-8 has also been identified at high levels in burn blister fluid and may be important in stimulating wound healing under these conditions (114). IL-12 inhibits angiogenesis in vivo, an action that is postulated to be mediated by interferon-γ (115). IL-6 and IL-2 are currently under investigation for their possible roles in angiogenesis. The varied effects of these interleukins suggest that the wound healing response could be moderated by subtle changes in a variety of signals.

Tumor Necrosis Factor-α

Tumor necrosis factor α (TNF-α) has been demonstrated to play a role in angiogenesis as well. It is a single-chain polypeptide (MW 17 kd) that is synthesized and secreted by macrophages and some tumor cells (for review see 116). TNF-α has biphasic actions both in vitro and in vivo; at high doses it inhibits angiogenesis, whereas at low doses it stimulates angiogenesis (117). TNF-α is found at low doses in serum where it may function as an angiogenesis promoter (23). However, locally high concentrations such as those at the site of macrophage release may serve to inhibit angiogenesis. TNF-α has also been shown to promote tissue debridement both through direct and indirect actions (111). Finally, hypoxia has been reported to stimulate TNF-α release as well as TNF-α receptor expression in a macrophage cell line in vitro (118). This may be an important regulatory mechanism for TNF-α availability at times of ischemic injury. All of these characteristics make TNF-α an important factor in the initial inflammation and tissue formation stages of wound healing.

Interferons

The interferons (IFNs) are a group of proteins with molecular weights ranging from 16 to 24 kd. Studies of the role of IFN-α have been motivated by its demonstrated efficacy in the treatment of pediatric hemangiomas (119). This cytokine had been shown to inhibit capillary EC migration in vitro (120), and its use was then expanded to the clinical arena. It is currently being used clinically as a chemotherapeutic agent in the treatment of advanced melanoma. IFN-γ has also been demonstrated to have anti-angiogenic actions in vitro (121), inhibiting growth factor–stimulated EC proliferation in a dose-dependent manner.

Experiments in which angiogenesis itself is inhibited (and not the actions of a particular growth factor) are necessary to directly assess the role of neovascularization in wound healing. The fungus-derived angiogenesis inhibitor, AGM-1470, inhibits wound healing in a dose-dependent manner (Brem and Folkman, manuscript in preparation), and it has been shown to inhibit EC proliferation and migration in culture (122). Other reagents that appear to act "downstream" of the angiogenic factors themselves to block vessel formation should be useful in these studies. For instance, inhibition of the integrin $\alpha_v\beta_3$ has been shown to prevent new vessel growth (123), and the endothelial inhibitor angiostatin appears to block blood vessels independent of the nature of the stimuli (124). Although additional investigations will be necessary to be certain that these agents act only on forming vessels, they represent potential approaches to determining the precise role of angiogenesis in the wound healing process.

Summary

In spite of the well-accepted fact that angiogenesis is a critical component of wound healing, to our knowledge no studies have been published that definitively demonstrate this point. Numerous growth factors and cytokines with angiogenic potential have been shown to accelerate or otherwise improve wound healing; however, virtually all of these factors have many other effects and it is impossible to assign the improved wound healing solely to its effects on angiogenesis. The development of models that permit a quantitative assessment of the angiogenesis during wound repair (125,

126) will facilitate these investigations and permit a systematic examination of the role of angiogenesis in wound healing.

References

1. Clark RAF. Wound repair. Curr Opinion Cell Biol 1989;1:1000–8.
2. Cohen IK. In: Cohen IK, Diegelmann RF, Lindblad WJ, eds. Wound healing: biochemical and clinical aspects. Philadelphia: W.B. Saunders, 1992.
3. Arnold F, West DC. Angiogenesis in wound healing. Pharmacol Ther 1991; 52:407–22.
4. Furie B, Furie BC. The molecular basis of blood coagulation. Cell 1988; 53:505–18.
5. Santoro S. Identification of a 160,000 dalton platelet membrane protein that mediates the initial divalent cation-dependent adhesion of platelets to collagen. Cell 1986;46:913–20.
6. Plow EF, McEver RP, Coller BS, Woods VL, Marguerie GA, Ginsberg MH. Related binding mechanisms for fibrinogen, fibronectin, von Willebrand factor, and thrombospondin on thrombin-stimulated human platelets. Blood 1988;66:724–7.
7. Grinnel F, Billingham RE, Burgess L. Distribution of fibronectin during wound healing in vivo. J Invest Dermatol 1981;76:181–9.
8. Clark RA, Lanigan JM, DellaPelle P, Manseau E, Dvorak HF, Colvin RB. Fibronectin and fibrin provide a provisional matrix for epidermal cell migration during wound reepithelialization. J Invest Dermatol 1982;79:264–9.
9. Hibbs MS, Masty KA, Seyer JM, Kang AH, Mainardi CL. Biochemical and immunological characterization of the secreted forms of human neutrophil gelatinase. J Biol Chem 1985;260:2493–500.
10. Leibovich S, Ross R. The role of the macrophages in wound repair. Am J Pathol 1975;78:71–100.
11. Nathan C. Secretory products of macrophages. J Clin Invest 1987;79:319–26.
12. Winter G. Formation of the scab and the rate of epithelialization of superficial wounds in the skin of the young domestic pig. Nature 1962;193:293–4.
13. Stanley JR, Alaverz OM, Bere ER, Eaglstein WH, Katz SI. Detection of basement membrane zone antigens during epidermal wound healing in pigs. J Invest Dermatol 1981;77:240–3.
14. Grondahl-Hansen J, Lung LR, Ralfkiaer E, Ottevanger V, Dano K. Urokinase and tissue-type plasminogen activators in keratinocytes during wound reepithelialization in vivo. J Invest Dermatol 1988;90:790–5.
15. Woodley DT, Kalebec T, Banes AJ, Link W, Prunieras M, Liotta L. Adult human keratinocytes migrating over non-viable dermal collagen produce collagenolytic enzymes that degrade type I and IV collagen. J Invest Dermatol 1986;86:418–23.
16. Gabbiani G, Chaponnier C, Huttner I. Cytoplasmic filaments and gap junctions in epithelial cells and myofibroblasts during wound healing. J Cell Biol 1978;76:561–8.
17. Forrest L. Current concepts in soft connective tissue wound healing. Br J Surg 1983;70:133–40.

18. Gabbiani G, Hirschel BJ, Ryan GB, Statkov PR, Majno G. Granulation tissue as a contractile organ. A study of structure and function. J Exp Med 1972;135:719-33.

19. Ausprunk DH, Folkman J. Migration and proliferation of endothelial cells in preformed and newly formed vessels during tumor angiogenesis. Microvasc Res 1977;14:53-65.

20. Mignatti P, Tsuboi R, Robbins E, Rifkin DB. In vitro angiogenesis on the human amniotic membrane: requirement for basic fibroblast growth factor-induced proteinases. J Cell Biol 1989;108:671-82.

21. Folkman J, Shing Y. Angiogenesis. J Biol Chem 1992;267:10931-4.

22. Thompson WD, Harvey JA, Kazmi MA, Stout AJ. Fibrinolysis and angiogenesis in wound healing. J Pathol 1991;165:311-8.

23. Klagsbrun M, D'Amore PA. Regulators of angiogenesis. Annu Rev Physiol 1991;53:217-39.

24. Vlodavsky I, Folkman J, Sullivan R, Fridman R, Ishai-Michaeli R, Sasse J, Klagsbrun M. Endothelial cell-derived basic fibroblast growth factor: synthesis and deposition into subendothelial extracellular matrix. Proc Natl Acad Sci USA 1987;84:2292-6.

25. Baird A, Esch F, Mormede P, et al. Molecular characterization of fibroblast growth factor: distribution and biological activities in various tissues. Recent Prog Horm Res 1986;42:143-205.

26. Muthukrishnan L, Warder E, McNeil PL. Basic fibroblast growth factor is efficiently released from a cytosolic storage site through plasma membrane disruptions of endothelial cells. J Cell Physiol 1991;148:1-16.

27. Villaschi S, Nicosia RF. Angiogenic role of endogenous basic fibroblast growth factor released by rat aorta after injury. Am J Pathol 1993;143:181-90.

28. Leek R, Harris A, Lewis C. Cytokine networks in solid human tumors: regulation of angiogenesis. J Leukoc Biol 1994;56:423-55.

29. Abraham JA, Whang JL, Tumolo A, et al. Human basic fibroblast growth factor: nucleotide sequence and genomic organization. EMBO J 1986; 5:2523-8.

30. McNeil PL, Muthukrishnan L, Warder E, D'Amore PA. Growth factors are released by mechanically wounded endothelial cells. J Cell Biol 1989; 109:811-22.

31. Ku P, D'Amore P. Regulation of basic fibroblast growth factor (bFGF) gene and protein expression following its release from sublethally injured cells. J Cell Biochem 1995;58:328-43.

32. Mignatti P, Morimoto T, Rifkin DB. Basic fibroblast growth factor, a protein devoid of secretory signal sequence, is released by cells via a pathway independent of the endoplasmic reticulum-Golgi complex. J Cell Physiol 1992;151:81-93.

33. D'Amore PA, Brown RH Jr, Ku P-T, et al. Elevated basic fibroblast growth factor in the serum of patients with Duchenne muscular dystrophy. Ann Neurol 1994;35:362-5.

34. Montesano R, Vassali JD, Baird A, Guillemin R, Orci L. Basic fibroblast growth factor induces angiogenesis in vitro. Proc Natl Acad Sci USA 1986;83:7297-301.

35. Hoppenreijs VP, Pels E, Vrensen GF, Treffers WF. Basic fibroblast growth factor stimulates corneal endothelial cell growth and endothelial wound healing of human corneas. Invest Ophthalmol Vis Sci 1994;35:931–44.
36. Bhora FY, Dunkin BJ, Batzri S, et al. Effect of growth factors on cell proliferation and epithelialization in human skin. J Surg Res 1995; 59:236–44.
37. Shing Y, Folkman J, Haudenschild C, Lund D, Crum R, Klagsbrun M. Angiogenesis is stimulated by a tumor-derived endothelial growth factor. J Cell Biochem 1985;29:275–87.
38. Davidson JM, Broadley KN. Manipulation of the wound-healing process with basic fibroblast growth factor. Ann NY Acad Sci 1991;638:306–15.
39. Broadley KN, Aquino AM, Woodward SC, et al. Monospecific antibodies implicate basic fibroblast growth factor in normal wound repair. Lab Invest 1989;61:571–5.
40. Lindner V, Reidy MA. Proliferation of smooth muscle cells after vascular injury is inhibited by an antibody against basic fibroblast growth factor. Proc Natl Acad Sci USA 1991;88:3739–43.
41. Reidy M. Neointimal proliferation: the role of basic FGF on vascular smooth muscle cell proliferation. Thromb Haemost 1993;70:176–6.
42. Anderson JE, Mitchell CM, McGeachie JK, Grounds MD. The time course of basic fibroblast growth factor expression in crush-injured skeletal muscles of SJL/J and BALB/c mice. Exp Cell Res 1995;216:325–34.
43. Kostyk SK, D'Amore PA, Herman Im, Wagner JA. Optic nerve injury alters basic fibroblast growth factor localization in the retina and optic tract. J Neurosci 1994;14:1441–9.
44. Finklestein SP, Apostolides PJ, Caday CG, Prosser J, Philips MF, Klagsbrun M. Increased basic fibroblast growth factor (bFGF) immunoreactivity at the site of focal brain wounds. Brain Res 1988;460:253–9.
45. Padua RR, Kardami E. Increased basic fibroblast growth factor (bFGF) accumulation and distinct patterns of localization in isoproterenol-induced cardiomyocyte injury. Growth Factors 1993;8:291–306.
46. Szabo S, Folkman J, Vattay P, Morales RE, Pinkus GS, Kato K. Accelerated healing of duodenal ulcers by oral administration of a mutein of basic fibroblast growth factor in rats. Gastroenterology 1994;106:1106–11.
47. Nguyen M, Watanabe H, Budson AE, Richie JP, Folkman J. Elevated levels of an angiogenic peptide, basic fibroblast growth factor, in urine of patients with a wide spectrum of cancers. J Natl Cancer Inst 1993;86:356–61.
48. Li V, Folkerth R, Watanabe H, Yu C, Rupnick M, Barnes P, Scott R, et al. Microvessel count and cerebrospinal fluid basic fibroblast growth factor in children with brain tumors. Lancet 1994;344:82–6.
49. Rohovsky S, Kearney M, Peiczek A, et al. Elevated levels of basic fibroblast growth in patients with limb ischemia. Am Heart J, in press.
50. Ross R, Raines E, Bowen-Pope D. The biology of platelet-derived growth factor. Cell 1986;46:155–69.
51. Bowen-Pope DF, Malpass TW, Foster DM, Ross R. Platelet-derived growth factor in vivo: levels, activity, and rate of clearance. Blood 1984;64:458–69.
52. Bar RS, Boes M, Booth BA, Dake BL, Henley S, Hart MN. The effects of

platelet-derived growth factor in cultured microvessel endothelial cells. Endocrinology 1989;124:1841–8.

53. Singh JP, Chaikin MA, Stiles CD. Phylogenetic analysis of platelet-derived growth factor by radio-receptor assay. J Cell Biol 1982;95:667–71.

54. Shimokado K, Raines EW, Madtes DK, Barrett TB, Benditt EP, Ross RA. Significant part of macrophage-derived growth factor consists of at least two forms of PDGF. Cell 1985;43:277–86.

55. DiCorleto PE, Bowen-Pope DF. Cultured endothelial cells produce a platelet-derived growth factor-like protein. Proc Natl Acad Sci USA 1983; 80:1919–23.

56. Seifert RA, Schwartz SM, Bowen-Pope DF. Developmentally regulated production of platelet-derived growth factor-like molecules. Nature 1984; 311:669–71.

57. Deuel TF, Senior RM, Huang JS, Griffin GL. Chemotaxis of monocytes and neutrophils to platelet-derived growth factor. J Clin Invest 1982;69:1046–9.

58. Seppa H, Grotendorst G, Seppa S, Schiffmann E, Martin G. Platelet-derived growth factor is chemotactic for fibroblasts. J Cell Biol 1982;92:584.

59. Grotendorst GR, Chang T, Seppa HE, Kleinman HK, Martin GR. Platelet-derived growth factor is a chemoattractant for vascular smooth muscle cells. J Cell Physiol 1982;113:261–6.

60. Huang J, Olsen T, Huang S. The role of growth factors in tissue repair I. The molecular and cellular bio of wound repair. 1988;243–51.

61. Berk BC, Alexander RW, Brock TA, Gimbrone MA, Webb RC. Vasoconstriction: a new activity for platelet-derived growth factor. Science 1986;232:87–90.

62. Risau W, Drexler H, Mironov V, et al. Platelet-derived growth factor in angiogenic in vivo. Growth Factors 1992;7:261–6.

63. D'Amore PA, Smith SR. Growth factor effects on cells of the vascular wall: a survey. Growth Factors 1993;8:61–75.

64. Nicosia R, Nicosia S, Smith M. Vascular endothelial growth factor, platelet-derived growth factor, and insulin-like growth factor-1 promote rat aortic angiogenesis in vitro. Am J Pathol 1994;145:1023–9.

65. Sato N, Beitz J, Kato J, et al. Platelet-derived growth factor indirectly stimulates angiogenesis in vitro. Am J Pathol 1993;142:1119–30.

66. Battegay EJ, Rupp J, Iruela-Arispe L, Sage EH, Pech M. PDGF-BB modulates endothelial proliferation and angiogenesis in vitro via PDGF β-receptors. J Cell Biol 1994;125:917–28.

67. Lepisto J, Peltonen J, Vaha-Kreula M, Ninikoski J, Laato M. Platelet-derived growth factor isoforms PDGF-AA, -AB and -BB exert specific effects on collagen gene expression and mitotic activity of cultured human wound fibroblasts. Biochem Biophys Res Commun 1995;209:393–9.

68. Murali S, Hardten DR, DeMartelaere S, et al. Effect of topically administered platelet-derived growth factor on corneal wound strength. Curr Eye Res 1994;13:857–62.

69. Campochiaro PA, Hackett SF, Vinores SA, et al. Platelet-derived growth factor is an autocrine growth stimulator in retinal pigmented epithelial cells. J Cell Sci 1994;107:2459–69.

70. Khouri R, Hong S, Deune E, et al. De novo generation of permanent

neovascularized soft tissue appendages by platelet-derived growth factor. J Clin Invest 1994;94:1757–63.

71. Doxey DL, Ng MC, Dill RE, Iacopino AM. Platelet-derived growth factor levels in wounds of diabetic rats. Life Sci 1995;57:1111–23.

72. Steed DL, Group DUS. Clinical evaluation of recombinant human platelet-derived growth factor for the treatment of lower extremity diabetic ulcers. Vasc Surg 1995;21:71–81.

73. Pierce GF, Tarpley JE, Allman RM, et al. Tissue repair processes in healing chronic pressure ulcers treated with recombinant platelet-derived growth factor BB. Am J Pathol 1994;145:1399–410.

74. Pierce GF, Tarpley JE, Tseng J, et al. Detection of platelet-derived growth factor (PDGF)-AA in actively healing human wounds treated with recombinant PDGF-BB and absence of PDGF in chronic nonhealing wounds. J Clin Invest 1995;96:1336–50.

75. Sporn MB, Roberts AB. Transforming growth factor-β: recent progress and new challenges. J Cell Biol 1992;119:1017–21.

76. Border WA, Okuda S, Languino LR, Sporn MB, Ruoslahti E. Suppression of experimental glomerulonephritis by antiserum against transforming growth factor-beta 1. Nature 1990;346:371–4.

77. Shull MM, Ormsby I, Kier AB, et al. Targeted disruption of the mouse transforming growth factor-β1 gene results in multifocal inflammatory disease. Nature 1992;359:693–9.

78. Letterio J, Geiser A, Kulkarni A, Roche N, Sporn M, Roberts A. Maternal rescue of transforming growth factor-β1 null mice. Science 1994;264:1936–8.

79. Border WA, Noble NA. Transforming growth factor beta in tissue fibrosis. N Engl J Med 1994;331:1286–92.

80. Harper JR, Spiro RC, Gaarde WA, et al. Role of transforming growth factor beta and decorin in controlling fibrosis. Methods Enzymol 1994;245:241–54.

81. Heimark RL, Twardzik DR, Schwartz SM. Inhibition of endothelial cell regeneration by type-beta transforming growth factor from platelets. Science 1986;233:1078–80.

82. Antonelli-Orlidge A, Saunders KB, Smith SR, D'Amore PA. An activated form of TGF-β is produced by cocultures of endothelial cells and pericytes. Proc Natl Acad Sci USA 1989;86:4544–8.

83. Sato Y, Rifkin DB. Inhibition of endothelial cell movement by pericytes and smooth muscle cells: activation of a latent transforming growth factor-beta 1-like molecule by plasmin during co-culture. J Cell Biol 1989;109:309–15.

84. Fajardo LF, Prionas SD, Kwan HH, Kowalski J, Allison AC. Transforming growth factor-beta-1 induces angiogenesis in vivo with a threshold pattern. Lab Invest 1996;74:600–8.

85. Wahl SM, Hunt DA, Wakefield IM, et al. Transforming growth factor-beta (TGF-β) induces monocyte chemotaxis and growth factor production. Proc Natl Acad Sci USA 1987;84:5788–92.

86. Merwin JR, Anderson JM, Kocher O, Van Itallie CM, Madri JA. Transforming growth factor beta$_1$ modulates extracellular matrix organization and cell-cell junctional complex formation during in vivo angiogenesis. J Cell Physiol 1990;142:117–28.

87. Senger DR, Van De Water L, Brown LF, et al. Vascular permeability factor (VPF, VEGF) in tumor biology. Cancer Metastasis Rev 1993;12:303–24.
88. Senger DR, Galli SJ, A.M. D, Perruzzi CA, Harvey VS, Dvorak HF. Tumor cells secrete a vascular permeability factor that promotes accumulation of ascites fluid. Science 1993;219.
89. Ferrara N, Henzel WJ. Pituitary follicular cells secrete a novel heparin-binding growth factor specific for vascular endothelial cells. Biochem Biophys Res Commun 1989;161:851–5.
90. Gospadarowicz D, Abraham JA, Schilling J. Isolation and characterization of a vascular endothelial cell mitogen produced by pituitary-derived folliculostel-late cells. Proc Natl Acad Sci USA 1989;86:7311–5.
91. Higashiyama S, Abraham JA, Klagsbrun M. Heparin-binding EGF-like growth factor stimulation of smooth muscle cell migration: dependence of interactions with cell surface heparan sulfate. J Cell Biol 1993;122:933–40.
92. Klagsbrun M. Mediators of angiogenesis: the biological significance of basic fibroblast growth factor (bFGF)-heparin and heparan sulfate interactions. Cancer Biol 1992;3:81–7.
93. Tessler S, Rockwell P, Hicklin D, et al. Heparin modulates the interaction of $VEGF_{165}$ with soluble and cell associate flk-1 receptors. J Biol Chem 1994;269:12456–61.
94. Ferrara N, Carver-Moore K, Chen H, et al. Heterozygous embryonic lethality induced by targeted inactivation of the VEGF gene. Nature 1996;380:439–42.
95. Carmeliet P, Ferriera V, Brier G, et al. Abnormal blood vessel development and lethality in embryoes lacking a single VEGF allele. Nature 1996;380:435–9.
96. Fong G-H, Rossant J, Gertsenstein M, Breitman ML. Role of the flt-1 receptor tyrosine kinase in regulating the assembly of vascular endothelium. Nature 1995;376:66–8.
97. Shweiki D, Itin A, Soffer D, Keshet E. Vascular endothelial growth factor induced by hypoxia may mediate hypoxia-initiated angiogenesis. Nature 1992;359:843–5.
98. Shima DT, Adamis AP, Yeo K-T, et al. Hypoxic induction of endothelial cell growth factors in retinal cells: identification and characterization of vascular endothelial growth factor (VEGF) as the mitogen. Mol Med 1995;1:182–93.
99. Connolly DT, Heuvelman DM, Nelson R, et al. Tumor vascular permeability factor stimulates endothelial cell growth and angiogenesis. J Clin Invest 1989;84:1470–8.
100. Leung DW, Cachianes G, Kuang WJ, Goeddel DV, Ferrara N. Vascular endothelial growth factor is a secreted angiogenic mitogen. Science 1989;246:1306–9.
101. Kim KJ, Li B, Winer J, et al. Inhibition of vascular endothelial growth factor-induced angiogenesis suppresses tumor growth in vivo. Nature 1993;362:841–4.
102. Millauer B, Shawver LK, Risau W, Ullrich A. Glioblastoma growth inhibited in vivo by a dominant-negative Flk-1 mutant. Nature 1994;367:576–9.
103. Miller JW, Adamis AP, Shima DT, et al. Vascular permeability factor/ vascular endothelial cell growth factor is temporally and spatially correlated with ocular angiogenesis in a primate model. Am J Pathol 1994;145:574–84.

104. Pierce EA, Avery RL, Foley ED, Aiello LP, Smith LEH. Vascular endothelial growth factor/vascular permeability factor expression in a mouse model of retinal neovascularization. Proc Natl Acad Sci USA 1995;92:905–9.
105. Pepper MS, Ferrara N, Orci L, Montesano R. Vascular endothelial growth factor (VEGF) induces plasminogen activators and plasminogen activator inhibitor-1 in microvascular endothelial cells. Biochem Biophys Res Commun 1991;181:902–6.
106. Unemori EN, Ferrara N, Bauer EA, Amento EP. Vascular endothelial growth factor induces interstitial collagenase expression in human endothelial cells. J Cell Physiol 1992;153:557–62.
107. Clauss M, Gerlach M, Gerlach H, et al. Vascular permeability factor: a tumor-derived polypeptide that induces endothelial cell and monocyte procoagulant activity, and promotes monocyte migration. J Exp Med 1990; 172:1535–45.
108. Brown LF, Yeo K-T, Berse B, et al. Expression of vascular permeability factor (vascular endothelial growth factor) by epidermal keratinocytes during wound healing. J Exp Med 1992;9:1375–9.
109. Peters KG, De Vries C, Williams LT. Vascular endothelial growth factor ·receptor expression during embryogenesis and tissue repair suggests a role in endothelial differentiation and blood vessel growth. Proc Natl Acad Sci USA 1993;90:8915–9.
110. Frank S, Hubner G, Breier G, Longaker MT, Greenhalgh DG, Werner S. Regulation of vascular endothelial growth factor expression in cultured keratinocytes. J Biol Chem 1995;270:12607–13.
111. Appleton I. Wound repair: the role of cytokines and vasoactive mediators. J R Soc Med 1994;87:500–2.
112. Lowry S. Cytokine mediators of immunity and inflammation. Arch Surg 1993;128:1235–41.
113. Hu D, Hori Y, Presta M, Gresham G, Fan T. Inhibition of angiogenesis in rats by IL-1 receptor antagonist and selected cytokine antibodies. Inflammation 1994;18:45–58.
114. Ono I, Gunji H, Zhang JZ, Maruyama K, Kaneko F. A study of cytokines in burn blister fluid related to wound healing. Burns 1995;21:352–5.
115. Voest E, Kenyon B, O'Reilly M, Truitt G, D'Amato R, Folkman J. Inhibition of angiogenesis in vivo by interleukin 12. J Natl Cancer Inst 1995; 87:581–6.
116. Jaattela M. Biologic activities and mechanisms of action of tumor necrosis factor-α/cachetin. Lab Invest 1991;64:724–42.
117. Fajardo LF, Kwan HH, Kowalski J, Prionas SD, Allison AC. Dual role of tumor necrosis factor-α in angiogenesis. Am J Pathol 1992;140:539–44.
118. Scannell G, Waxman F, Kamal GJ, et al. Hypoxia induces a human macrophage cell line to release tumor necrosis factor-α and its soluble receptors in vitro. J Surg Res 1993;54:281–5.
119. White CW, Sondheimer HM, Crouch EC, Wilson H, Fan LL. Treatment of pulmonary haemonagiomatosis with recombinant interferon alfa-2a. N Engl J Med 1989;320:1197–200.
120. Stinson WG, Miller JW, Puliafito CA, Folkman J. Alpha interferon treatment

of experimental iris neovascularization. Invest Ophthalmol Vis Sci 1991; 32:1046.

121. Friesel R, Komoriya A, Maciag T. Inhibition of endothelial cell proliferation by gamma-interferon. J Cell Biol 1987;104:689-96.

122. Ingber D, Fujita T, Kishimoto S, et al. Synthetic analogues of fumagillin that inhibit angiogenesis and suppress tumor growth. Nature 1990;348:555-7.

123. Brooks PC, Clark AF, Cheresh DA. Requirement of vascular integrin a vb3 for angiogenesis. Science 1994;264:569-71.

124. O'Reilly MS, Holmgren L, Shing Y, et al. Angiostatin: a novel angiogenesis inhibitor that mediates the suppression of metastases by a Lewis lung carcinoma. Cell 1994;315-28.

125. Roesel JF, Nanney LB. Assessment of differential cytokine effects on angiogenesis using an in vivo model of cutaneous wound repair. J Surg Res 1995;58:449-59.

126. Clauss M, Gerlach M, Gerlach H, et al. Vascular permeability factor: a tumor-derived polypeptide that induces endothelial and monocyte procoagulant activity and promotes monocyte migration. J Exp Med 1990; 172:1535-1545.

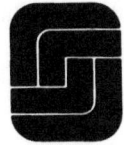

3

The Regulation of Basic Fibroblast Growth Factor (FGF-2) Through Limited Bioavailability

ANDREW BAIRD

There are at least nine distinct but structurally related members of the fibroblast growth factor (FGF) family of growth factors (1–5), and they are presented in schematic form in Figure 3.1. They include acidic FGF (FGF-1), basic FGF (FGF-2), int-2 (FGF-3), Kaposi-FGF or hst-1 (FGF-4), FGF-5, FGF-6, keratinocyte growth factor (FGF-7), androgen inducible growth factor (FGF-8), and glia activating factor (FGF-9). The superfamily also includes the cytokines interleukin (IL)-1α and IL-1β (not shown) that are homologous albeit not considered direct members of the family. Although the FGFs have numerous common characteristics, they also have significant differences. For example, while most FGFs are potent mitogens for cells derived from the mesoderm and neuroectoderm, KGF (FGF-7) is specific for epithelial cells.

All nine members of the FGF family contain a common domain in which most of their structural homology can be found. There are two FGFs that are dramatically distinct from other members of the family: FGF-1 and FGF-2. Their precursors do not have a single peptide that might account for their secretion, although both are found outside cells. Unlike the FGFs 3 to 9, FGF-1 and -2 are widely distributed in tissues, and are expressed by a large number of cells in culture. Like all FGFs, however, they can stimulate the proliferation and differentiation of numerous cell types, presumably because they act through a common family of high-affinity receptors (3).

Numerous studies have shown that despite the absence of a known mechanism to account for basic FGF (FGF-2) export from cells, it appears to be translocated to the cell surface. For example, immunohistochemical studies show FGF-2 localizes to the basement membrane in vivo and to the extracellular matrix of numerous tissues, suggesting it is sequestered outside of the target cell. If so, then it is in a biologically inert form, because the

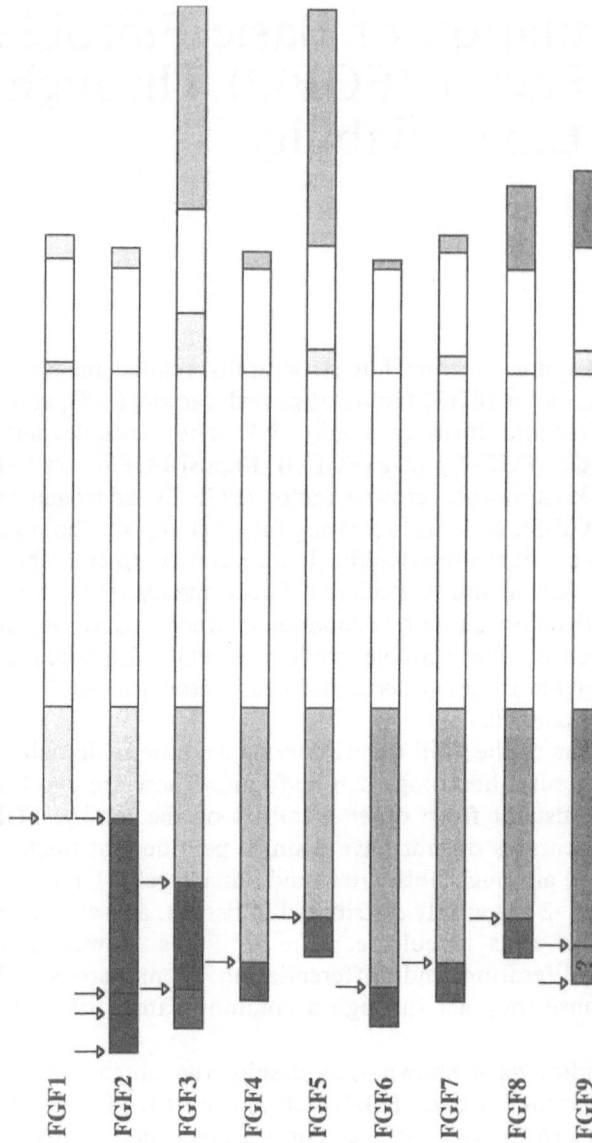

FIGURE 3.1. The FGF family of growth factors. The nine known members are illustrated as bars. The area containing the most homology is presented in the clear bar. In some of the FGFs, an intervening sequence interrupts this homology. This is the site identified as the receptor binding domain in FGF-2.

cells surrounding this FGF are quiescent and often unresponsive to the growth factor when infused (6).

A number of investigators observed when FGF-2 (or FGF-1) is conferred with the ability to enter the secretory pathway (by engineering a signal peptide into its primary sequence), it becomes a transforming molecule (7–9). These findings were largely interpreted to mean that, under the right circumstances, FPF-2 could have oncogenic potential. Alternatively, the absence of a signal peptide in FGF-2 could reflect the cell's desire to limit FGF-2 action by preventing secretion. To account for this observation, and in consideration of the fact that FGF-2 can be found outside cells, Florkiewicz et al. (10) suggested specific mechanisms must exist to "export" FGF outside cells. This hypothetical mechanism of export translocates FGF-2 from the cytoplasm to the cell surface. The mechanism would be tightly controlled, independent of the Golgi–endoplasmic reticulum secretion pathway, and protect the cell from the transforming potential of a secreted FGF described above. In any case, this selective release of FGF-2 (which also applies to FGF-1) is most likely a process that tightly regulates the growth factors' activities by limiting their respective bioavailability.

Because a molecule like FGF-2 stimulates the growth responses of a broad range of cell types, it was initially not clear how a molecule that is so pleiotropic could play a physiologic role in the control of cell growth and differentiation. This activity was further complicated by the observation that the growth factor could be purified from almost any tissue in which the target cells are found. If this protein is important in vivo, how could it be present in so many tissues in which the target cells are essentially quiescent? One possibility is that it is not a growth factor in vivo, and plays some other function (11). Yet it is found in the extracellular matrix, where it is presumably sequestered and stored in an inactive form. Three mechanisms regulating this bioavailability have been proposed: through its receptors, by limited proteolysis, or by structural modification (1, 12). These possibilities are described here.

Regulation of FGF Activities by Its Low- and High-Affinity Receptor

The high-affinity receptors for FGF-2 (of which there are four known genes) are tyrosine kinases and ligand binding, extracellular domains of the immunoglobulin G (IgG) superfamily. Alterative splicing leads to the expression of numerous forms of the high affinity receptors encoded by any one gene. It is generally assumed the expression of different combinations of receptor isoforms predetermines ligand action.

The low-affinity proteoglycan FGF receptors also play a major role in regulating FGF action (7–9). But it is important to note first that there are at least three types of low affinity FGF receptors: syndecans, β-glycan, and glypican. Syndecans are transmembrane receptors with heparan sulfate attached to a protein core sequence encoded by one of four genes. β-Glycan is also a transmembrane heparan sulfate proteoglycan that is better known for its ability to bind transforming growth factor-β (TFG-β). Glypican, on the other hand, is an FGF-binding proteoglycan that is not a transmembrane, but is linked to the cell surface through a phosphoinositol. In contrast, perfecan is a heparan sulfate proteoglycan that is not associated with the cell surface, but localizes to the extracellular matrix (ECM). It is assumed all of these heparan sulfate proteoglycans bind FGF, and their role is to deliver FGF to high affinity receptors (13–15).

High-Affinity Receptor Regulation of FGF Activity

If the high-affinity receptors for FGF are involved in the regulation of FGF-2 activities, it is most likely mediated through their restricted expression in vivo (Fig. 3.2). Recent studies have now shown these receptors are present during embryonic development. Their distribution is also cell type specific (16). In normal adult tissues there is little expression, but expression is readily detectable after injury, in tumors, or in proliferative disease. There are also certain exceptions to this observation: in the central nervous system, there are focal sites of FGF synthesis that include the hippocampus, ependymal cells of the lateral and third ventricles, and the subfornical organ, to name a few. Generally, however, receptor expression is low in peripheral tissues.

If there is indeed limited receptor expression, then FGF-2 may have a specificity in spite of it being both multifunctional, pluripotent, and ubiquitous. For example, there is compelling evidence that cells have specific signatures of high-affinity receptor isoform expression on their cell surface (16). Increased receptor concentrations at the cell surface could also, by mass action, promote the transfer of the ligand from low-affinity to high-affinity sites of binding. These hypotheses are supported in part by the findings that the infusion of FGF-2 into animals does not appear to have impact on the function of many of its target cells (6). Furthermore, when FGF-2 is made cytotoxic by linking it to the ribosomal inactivating protein saporin, the mitotoxin is highly specific in vivo for proliferating cells, but not to all of its presumed cell targets (17–19). That being the case, cells can be seen as refractory to FGF, unless there is an injury that activates the FGF high-affinity receptor system. Similarly, numerous cells are responsive to FGF in vitro, because under the conditions of cell culture, they have an injured and activated phenotype with an activated FGF receptor system.

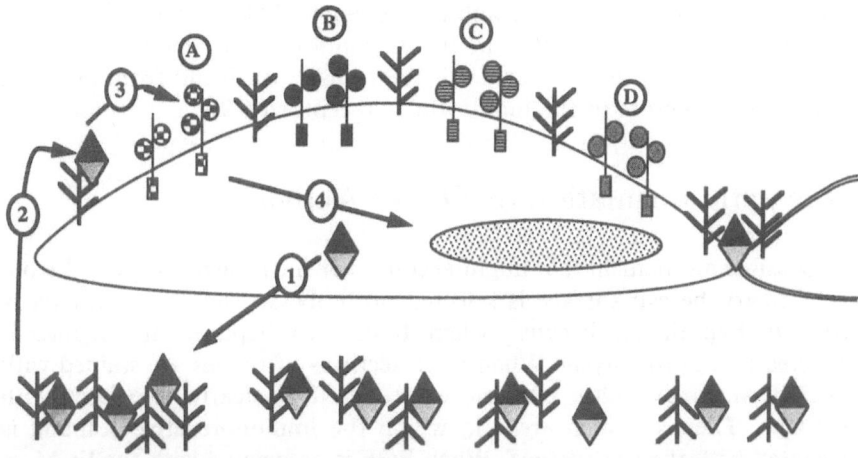

FIGURE 3.2. Complexity of FGF regulation. Shown are the high affinity receptors for FGF (labeled A–D) on the cell surface. FGF-2 is represented by the diamonds made up of solid and shaded triangles. Heparan sulfate proteoglycans are represented by the tree-like structures. After expression of the FGF-2 gene (an event highly regulated in its own right) and the translation of its mRNA (another highly regulated event) into the appropriate molecular form of FGF-2 (see ref. 10), FGF-2 is presumably exported from cells where it is sequestered in the extracellular matrix (step 1). From the matrix, it must be translocated to low-affinity heparan sulfate proteoglycans on the cell surface (step 2), which then have to present it to the appropriate high-affinity receptor (step 3). Upon formation of a receptor complex, the ligand triggers intracellular tyrosine kinase phosphorylation, sets off a cellular response, and is internalized (step 4). (Adapted from Klagsbrun and Baird [15].)

Low-Affinity Receptor Regulation of FGF Activity

There are many possible mechanisms through which proteoglycan low-affinity receptors might regulate FGF activity. The most likely is they serve a dual function to sometimes sequester, and other times deliver (after the appropriate signal), FGF to its high-affinity receptor. The nature of the signal that elicits the transfer is not known (see below). Accordingly, the low-affinity receptor complex should be viewed as another step in the regulation of FGF action.

Because there are several different types of low-affinity receptor protein cores, and each may have multiple patterns of complexity (depending on the extent of heparan sulfate glycosylation and sulfation), it is exceedingly difficult to dissect a specific function for any one low-affinity receptor proteoglycan. Each isoform may have different effects on FGF specificity and function, some inhibiting FGF action and others promoting it. Certainly it appears that the sites of sequestration where a cell deposits its FGF-2 appear to be different from the low-affinity binding sites where exogenous FGF-2 binds. Some cells that synthesize FGF-2 do not recognize their own FGF-2, but respond well to exogenous FGF-2. Thus, it appears that one of the key processes in the formation of a functional ligand-receptor complex at the cell surface is the transfer of ligand from different low-affinity receptors to the high-affinity receptor (7–9).

Proteolytic Regulation of FGF-2 Activity

One possible mechanism that might account for the transfer of FGF-2 from the ECM to the cell surface is selected proteolysis. This is a particularly attractive hypothesis, because when bound to heparin, the ligand is protected from proteolysis. When fixed sections of tissues are stained with anti-FGF antibodies (20), immunoreactive FGF is clearly associated with the ECM. There are also areas in which the immunoreactive staining is associated with the cell surface. When FGF is associated with the ECM, it can be released in a soluble form by proteolysis (21–23). Brem et al (24) also showed an immunoreactive FGF-2 (when assayed by enzyme- linked immunosorbent assay [ELISA]) is detected in the fluids of partial-thickness and full-thickness wounds, suggesting the FGF present in these fluids may have been released because of degradation of the ECM during wounding. In the retina where FGF-2 staining can be observed in the basement membranes of the retinal pigmented epithelial (RPE) cells, heparinase treatment eliminates FGF staining (25). FGF-2 can also be released from the cell surface by the treatment of cells with phospholipase C (26), suggesting there is an active release of the growth factor and translocation between the ECM and its tyrosine kinase receptors.

If limited proteolysis is a physiologic mechanism regulating the release of FGF-2 from the ECM, there should be instances in vivo where FGF is detectable in serum or biologic fluids. Over the course of the last several years, there have been isolated reports that have described the presence of FGF-like molecules in urine, vitreous, and blood. Most recently, the availability of a highly sensitive ELISA for FGF has resulted in the systematic analysis of FGF in cancer patients (27). Whether this FGF derives directly from tumor cells or after the proteolysis that accompanies tissue remodeling remains to be determined.

Regulation of FGF by Posttranslational Modification

The low-affinity FGF receptor is not just a means of sequestering the growth factor, as it participates in the regulation of FGF-2 activity. The next question that arises is to understand how the growth factor translocates from one receptor to another. As described above, there could be a release of soluble FGF that would then be available to the general circulation (as described above). Yet there are a number of instances when FGF-2 is available to cells that have both low-affinity and high-affinity receptors on their surfaces, yet they do not seem to utilize their endogenous growth factor. These same cells respond to exogenous FGF. How can a cell that synthesizes FGF (presuming it translocates it onto the cell surface) be unable to respond to this same growth factor?

To explain this observation, we hypothesized that there might exist a specific extracellular process to catalyze the growth factor's shift from low-affinity receptors of sequestration toward low-affinity receptors of delivery, and ultimately toward high-affinity receptors of signal transduction. This is illustrated in Figure 3.3. We also reasoned this molecular event might involve a posttranslational modification of the growth factor. In particular, we observed FGF-2 could be phosphorylated, so we examined whether FGF could be phosphorylated extracellularly (28). We also reported the detection of a non–adenosine 3′,5′-cyclic monophosphate (cAMP) activated protein kinase capable of phosphorylating FGF-2 on the outer cell surface of human hepatoma cells (SK-Hep cells). During the course of its characterization, we also detected a second, distinct kinase that is cAMP independent. The addition of $[\gamma\text{-}^{32}P]$–adenosine triphosphate (ATP) results in a rapid (<5 min) incorporation of $[^{32}P]$ into FGF-2. The reaction is time, ATP, and substrate dependent. It is unaffected by inhibitors of cAMP-dependent phosphorylation (PKI, K562b), but is modulated by calcium, magnesium, and manganese. Heparin also modulates phosphorylation on FGF-2. Gel permeation chromatography of SK-Hep cell membranes identifies two constitutes of 350 and 90 kd. From these results, we have developed our current working hypothesis that a cell surface protein kinase is a potential signal that modifies FGF-2 such that it

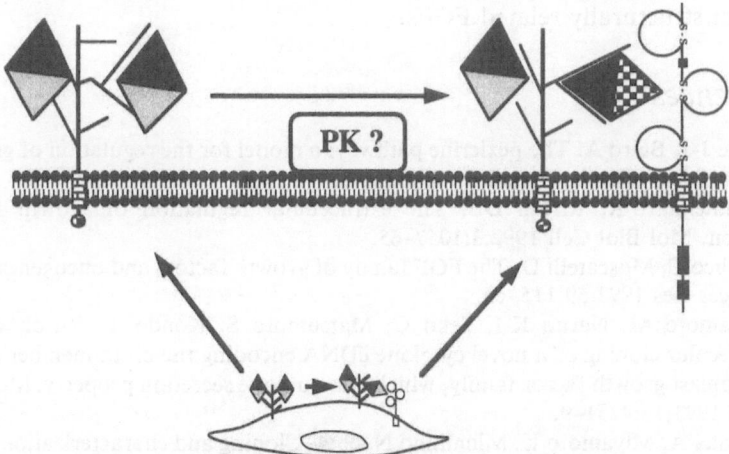

FIGURE 3.3. Potential role of ecto-phosphorylation in the regulation of FGF activity. Establishing that FGF-2 is the physiologic cell surface substrate for this kinase remains to be shown. (Adapted from Klagsbrun and Baird [15].)

can be translocated from extracellular sites of sequestration and recognized by its signal transducing high-affinity receptor. The structural characterization of this molecule, which will be the ultimate test of this hypothesis, is under way to determine whether its physiologic substrate on the cell surface is FGF, whether it is involved in FGF regulation, and what its function might be.

Conclusion

The physiology of FGF regulation is complex and far from understood. It involves extracellular low- and high-affinity receptors, sequestered and active forms of extracellular FGF, and potentially various posttranslational modifications of FGF including phosphorylation. FGF appears to be regulated at numerous steps: (1) at the level of its synthesis, where gene expression (in peripheral tissues) is low and activated by injury and/or physicochemical insult; (2) at the level of its export from cells, where it appears to remain cell-associated with heparan sulfate–related proteoglycans; (3) at the level of these matrix proteoglycans, which can serve to sequester the growth factor and keep it away from the target cell; (4) at the level of cell-associated proteoglycans, which can serve to deliver the growth factor to its signal transducing high-affinity receptor; (5) at the level of the high-affinity receptor, whose expression is exceedingly low in normal quiescent tissues; and (6) by the sheer complexity of the ligand receptor complex, that can include four genes encoding numerous isoforms of high-affinity receptors, seven genes encoding low-affinity receptors that are differentially sulfated and glycosylated, and at least nine genes encoding different structurally related FGFs.

References

1. Feige J-J, Baird A. The pexicrine pathway: a model for the regulation of growth factor bioavailability. Med Sci 1992;8:805–10.
2. Flaumenhaft R, Rifkin DB. The extracellular regulation of growth factor action. Mol Biol Cell 1992;3:1057–65.
3. Basilico C, Moscatelli D. The FGF family of growth factors and oncogenes. Adv Cancer Res 1992;59:115–65.
4. Miyamoto M, Naruo K-I, Seko C, Matsumoto S, Kondo T, Kurokawa T. Molecular cloning of a novel cytokine cDNA encoding the ninth member of the fibroblast growth factor family, which has a unique secretion property. Mol Cell Biol 1993;13:4251–9.
5. Tanaka A, Miyamoto K, Minamino N, et al. Cloning and characterization of an androgen-induced growth factor essential for the androgen-dependent growth of mouse mammary carcinoma cells. Proc Natl Acad Sci USA 1992;89:8928–32.
6. Whalen FG, Shing Y, Folkman J. The fate of intravenously administered bFGF and the effect of heparin. Growth Factors 1989;1:157–64.
7. Blam SB, Mitchell R, Tischer E, et al. Addition of growth hormone secretion

signal to basic fibroblast growth factor results in cell transformation and secretion of aberrant forms of the protein. Oncogene 1988;3:129–36.

8. Rogelj S, Weinberg RA, Fanning P, Klagsbrun M. Basic fibroblast growth factor fused to a signal peptide transforms cells. Nature 1988;331:173–5.

9. Brill G, Vaisman N, Neufeld G, Kalcheim C. BHK-21-derived cell lines that produce basic fibroblast growth factor, but not parallel BHK-21 cells, initiate neuronal differentiation of neural crest progenitors. Development 1992; 115:1059–69.

10. Florkiewicz RA, Baird A, Gonzalez A-M. Multiple forms of bFGF: differential nuclear and cell surface localization. Growth Factors 1991;4:265–75.

11. Baird A. Fibroblast growth factors: What's in a name? Endocrinology 1993; 132:487–8.

12. Baird A, Walicke PA. Fibroblast growth factors. Br Med J 1989;45:438–52.

13. Orintz DM, Yayon A, Flanagan JG, Svahn CM, Levi E, Leder P. Heparin is required for cell-free binding of basic fibroblast growth factor to a soluble receptor and for mitogenesis in whole cells. Mol Cell Biol 1992;12:240–7.

14. Rapraeger AC, Krufka A, Olwin BB. Requirement of heparan sulfate for bFGF-mediated fibroblast growth and myoblast differentiation. Science 1991; 252:1705–8.

15. Klagsbrun M, Baird A. A dual receptor system is required for basic fibroblast growth factor activity. Cell 1991;67:229–31.

16. Patstone G, Pasquale EB, Maher PA. Different members of the fibroblast growth factor receptor family are specific to distinct cell types in the developing chicken embryo. Dev Biol 1993;155:107–23.

17. Lappi DA, Baird A. Mitotoxins: growth factor targetted cytotoxic molecules. Prog Growth Factor Res 1991;2:22–36.

18. Beitz JG, Davol P, Clark JW, et al. Antitumor activity of basic fibroblast growth factor-saporin mitotoxin in vitro and in vivo. Cancer Res 1992; 52:227–30.

19. Lindner V, Lappi DA, Baird A, Majack RA, Reidy MA. Role of basic fibroblast growth factor in vascular lesion formation. Circ Res 1991;68:106–13.

20. Gonzalez AM, Buscaglia M, Ong M, Baird A. Immunolocalization of basic FGF in the 18 day rat fetus: association with the basement membrane of various tissues. J Cell Biol 1990;110:753–65.

21. Baird A, Ling N. Fibroblast growth factors are present in the extracellular matrix produced by endothelial cells in vitro: implication for a role of heparinase-like enzymes in the neovascular response. Biochem Biophys Res Commun 1987;142:428–35.

22. Vlodavsky I, Folkman J, Sullivan R, et al. Endothelial cell-derived basic fibroblast growth factor: synthesis and deposition into subendothelial extracellular matrix. Proc Natl Acad Sci USA 1987;84:2292–6.

23. Folkman J, Klagsbrun M, Sasse J, Wadzinski MG, Ingber D, Vlodavsky I. A heparin-binding angiogenic protein—basic fibroblast growth factor—is stored within basement membrane. Am J Pathol 1988;130:393–400.

24. Brem S, Tsanaclis AMC, Gately S, Gross JL, Herblin WF. Immunolocalization of basic fibroblast growth factor to the microvasculature of human brain tumors. Cancer 1992;70:2673–80.

25. Hanneken A, De Juan E Jr, Lutty GA, Fox GM, Schiffer S, Hjelmeland LM. Altered distribution of basic fibroblast growth factor in diabetic retinopathy. Arch Ophthalmol 1991;109:1005–11.

26. Brunner G, Gabrilove J, Rifkin DB, Wilson EL. Phospholipase C release of basic fibroblast growth factor from human bone marrow cultures as a biologically active complex with a phosphatidylinositol-anchored heparan sulfate proteoglycan. J Cell Biol 1991;114:1275–83.
27. Nguyen M, Watanabe H, Budson AE, Richie JP, Folkman J. Elevated levels of the angiogenic peptide basic fibroblast growth factor in urine of bladder cancer patients. J Natl Cancer Inst 1993;85:241–2.
28. Vilgrain I, Baird A. Phosphorylation of basic fibroblast growth factor by a protein kinase associated with the outer surface of a target cell. Mol Endocrinol 1991;5:1003–12.

4

Cultured Skin Cells for Wound Closure and for Promoting Wound Healing

JOHN F. HANSBROUGH AND HANS OLIVER RENNEKAMPFF

The Need for Accelerating Wound Closure

Burn clinicians have developed great expertise in treating patients with severe burns, and survival of extensively burned patients has markedly improved in the past several decades (1, 2). However, technologies are greatly needed to improve the functional and cosmetic outcomes of burn injury. For example, although meshing and stretching of skin grafts permit wider areas of skin coverage, the cosmetic and functional results of meshed skin grafting are frequently unsatisfactory. We must develop technologies and expertise to decrease scar formation and improve the quality of life of burn patients. We hope that biotechnology research and the biotechnology industry can help us to achieve these goals.

If we examine the refinements in burn care over the past three decades, it appears that excisional therapy has been associated with the most significant increase in survival of seriously burned patients (2, 3). Increasingly early after injury and stabilization of the patient, patients are moved to the operating room where their wounds are surgically excised (4, 5) (Fig. 4.1). Burn wound excision has important benefits in terms of reducing the dead tissue that can serve as a culture medium for microorganisms (6), and perhaps decreasing the metabolic responses to burn injury (7). However, surgical excision creates extensive open wounds that in many patients cannot be immediately closed with autologous skin. We must develop improved technologies for closing these wounds with both temporary and permanent skin replacements.

A number of skin replacements have been tested, and several are currently clinically available. These include both temporary and permanent skin replacements, epidermal and dermal skin replacements, and synthetic/biosynthetic and biologic skin replacements (8).

The gold standard for providing temporary wound coverage following

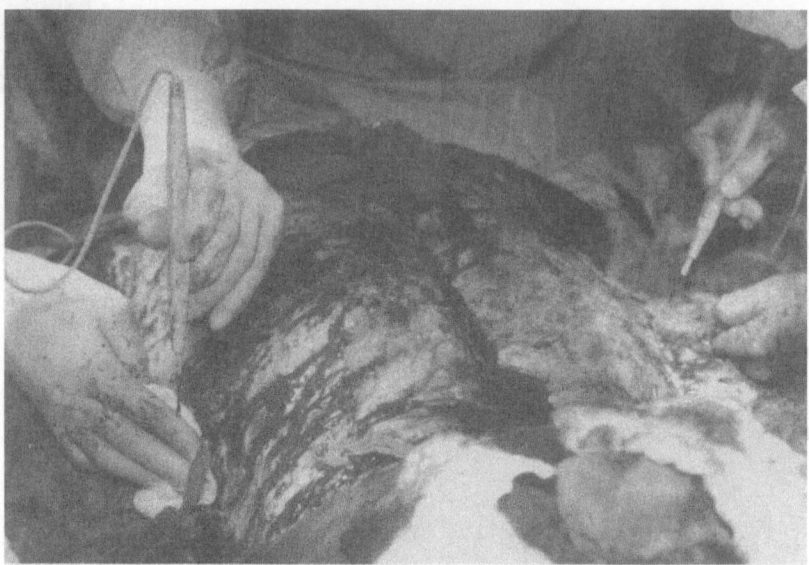

FIGURE 4.1. Within days of admission, this patient, who had sustained extensive burns, is taken to the operating room where burned tissue is surgically excised. In this case, two separate operating teams are working to speed the process.

surgical excision is cadaver allograft skin. Allograft skin is utilized by most burn centers in this country for this purpose. Cadaver skin is effective for providing temporary closure of these wounds and it can be lifesaving for patients with massive burn injuries. Allograft effectively closes the wound and prepares the wound for subsequent definitive autografting. When viable allograft skin has adhered to the wound and is subsequently removed, a well-vascularized wound base remains behind that can then readily accept skin autografts. However, there are significant problems with cadaver skin that will be addressed later, including the very serious problem of the danger of infectious disease transmission. These problems make it important that effective replacements for cadaver skin be developed.

A larger patient population than that of burn patients is those individuals who have developed chronic wounds that are slow to heal, or that completely fail to heal over a long time period. This population includes patients with venous stasis skin ulcers, with diabetic and vascular ulcers, and with pressure ulcers (decubiti). Trials of various products have been performed or are under way in attempts to improve healing of these wounds. One approach has been to apply biologic agents such as growth factors or tissue extracts to these wounds to attempt to accelerate wound closure. Another method has been to apply various types of cultured grafts to these wounds, with the hypothesis that the cultured cells will elaborate various cytokines that will stimulate the wound and accelerate wound closure. Some of these biologic agents and graft materials will be briefly discussed.

Cultured Epithelium

One method to permanently close the wound is to culture the epithelial cells, the keratinocytes, after separation of the epidermis from the dermis with the use of enzymatic digestion. Over 15 years ago, successful technologies to rapidly propagate human keratinocytes in tissue culture were developed (9, 10), utilizing several different methods of tissue culture. Cultured keratinocyte sheets were then applied to burn wounds (11), with varied success. Numerous trials have been subsequently performed to determine the ability of cultured epithelium to permanently close full-thickness wounds (8, 12, 13). Reports of clinical trials from multiple burn centers are contained in the January/February 1992 issue of the *Journal of Burn Care and Rehabilitation,* and the results were summarized (12). Cultured epithelial sheets are exceedingly fragile, they are difficult to handle and affix to the wound, and their transport from the laboratory to the site for transplantation can be complex. The subsequent wound care must be meticulous and cultured grafts appear to be highly susceptible to infection. The success of cultured epithelium for closing wounds is quote variable. Rives's group (14) from France has reported some of the best results; however, the intensity of wound care that is required to apparently achieve these results can be extraordinary in terms of time and personnel. In addition, several studies have reported that the healed epithelium can be quite fragile and the skin is prone to breakdown and contractions (15–18). Clinical results following grafting of cultured epithelium appear to be optimized when the grafts are placed over cadaver dermis, following previous application of cadaver skin to the wounds and mechanical removal of the epidermis (12, 19, 20). Removal of the epidermal layer is facilitated by the rejection response of the host to the epidermis. In contrast, dermis is relatively nonantigenic and may remain attached to the wound bed following sloughing of the epidermis.

Culturing keratinocytes on flexible, biocompatible membranes can theoretically facilitate the transfer of cell sheets to the wound bed, by eliminating the need to cleave the attachments between cells and the culture surface with proteolytic enzymes prior to transfer of grafts. In addition, the handling of delicate cultured epithelium is difficult and labor intensive, and the simple transfer of cell-coated membranes to the wound would greatly simplify graft transfer, operative surgery, and wound care, particularly if the membrane could be left in place postoperatively to secure the cells to the wound surface. These experiments are under way in our own laboratory (21) and will be described in a following section.

When cultured epithelial sheets are placed on the full-thickness wound,

which by definition lacks dermis elements, there is delayed basement
membrane formation with initial development of a flat dermal-epidermal
junction (Fig. 4.2). This may have very important consequences for wound
healing. In normal skin, rete ridges are present that result in interdigitation
of epidermis and dermis; this markedly increases the surface area of the
dermal-epidermal junction that furnishes strength and durability of the skin
(22). On a molecular level, the dermis is important for epithelial development and maturation (23), including the development of ultrastructural
elements such as anchoring fibrils that help attach epidermis to the dermis.
Because the full-thickness wound by definition lacks dermis, and dermis
does not regenerate or does so very slowly, developing of attachment
structures is delayed (24). This may account for the disappointing take of
epithelial sheet grafts. One of the largest clinical series published 3 years ago
from the U.S. Army Burn Center showed disappointingly poor take of
cultured epithelial autograft (25). A take rate as low as 13% to 20% was
found in deeper wounds that had been excised to the level of the fascia. It
is disastrous to wait 3 to 4 weeks and spend many thousands of dollars for
cultured epithelium only to achieve limited take of the grafts. Other reports
describe an adequate initial take of cultured epithelium but later wound
problems such as shearing and wound contraction (15).

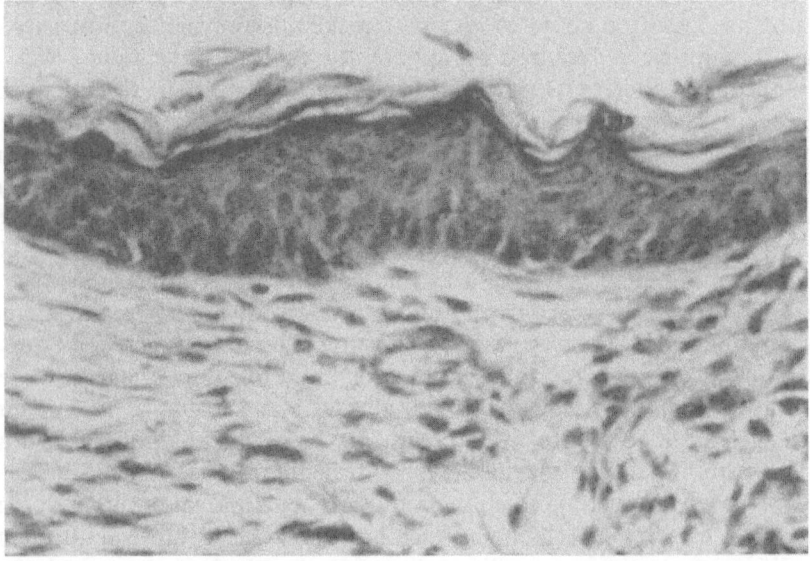

Figure 4.2. Two weeks after application of cultured epithelial grafts to full-
thickness wounds on athymic mice, a flat dermal-epidermal junction is found
without evidence of rete ridge interdigitations that occur between epidermis and
dermis in normal skin. Formation of basement membrane structures, in the absence
of dermis, is very slow to occur in this situation.

Development of Composite (Epidermal-Dermal) Skin Grafts

We and increasingly other groups believe that it is necessary to replace the dermal layer of the skin, as well as the epidermis, for achieving optimal results for covering full-thickness wounds. The best means to accomplish this remains to be determined. Several years ago our group developed a dermal analogue composed of human fibroblasts cultured in a collagen-glycosaminoglycan (GAG) membrane (26, 27). We found that inclusion of fibroblasts in the membrane was necessary to obtain confluent growth of keratinocytes on the surface of the dermal substrate. Without the inclusion of fibroblasts, we were not able to achieve satisfactory epithelial growth on the surface. We subsequently showed that levels of collagen type IV, a structural protein component of basement membrane, were far higher in the culture medium when keratinocytes were cultured together compared with cultures of the individual cell types (28). Keratinocytes cultured alone produced little laminin, another structural protein component of basement membrane, while fibroblasts as well as composite cultures produced high amounts of laminin. Clearly, fibroblasts play an important role in the development of the basement membrane.

These composite grafts reproducibly closed full-thickness, excised wounds in athymic mice (29). When we placed the composite grafts on patients following burn wound excision (30), we found some areas of excellent wound take with good skin appearance and minimal hypertrophic scar formation. As early as 10 days postgrafting, we found extensive rete ridge interdigitation, far different from the flat dermal-epidermal junction that occurs when cultured epithelial sheets are applied to wounds. This was a very uniform finding in our seven patients. Basement membrane proteins laminin and type IV collagen were identified immunohistochemically in all patients. We believe that early formation of normal anatomic structures is facilitated in these composite grafts that contain both epidermal and dermal components.

However, overall take of this composite skin was approximately 50%, not successful enough to make this a routinely acceptable skin replacement. We believe that graft take was limited for several reasons. The wounds that receive autologous cultured grafts are really chronic wounds, since we must wait 3 to 4 weeks after injury to produce the cultured grafts. Many of these wounds probably contain high levels of proteases, which probably attack the collagen-GAG membrane. In addition, many of the wounds have high bacterial counts (31), which also limits the success of the fragile grafts.

We have evaluated a variety of dermal replacements, including fibroblasts cultured on polyglyactin mesh. Surgeons routinely utilize sutures and grafts composed of these biodegradable fibers. We have worked with

Advanced Tissue Sciences, Inc. (La Jolla, CA) to develop living dermal replacements by culturing human neonatal fibroblasts on polyglactin mesh (32, 33). Because the polyglactin fibers undergo hydrolysis in the wound, rather than degradation by proteases and inflammatory cells, we believe that these materials will be noninflammatory when placed on the wound. The cultured fibroblasts secrete matrix proteins that are deposited in the dermal analogue during the culture process. This material, Dermagraft, is undergoing clinical evaluation as a replacement for human dermis (34). We and others are also investigating the attributes of other biodegradable matrix supports.

We have cultured keratinocytes on the surface of Dermagraft, and have achieved confluent growth of the keratinocytes resulting in a multilayered epithelium (Fig. 4.3). These composite grafts successfully closed wounds on athymic mice and resulted in early formation of basement membrane structures including appearance of laminin and type IV collagen (35).

Very importantly, these composite grafts are easy to handle, which benefits the cell culture technician as well as the surgeon. The grafts are easy to remove from the culture vessel since they have good structural integrity and they do not require enzymatic treatment to release them from the

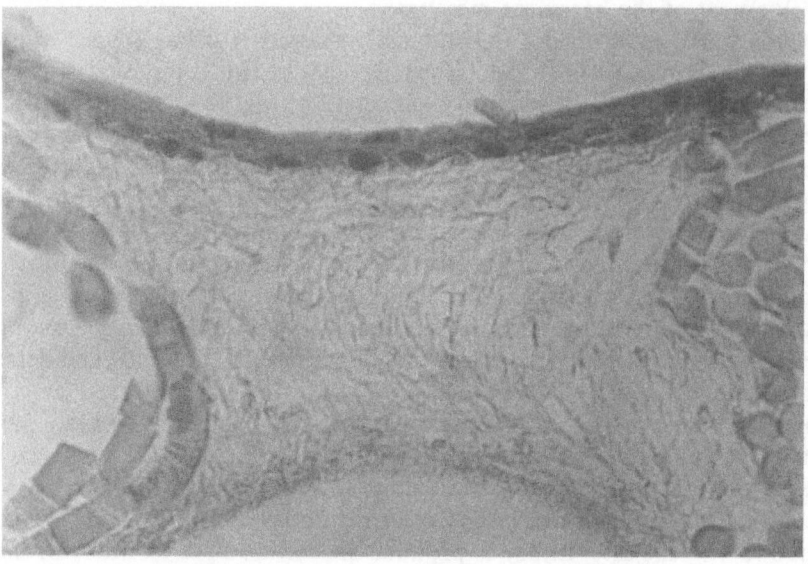

FIGURE 4.3. A composite graft composed of keratinocytes cultured for 17 days on a polyglactin biodegradable mesh (Vicryl, Ethicon, Inc., Somerville, NJ) containing fibroblasts (Dermagraft, Advanced Tissue Sciences, Inc.), ready for graft placement. The polyglactin fibers are cut transversely; spaces between the fibers are filled with fibroblasts and secreted collagen and other matrix proteins, while the keratinocytes form a multilayered epithelium. H&E, ×200.

culture vessel (Fig. 4.4). The grafts drape easily and can be moved around on the wound bed, they have good resistance to tearing, and they can be easily sutured or stapled to the wound. Thus, an important advantage of using a dermal replacement in conjunction with the cultured cell epithelium is that graft handling and placement are greatly facilitated.

Bell et al. (36) developed one of the first composite skin replacements, comprising fibroblasts cast in bovine collagen lattices that were allowed to contract and then seeded with dispersed, noncultured epidermal cells. A multilayered keratinizing epidermis with desmosomes, tonofilaments, and hemidesmosomes developed with formation of basement membrane within 2 weeks. It was suggested that the dermal replacement could provide better interactions between fibroblasts and other cell types in vitro, compared with cells cultured on a plastic or glass surface. Organogenesis, Inc. (Canton, MA) has further developed this composite skin replacement (Graftskin). In our laboratory (37, 38), Graftskin placed on full-thickness excised wounds on athymic mice persisted for the 60-day study period with minimal contraction and resulted in well-differentiated epidermis with stratum

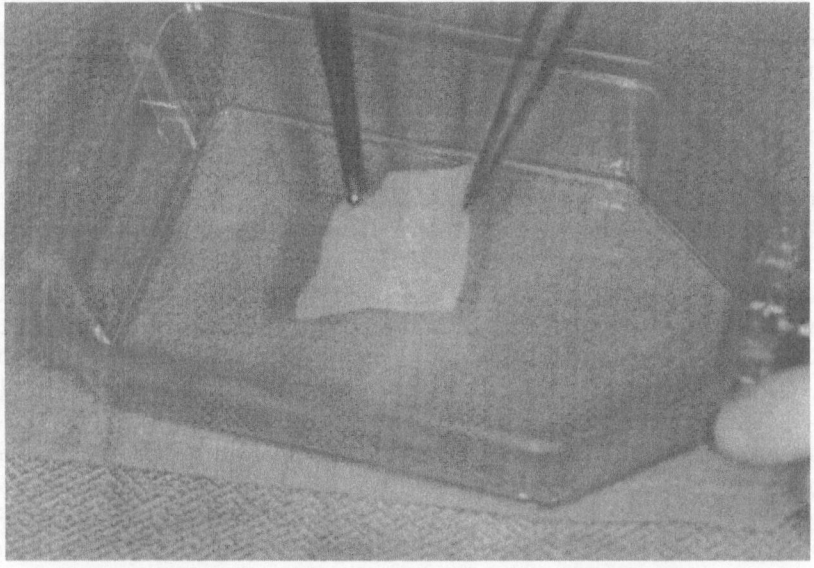

FIGURE 4.4. When epithelial cells are cultured on a dermal support that has structural integrity, the composite grafts can be easily handled and transported from the culture flask to the wound. This is in contrast to the difficulty involved in manipulating and transporting delicate epithelial sheet grafts. The cultured grafts are easy to handle because of the inherent strength of the polyglactin mesh, and enzymatic release of the cultured epithelium, which can damage the cells and results in shrinkage of the epithelial sheets, is not required prior to placement of the grafts on wounds.

corneum. Basement membrane proteins were identified by immunohisto-chemical staining and electron microscopy within 2 weeks of placement. Graftskin is currently under investigation in clinical trials as a temporary skin replacement for burn wounds, and as a dressing to facilitate the closure of cutaneous ulcers (39).

Cultured Grafts for Delivery of Cytokines for Accelerating Wound Healing

Several types of cultured grafts have been utilized in clinical care to deliver cytokines to wounds. These include Dermagraft, (Advanced Tissue Sciences, Inc.), which is composed of human neonatal foreskins cultured on a polyglactin mesh, and Graftskin (Organogenesis, Inc.), containing both keratinocytes and fibroblasts, and which is described above. These grafts are used primarily with the idea that the cultured cells will elaborate growth peptides into the underlying wounds. Both materials are currently in clinical trials for treating chronic nonhealing wounds.

Regulatory peptides such as cytokines and growth factors are multifunc-tional molecules with both stimulatory and inhibitory actions, depending on the cellular context. All peptide growth factors initiate their effects by binding to and activating specific, high-affinity receptor proteins located in the plasma membrane of the target cells. Thereby they may act in autocrine, paracrine, juxtacrine, or endocrine fashions.

There are five major growth factor families that appear to contribute significantly to the wound healing process: epidermal growth factor (EGF), transforming growth factor-β (TGF-β), insulin-like growth factor (IGF), platelet-derived growth factor (PDGF), and the fibroblast growth factor (FGF) family (40). In addition a number of keratinocyte-derived cytokines are critically involved in the wound healing process: interleukin (IL)-1β, IL-6, IL-10, chemokines, and the colony stimulating factors (41).

In contrast to EGF, TGF-α is detected in normal skin. TGF-α expression is markedly increased in healing skin wounds (42). Like EGF, TGF-α is highly mitogenic for keratinocytes. Furthermore, it was shown that TGF-α can stimulate additional TGF-α release and also its own receptor expression (43). These in vitro findings for mitogenicity and positive autoregulation underline the importance of TGF-α as a major autocrine mitogen in the epidermis. In a number of studies, topically applied EGF and TGF-α have been shown to accelerate the healing of cutaneous wounds (44, 45). Moreover, TGF-α is angiogenic and has been shown to increase the number of dermal fibroblasts and granulation tissue (42). Therefore, beneficial effects of TGF-α on epithelialization are not simple to associate with epidermal proliferation alone.

Interestingly these studies have found rather limited, albeit significant improvements in healing over placebo controls. This is likely due to the fact that multiple other growth peptides are present in the healing wound. Synergistic, additive, and converse findings with combinations of growth factors are reported (46). The importance of the combination of growth factors to control an appropriate healing is underlined by our findings (44) that synergistically applied basic FGF (bFGF) reduced the effect of EGF on the rate of epithelialization in experimental wounds.

A number of autocrine functioning interleukins have gained new attention. Interleukin-6 is a multifunctional cytokine produced at high levels by activated keratinocytes. It stimulates the proliferation of human keratinocytes (47). Recent findings demonstrated transient upregulation of the integrin $\alpha_5\beta_1$, the major fibronectin receptor on keratinocytes (48). This integrin is critically involved in the migration process of keratinocytes. As two major processes in wound healing are affected by IL-6, it is not surprising that IL-6 has been shown to facilitate wound healing in vivo (49).

A new superfamily of chemokines, apparently encoding chemotactic and inflammatory cytokines—hence their name—has been described in recent years (50). One of the most recently described and important chemokines that may be particularly important to the skin is interleukin-8. IL-8 has been detected in large quantities in psoriasis (51), a hyperproliferative benign skin disease. Furthermore, a gradient of IL-8 release was detected in partial thickness burn wounds (52). IL-8 is produced by keratinocytes under the influence of various stimuli. Our own studies (53) and those of others (54) demonstrated that the chemokines IL-8 and melanoma growth stimulating activity/gro (MGSA/gro) are mitogenic for keratinocytes, but not for fibroblasts. In addition, we demonstrated that chemokines can induce overexpression of various integrin receptors, critically involved in wound healing processes. Functionally this is underlined by the chemotactic response of keratinocytes to IL-8 (55). Furthermore, IL-8 was found to be angiogenic (56).

While many growth factors and cytokines enhance healing in acute experimental wounds in animals, their topical application in human chronic wounds frequently does not achieve the same success (57). This indicates that chronic wounds may lack an orderly progression of growth peptides, and this may not be remedied by the application of a single growth factor. Cultured keratinocytes either as an autologous or allogeneic sheet graft may provide growth factors in the appropriate type, amounts, and sequence most favorable for promoting wound healing. Application of cultured cells to wounds may also provide matrix material for cell growth. While autologous keratinocyte sheets may generate growth peptides and provide tissue for permanent wound closure, the major action of keratinocyte allografts would be to provide a growth peptide stimulation of the healing process even though the cells would be ultimately rejected. A number of reports of accelerated healing by grafting of leg ulcers and partial-thickness burns and donor sites with allogeneic epidermis are evidence for the action of keratinocyte-derived growth peptides. Grafting of donor sites and partial-thickness wounds with allogeneic epidermis accelerated healing compared with mirror image control sites (58). The treatment of leg ulcers with autologous and allogeneic cultured keratinocyte sheets showed improved healing of otherwise unresponsive wounds (59). However, time requirements and costs for fabricating these grafts have limited their application. Furthermore, basal keratinocytes and parabasal keratinocytes depict an activated state and release cytokines such as TGF-α (60).

Viability of cultured epithelial sheets, evaluated with propidium iodide exclusion combined with fluorescence activated cell sorting (FACS) analysis, is linked to basal and immediately suprabasal cells and may be as low as 20% (unpublished data). Therefore, it seems obvious that a single layer of active, proliferating keratinocytes may be a sufficient method to deliver growth peptides. The application of cultured keratinocytes dispersed in a fibrin glue (61) or cultured to subconfluent stage on a polyurethane film inverted onto the wound bed (21, 62) are methods in favor of this approach. As described above, certain polyurethane membranes have been shown to serve as excellent surfaces for supporting the growth of epithelial cells. These membranes have been considered as "intelligent" dressings, allowing control of moisture vapor permeability according to their degree of hydration following placement on the wound. These polyurethane membranes in combination with seeded keratinocytes can be considered as an analogue to the stratified layers in cultured keratinocyte sheets, which may provide a barrier function for the wound. We have seeded human keratinocytes onto the surface of such membranes (Fig. 4.5). The keratinocytes readily attach to the membrane and proliferate, and they can be transferred to the wound in a subconfluent state without the necessity of removing them from the membrane.

As shown in Figure 4.6, polyurethane membranes with a confluent layer of keratinocytes released substantial amounts of interleukin-6 into the culture medium. These cytokine levels have been shown by others to promote wound healing (49). Substantial levels (TGF-α) were also released into the culture medium, as shown in Figure 4.7.

A Laboratory-Prepared Replacement for Cadaver Allograft Skin

As noted earlier, cadaver allograft skin is the standard material for temporary skin replacement in patients with extensive burns (8, 63). However, allograft skin is not without its problems. There is high demand for allograft skin and it frequently is unavailable at individual burn centers. Since the U.S. Food and Drug Administration has recently increased its regulations regarding skin banking, the supply of cadaver skin has become

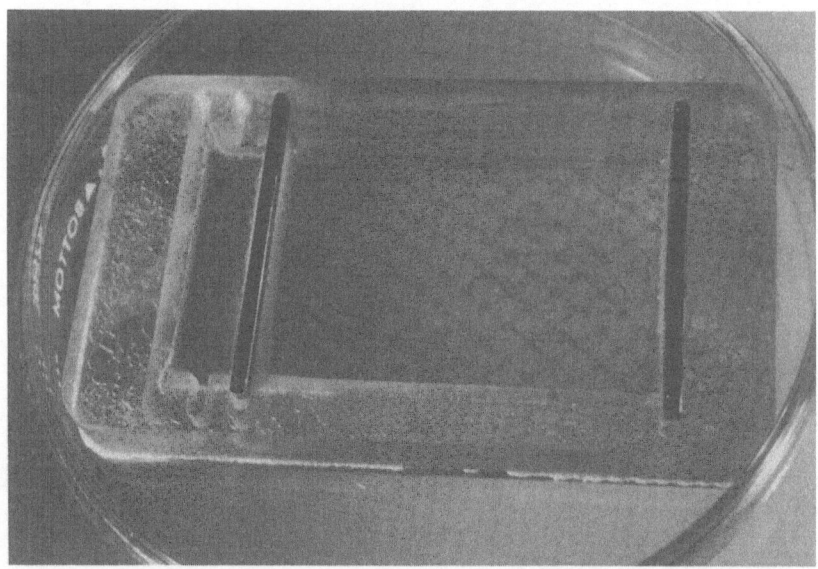

FIGURE 4.5. We have developed a technique of culturing human keratinocytes on a hydrophilic polyurethane membrane (Hydroderm, Wilshire Medical, Inc.), which is shown in a device designed to hold the membrane taut while it is submerged in culture medium. The cells attach and proliferate on the membrane; following inversion and transfer to the wound, the membrane provides a moisture vapor barrier to protect the cells and the wound while keratinocytes continue to proliferate and close the wound.

even more limited. In addition the quality is variable, since donors may be quite elderly and sometimes only limited areas of the body are able to be harvested. The potential for infection, both bacterial and viral, is always present. It will probably never be possible to ensure that allograft skin is free of contaminating viruses. The donor of the skin may be recently infected but actually be seronegative, and the donor of skin, unlike the blood donor, can obviously not be serologically retested at a later time point.

Allograft skin is rejected within several weeks of placement on the wound. Twenty years ago, allograft skin routinely survived a month or even longer. However, as our overall care for burn patients has improved, particularly in the area of early excision and nutritional support, immune function is greatly improved so that allograft skin is rejected much more quickly.

Utilizing our experience with cultured fibroblasts and Dermagraft, we are attempting to develop a laboratory-grown temporary replacement for human skin. An important aspect of human fibroblasts is that they are relatively nonimmunogenic, so they do not stimulate a rejection response in the allogeneic host. Thus, allogeneic fibroblasts can be utilized to produce

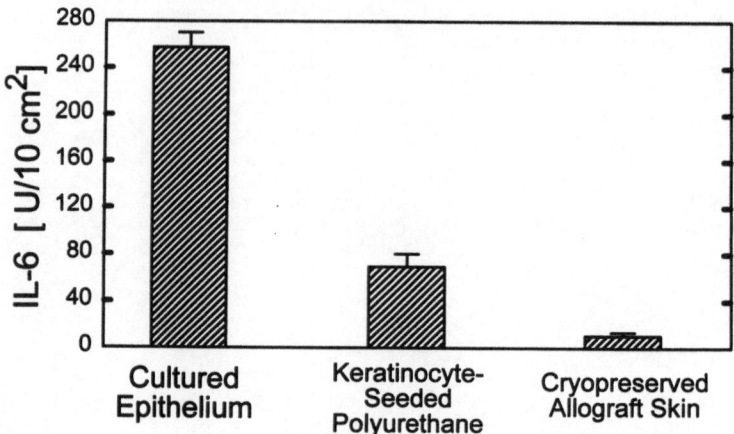

FIGURE 4.6. Similarly to the previous figure, culture medium was assayed for IL-6 levels using a bioassay.

a storable tissue culture product that can be used immediately after injury on the patient. We utilized a biosynthetic dressing, Biobrane (Dow Hickam Inc., SugarLand, TX), which had been moderately successful as a temporary skin replacement, and have attempted to improve its performance as a biologic skin replacement. Biobrane is composed of nylon fibers that are bonded to a thin silicone membrane; the membrane provides a barrier against water-vapor transmission from the wound and bacterial invasion from the environment. Although Biobrane has been utilized as a temporary

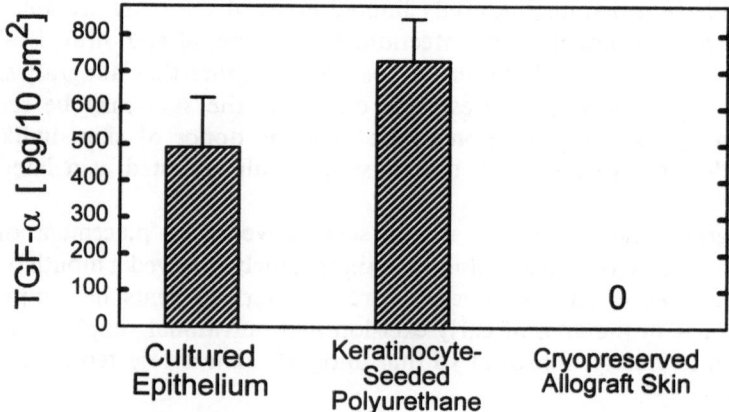

FIGURE 4.7. Culture medium from cultured epithelial sheets and keratinocytes cultured on Hydroderm polyurethane membrane and from allograft skin soaked in culture medium were assayed for transforming growth factor-α (TGF-α) using an enzyme-linked immunosorbent assay (ELISA) technique.

skin replacement by some burn centers, it does not encourage the excellent fibrovascular ingrowth that results following the application of human skin. As a result, Biobrane has not been universally accepted as a temporary skin replacement for excised wounds. We attempted to improve the biologic and clinical performance of Biobrane by seeding human fibroblasts in the nylon mesh of Biobrane. We found that the cells proliferated rapidly within the mesh and after several weeks a densely cellular "tissue" formed surrounding the nylon fibers (Fig. 4.8), which contained high levels of secreted human matrix proteins as well as multiple growth factors. Animal testing showed that this skin replacement could be used either fresh or cryopreserved (viable), or as a nonviable product, to close full-thickness wounds. We believe that the matrix proteins and growth factors contained in the "tissue" encourage fibrovascular ingrowth from the wound bed and decrease the inflammatory response to the foreign materials (nylon and silicone).

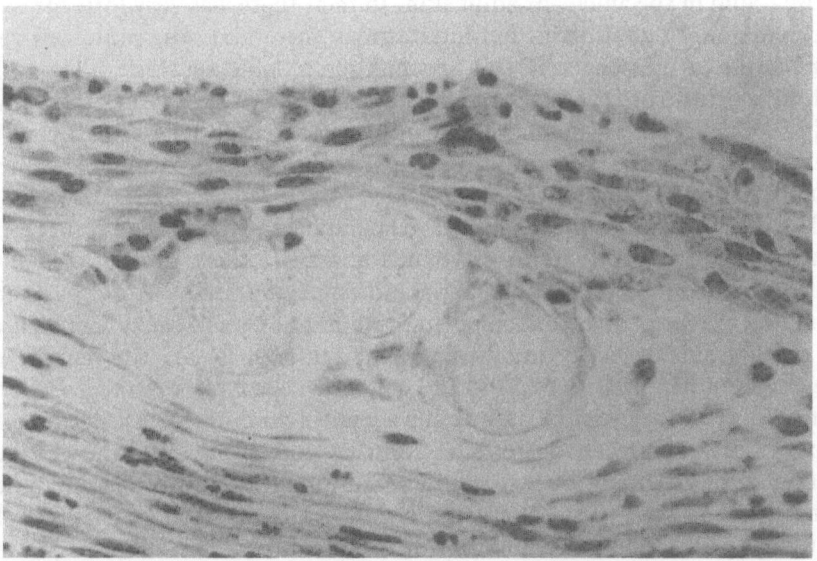

FIGURE 4.8. Histologic section of human fibroblasts cultured 2 weeks in the biosynthetic dressing Biobrane. Biobrane is composed of a nylon mesh covered with a thin silicone "epidermal" barrier. During cell culture a dense cellular "tissue" is formed, and human matrix proteins can be identified in the tissue that surrounds the nylon fibers, which are cut transversely in this section. In addition, messenger RNA encoding multiple growth factors has been identified. A thin silicone membrane layer, which provides a moisture vapor barrier for the graft, is faintly visible on the upper surface of this section. These grafts have been termed Dermagraft-Transitional Covering (Dermagraft-TC), and they are being tested in clinical trials in burn patients as a temporary covering (Advanced Tissue Sciences, Inc., La Jolla, CA) for excised burn wounds.

These grafts were successful in closing full-thickness wounds in athymic mice (64). Even though the human fibroblasts are nonimmunogenic in the allogeneic situation, they would quickly incite a rejection response in the heterograft situation. Thus we utilize athymic mice to test these grafts, since the animals lack a cell-mediated immune response. The grafts stimulated excellent fibrovascular ingrowth and also appeared to completely inhibit the wound contract process. In vivo a dense array of fibroblasts and blood vessels was visible 10 days after placement of grafts on the wound. We quantified the adherence of these grafts, working with our bioengineering colleagues. We found that this material, which is now termed Dermagraft-Transitional Covering (DG-TC), was actually more adherent to the wound over a 2-week-period compared with cryopreserved human allograft skin.

When we measured messenger RNAs (mRNAs) for various growth factors in the DG-TC, high levels of message was found for multiple cytokines including acidic and basic FGFs, keratinocyte growth factor, and TGF-α and -β (64). Levels of cytokine-specific message were far higher than those found in specimens of adult skin. In fact, there was very little message for cytokines in adult skin, but interestingly, neonatal skin contained very high levels of messenger RNAs for multiple trophic cytokines. Thus, the cytokine profile of DG-TC parallels that of neonatal skin rather than adult skin. We believe that the high levels of growth factors that are reflected by this mRNA profile will improve the physiologic performance of this temporary skin replacement.

Handling of skin replacements is very important for the burn surgeons, who must work with extensive wounds and close them rapidly. Many of these wounds are irregular in shape and configuration. DG-TC has good handling characteristics and can be moved on the wound easily and sutured or stapled quickly. Very importantly, the material is safe for human use since the mother, the baby, and the cultured cells can be screened over a period of time for multiple pathogenic agents including viruses. Because the donor and mother can be retested for viral infections after the cells are obtained, there should be essentially zero incidence of viral contamination with these grafts. This is very important, since as discussed above the potential for viral contamination with human cadaver skin is always present.

A material such as this can be stored "on the shelf" and utilized immediately to close excised wounds. Ready availability is very important for these patients because it has been shown that patients who are excised soon after admission have a better outcome than the former technique of waiting for the burn tissue or "eschar" to gradually separate over time (4). It is critically important to have a temporary graft material readily available for wound coverage. It would be a further advantage to have a skin replacement that will not be rejected. Because human fibroblasts appear to be nonimmunogenic in the allogeneic situation, this offers a further advantage to skin replacements that contain human fibroblasts. On the other hand, human keratinocytes are highly immunogenic. Although early studies suggested that the culture process would decrease their antigenicity, perhaps by decreasing expression of surface transplantation antigens, in clinical practice the cultured allogeneic epithelium is rapidly rejected.

Pilot clinical studies in ten patients with this temporary skin replacement, Dermagraft-TC, have been successfully completed. The material functioned well and in several patients it outperformed adjacent areas of cryopreserved cadaver skin, which developed early sloughing of the epidermal layer either from immunologic rejection or as a result of damage to the dermal-epidermal junction from the cryopreservation process.

Conclusion

There is much progress to be made to develop optimal laboratory-grown temporary and permanent skin replacements. It seems clear that replacement of both epidermal and dermal layers will be important for final optimal wound healing. Although the use of retained cadaver allodermis on the wound bed appears to improve the performance of cultured epithelium (12), utilization of this technique imposes complexities of care and timing on the part of the clinician. It is hoped the development of more complete unified skin replacements will improve and also simplify burn care in the future.

References

1. Pruitt BA Jr, ed. Symposium: progress in burn care. World J Surg 1992; 16:1-96.
2. Feller I, Tholen D, Cornell RG. Improvements in burn care, 1965 to 1979. JAMA 1980;244:2074-8.
3. Wolfe RA, Roi LD, Flora JD, et al. Mortality differences and speed of wound closure among specialized burn care facilities. JAMA 1983;250:763-6.
4. Sheridan RL, Tompkins RG, Burke JF. Management of the burn wound by prompt excision and immediate closure. J Intensive Care Med 1993;9:6-19.
5. Gray DT, Pine RW, Harnar TJ, et al. Early surgical excision versus conventional therapy in patients with 20 to 40 percent burns. Am J Surg 1982; 144:76-80.
6. Hansbrough JF. Burn wound sepsis. J Intensive Care Med 1987;2:313-27.
7. LaLonde C, Demling RH. The effect of complete burn wound excision and closure on postburn oxygen consumption. Surgery 1987;102:862-8.
8. Hansbrough JF. Wound coverage with biologic dressings and cultured skin substitutes. Austin: R.G. Landes, 1992.
9. Rheinwald JG, Green H. Serial cultivation of strains of human epidermal keratinocytes: the formation of keratinizing colonies from single cells. Cell 1975;6:331-43.
10. Green H, Kehinde O, Thomas J. Growth of cultured human epidermal cells into multiple epithelia suitable for grafting. Proc Natl Acad Sci USA 1979; 76:5665-8.

11. Gallico GG, O'Connor NE, Compton CC, et al. Permanent coverage of large burn wounds with autologous cultured human epithelium. N Engl J Med 1984;311:448–51.
12. Odessey R. Addendum: multicenter experience with cultured epidermal autograft for treatment of burns. J Burn Care Rehab 1992;13:174–80.
13. Compton CC. Wound healing potential of cultured epithelium. Wounds 1993;5:97–111.
14. Rives JM, Sellam P, Karcenty B, et al. Cultured epithelial autografts (CEA) management and colonization control in extensive burn injuries: "Thoughts on local dressing": 9th Congress, International Society of Burn Injuries Paris, 1994:152.
15. Desai MH, Mlakar JM, McCauley RL, et al. Lack of long-term durability of cultured keratinocyte burn-wound coverage: a case report. J Burn Care Rehab 1991;12:540–5.
16. Kumagai N, Nishina H, Tanabe H, Hosaka T, Ishida H, Ogino Y. Clinical application of autologous cultured epithelia for the treatment of burn wounds and burn scars. Plast Reconstr Surg 1988;82:99–108.
17. Herzog SR, Meyer A, Woodley D, Peterson HD. Wound coverage with cultured autologous keratinocytes: use after burn wound excision, including biopsy followup. J Trauma 1988;28:195–8.
18. Clugston PA, Snelling CFT, Macdonald IB, et al. Cultured epithelial autografts: three years of clinical experience with eighteen patients. J Burn Care Rehab 1991;12:533–9.
19. Cuono C, Langdon R, McGuire J. Use of cultured epidermal autografts and dermal allografts as skin replacement after burn injury. Lancet 1986; 1:1123–4.
20. Langdon RC, Cuono CB, Birchall N, et al. Reconstitution of structure and cell function in human skin grafts derived from cryopreserved allogeneic dermis and autologous cultured keratinocytes. J Invest Dermatol 1988;91:478–85.
21. Rennekampff HO, Hansbrough JF, Kiessig V, Abiezzi S, Woods V Jr. Wound closure with human keratinocytes cultured on a polyurethane dressing overlaid on a living dermal replacement. Surgery (submitted).
22. Briggaman RA, Wheeler CE Jr. The epidermal-dermal junction. J Invest Dermatol 1975;65:71–84.
23. Coulomb B, Lebreton C, Dubertret L. Influence of human dermal fibroblasts on epidermalization. J Invest Dermatol 1989;92:122–5.
24. Woodley DT, Peterson HD, Herzog SR, et al. Burn wounds resurfaced by cultured epidermal autografts show abnormal reconstitution of anchoring fibrils. JAMA 1988;259:2566–71.
25. Rue LW III, Cioffi WG, McManus WF, Pruitt BA Jr. Wound closure and outcome in extensively burned patients treated with cultured autologous keratinocytes. J Trauma 1993;34:662–8.
26. Boyce S, Hansbrough JF. A skin autograft substitute: biological attachment and growth of cultured human keratinocytes on a graftable collagen and chondroitin-6-sulfate substrate. Surgery 1988;103:421–31.
27. Boyce S, Christianson D, Hansbrough J. Structure of a collagen-GAG skin substitute optimized for cultured human epidermal keratinocytes. J Biomat Res 1988;22:939–57.
28. Cooper ML, Andree C, Hansbrough JF, et al. Direct comparison of a cultured composite skin substitute containing human keratinocytes to an epidermal sheet

graft containing human keratinocytes on athymic mice. J Invest Dermatol 1993;101:811-9.

29. Cooper ML, Hansbrough JF. Use of a composite skin graft composed of cultured human keratinocytes and fibroblasts and a collagen-GAG matrix to cover full-thickness wounds on athymic mice. Surgery 1991;109:198-207.

30. Hansbrough JF, Boyce ST, Cooper ML, Foreman TJ. Burn wound closure with cultured autologous keratinocytes and fibroblasts attached to a collagen-glycosaminoglycan substrate. JAMA 1989;262:2125-30.

31. Greenleaf G, Cooper ML, Hansbrough JF. Microbial contamination in allografted wound beds in burn patients. J Burn Care Rehab 1991;12:442-5.

32. Cooper ML, Hansbrough JF, Spielvogel RL, et al. In vivo optimization of a living dermal substitute employing cultured human fibroblasts on a biodegradable polyglycolic acid or polyglactin mesh. Biomaterials 1991;12:243-8.

33. Hansbrough JF, Cooper ML, Cohen R, et al. Evaluation of a biodegradable matrix containing cultured human fibroblasts as a dermal replacement beneath meshed skin grafts on athymic mice. Surgery 1992;111:438-46.

34. Hansbrough JF, Doré C, Hansbrough WN. Clinical trials of a living dermal tissue replacement placed beneath meshed, split-thickness skin grafts on excised burn wounds. J Burn Care Rehab 1992;13:519-29.

35. Hansbrough JF, Morgan JL, Greenleaf GE, Bartel R. Composite grafts of human keratinocytes grown on a polyglactin mesh-cultured fibroblast dermal substitute function as a bilayer skin replacement in full-thickness wounds on athymic mice. J Burn Care Rahab 1993;14:485-94.

36. Bell E, Ehrlich HP, Buttle DJ, Nakatsuji T. Living tissue formed in vitro and accepted as skin-equivalent tissue. Science 1981;211:1052-4.

37. Hansbrough JF, Morgan J, Greenleaf G, et al. Evaluation of Graftskin composite grafts on full-thickness wounds on athymic mice. J Burn Care Rehab 1994;15:346-53.

38. Nolte CJM, Oleson MA, Hansbrough JF, et al. Ultrastructural features of bilayered skin cultures grafted onto athymic mice. J Anat 1994;185:325-33.

39. Sabolinski ML, Rovee DT, Parenteau NL, et al. The efficacy and safety of Graftskin for the treatment of chronic venous ulcers. Abstract, Wound Healing Soc, April 1995, Minneapolis MN: Symposium on Advanced Wound Care, San Diego, CA, May 1995.

40. Bennett NT, Schultz GS. Growth factors and wound healing: biochemical properties of growth factors and their receptors. Am J Surg 1993;165:728-37.

41. Myers S, Navsaria H, Sanders R, et al. Transplantation of keratinocytes in the treatment of wounds. Am J Surg 1995;170:75-83.

42. Elder JT. Transforming growth factor-α and related growth factors. In: Luger TA, Schwarz T, eds. Epidermal growth factors and cytokines. New York: Marcel Dekker, 1993:205-40.

43. Gill GN, Bertics PJ, Santon JB. Epidermal growth factor and its receptor. Mol Cell Endocrinol 1987;51:169-86.

44. Cooper ML, Hansbrough JF, Foreman TJ, Sakabu SA, Laxer JA. The effects of epidermal growth factor and basic fibroblast growth factor on epithelialization of meshed skin graft interstices. Clinical and experimental approaches to dermal and epidermal repair: normal and chronic wounds. New York: Wiley-Liss 1991:429-42.

45. Nanney LB. Epidermal and dermal effects of epidermal growth factor during wound repair. J Invest Dermatol 1990;94:624-9.

46. Cook PW, Pittelkow MR, Shiley GD. Growth factor-independent proliferation of normal human neonatal keratinocytes: production of autocrine-and paracrine-acting mitogenic factors. J Cell Physiol 1991;146:277–89.
47. Grossmann RM, Kruger J, Yourish D, et al. Interleukin 6 is expressed in high levels in psoriatic skin and stimulates proliferation of cultured human keratinocytes. Proc Natl Acad Sci USA 1989;86:6367–71.
48. Ohashi H, Maeda T, Mishima H, Otori T, Nishida T, Sekiguchi K. Up-regulation of integrin $\alpha 5\beta 1$ expression by interleukin-6 in rabbit corneal epithelial cells. Exp Cell Res 1995;218:418–23.
49. Nishida T, Nakamura M, Mishima H, Otori T, Hikida M. Interleukin 6 facilitates corneal epithelial wound closure in vivo. Arch Ophthalmol 1992;110:1292–4.
50. Schröder J-M, Sticherling M, Smid P, Christophers E. Interleukin 8 and structurally related cytokines. In: Luger TA, Schwarz T, eds. Epidermal growth factors and cytokines. New York: Marcel Dekker, 1993:89–112.
51. Schröder J-M, Gregory H, Young J, Christophers E. Neutrophil-activating proteins in psoriasis. J Invest Dermatol 1992;98:241–7.
52. Garner WL, Rodriguez JL, Miller CG, Till GO, Rees RS, Smith DJ, Remick DG. Acute skin injury releases neutrophil chemoattractants. Surgery 1994;116:42–8.
53. Rennekampff HO, Hansbrough JF, Schröder JM, Kiessig V, Tenenhaus M, Woods V Jr. MGSA/gro modulates keratinocyte growth and promotes wound healing. J Invest Dermatol (submitted).
54. Reusch MK, Studtmann M, Schröder J-M, Sticherling M, Christophers E. NAP/interleukin 8 is a potent mitogen for human keratinocytes in vitro. J Invest Dermatol 1990;95A:485.
55. Michel G, Kemeny L, Peter RU, Beetz A, Ried C, Arenberger P, Ruzicka T. Interleukin-8 receptor-mediated chemotaxis of normal human epidermal cells. FEBS Lett 1992;305:241–3.
56. Hu DE, Hori Y, Fan TPD. Interleukin-8 stimulates angiogenesis in rats. Inflammation 1993;17:135–43.
57. Falanga V. Chronic wounds: pathophysiologic and experimental considerations. J Invest Dermatol 1993;100:721–5.
58. Madden MR, Finkelstein JL, Staiano-Coico L, et al. Grafting of cultured allogeneic epidermis on second- and third-degree burn wounds on 26 patients. J Trauma 1986;26:955–62.
59. Leigh IM, Purkis PE, Navsaria HA, Phillips TJ. Treatment of chronic venous ulcers with sheets of cultured allogenic keratinocytes. Br J Dermatol 1987;117:591–7.
60. Compton CC, Tong Y, Trookman N, Zhao H, Roy D, Ress W. Transforming growth factor alpha gene expression in cultured human keratinocytes is unaffected by cellular aging. Arch Dermatol 1995;131:683–90.
61. Kaiser HW, Stark GB, Kopp J, Balcerkiewicz A, Spilker G, Kreysel HW. Cultured autologous keratinocytes in fibrin glue suspension, exclusively and combined with STS-allograft (preliminary clinical and histological report of a new technique). Burns 1994;20:23–9.
62. Barlow YM, Burt AM, Clarke JA, McGrouther DA, Lang SM. The use of a polymeric film for the culture and transfer of sub-confluent autologous keratinocytes to patients. J Tiss Viability 1992;2:33–6.

63. Greenleaf G, Hansbrough JF. Current trends in the use of allograft skin for burn patients and reflections on the future of skin banking in the United States. J Burn Care Rehab 1995;15:428-31.
64. Hansbrough JF, Morgan J, Greenleaf G, Underwood J. Development of a temporary living skin replacement composed of human fibroblasts cultured in Biobrane, a synthetic dressing material. Surgery 1994;115:633-44.

5

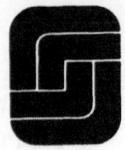

The Growth Hormone Insulin-Like Growth Factor-I Axis

ARVIND Y. KRISHNA AND LAWRENCE S. PHILLIPS

Growth Hormone

Somatotropin or growth hormone (GH) is the most abundant hormone in the human pituitary. GH is a peptide synthesized and secreted by the anterior pituitary, and is an important regulator of growth and differentiated function. Human GH differs from that of other species, including primates, making it unique among pituitary hormones; whereas adrenocorticotropic hormone (ACTH), prolactin, and thyroid stimulating hormone extracted from other species have bioactivity in humans, GH from other species has no effect in humans (1). As opposed to all other anterior pituitary hormones, which act only on specific target organs, GH has effects on multiple target tissues throughout the body. Interestingly, GH exerts its effects directly on some tissues, and on other tissues the insulin-like growth factors (IGFs, particularly IGF-I) mediate the growth-promoting and anabolic effects of GH.

Regulation of Growth Hormone Secretion

The release of GH is regulated by stimulatory and inhibitory hypothalamic drive, mediated through the release of growth hormone-releasing hormone (GHRH) and somatostatin/somatotropin release inhibiting factor (SRIF), respectively, by the hypothalamus. The interrelationship of specific neural centers controlling GH secretion and the modulation of these centers by metabolic events is complex (2). It is now thought that the secretion of GH is modulated by at least three neural centers: the ventromedial nucleus (VMN), the arcuate nucleus (AN), and the limbic system (LS) (1). Although the neural transmitters for each locus are different, the centers have a common final action—the discharge of GHRH from the median eminence into the hypophysial portal system. GHRH release thus is thought to act as the final pathway for the release of GH from the anterior pituitary. GH release is inhibited by somatostatin, a peptide released from the hypothalamus. Since somatostatin's actions are not specific for GH, somatostatin is considered as a more general neuroinhibitory agent (1).

Various stimuli induce or inhibit GH secretion, with final action through somatostatin or GHRH. However, the mechanisms for these actions are often complex, and not totally understood. At the VMN level, the major provocative stimuli appear to be hypoglycemia (3), and α-adrenergic agents. Vasopressin and arginine also are presumed to act at this level (1). L-dopa probably acts through the AN. The LS, which is activated during slow-wave sleep, has been suggested as an important center controlling the typical "spikes" of GH secretion that occur in deep sleep (1). Other hormones, most notably estrogen, can sensitize centers of this system to provocative stimuli, and thus enhance GH release (4).

Other stimuli of GH release have no clear locus of action. These include stress, exercise, and protein depletion. Evidence is emerging that the latter is probably mediated in part by decreased levels of IGF-I. There is even less understanding of underlying mechanisms in conditions of inhibited GH release, such as obesity, elevation of free fatty acid levels, and chronic glucocorticoid administration.

The secretion of GH is regulated at several levels via negative feedback pathways. An ultrashort-loop feedback mechanism refers to the negative feedback by GH at the level of the pituitary itself. Such a process is suggested by the presence of GH receptors on the pituitary gland (5). In human subjects in whom lipolysis and somatostatin (SRIF) secretion are blocked (6), the endogenous GH response to GHRH is blunted by exogenous GH, consistent with autoinhibition of GH secretion at the pituitary level. Exogenous GH therapy or elevations in endogenous GH secretion (7) also reduce pulsatile GH release (8) and GH responses to pituitary-acting stimuli [GHRH and thyrotropin-releasing hormone (TRH)] (8), indicating autoregulatory actions of GH at pituitary (or hypothalamic) sites.

Acting in a short loop, GH stimulates the release of somatostatin/SRIF and inhibits the release of GHRH by the hypothalamus. GH may also stimulate synthesis of IGF-I and IGF-II in the hypothalamus. These centrally produced IGFs inhibit GHRH synthesis (9) and release (10), and stimulate SRIF synthesis and release (9). It has been suggested that GH also exerts a direct inhibitory effect on GHRH production, independent of central IGF-I (9).

In addition to pituitary and central mechanisms participating in GH autoregulation, slower onset long-loop feedback pathways are also well established. These pathways are mediated by GH-induced IGF-I production in sites outside the central nervous system; these IGFs exert negative feedback at the level of the hypothalamus and the pituitary. In the hypothalamus, systemic IGF-I has been shown to stimulate SRIF synthesis and release and inhibit GHRH synthesis and release (9). In the pituitary, systemic IGF-I directly inhibits pituitary GH gene transcription (11), and inhibits both basal and adenosine 3',5'-cyclic monophosphate (cAMP)-, protein kinase C-, GHRH-, and TRH-induced GH release (12). However, IGF-I is relatively less effective than SRIF in inhibiting GH release (13), and may only inhibit GH release from a subpopulation of GH-secreting cells that are not responsive to SRIF inhibition (13). The involvement of IGFs in long-loop GH autoregulation is also indicated by the elevated circulating GH concentrations in Laron dwarfs (14), a condition in which GH is unable to induce IGF-I synthesis due to lack of functional GH receptors. GH levels are also high in patients with anorexia nervosa (15), cirrhosis (16), diabetes (17), or malnutrition (18), as GH is unable to induce adequate IGF-I production in these conditions. In contrast, GH secretion is impaired in disease states characterized by elevated IGF-I concentrations (19); the elevated IGF-I levels in obese children and patients with affective disorders may thus account for blunted GH responses to GHRH stimulation in these situations (20).

Direct Effects of Growth Hormone

Some effects of GH do not require the mediation of the IGFs and thus are direct effects of GH on target tissues. GH exerts an initial, transitory insulin-like effect on carbohydrate metabolism in humans, followed by an anti-insulin (diabetogenic) effect (21). The initial insulin-like effect of GH is probably mediated in part by increased substrate availability, due to increased glucose transport and also to changes in the content/activity of key enzymes in metabolic pathways (22). On the other hand, peripheral uptake and utilization of glucose are reduced by chronic administration of GH. GH lowers the apparent sensitivity/responsiveness of adipose tissue to insulin, downstream from the insulin receptor (22). In vitro studies suggest that chronic exposure to GH decreases the synthesis of Glut 1, the major glucose transporter in the plasma membranes of adipocytes, thereby exerting an anti-insulin action (23).

Chronic exposure of adipose tissue to GH results in lipolysis (hydrolysis of triglyceride to free fatty acids and glycerol). This appears to be a direct action of GH (24). There is evidence that GH can also increase the sensitivity and/or responsiveness of adipose tissue to agents such as epinephrine and norepinephrine that influence lipolysis (25, 26). GH may be exerting these effects by increasing the β_3-adrenergic receptor number, or reducing inhibitory influences. GH also exerts an antilipogenic/anti-insulin effect in reducing fatty acid synthesis in the presence of insulin or insulin and dexamethasone (27, 28).

GH exerts a protein anabolic action and leads to muscle protein synthesis. The GH-induced restraint on proteolysis and promotion of lipolysis spares nitrogen and facilitates use of alternate metabolic fuels. IGF-I acts as an important mediator of this protein anabolic action of GH, but at high physiologic concentrations GH has been shown to stimulate muscle protein synthesis directly as well (29).

GH exerts a modulatory role in human reproduction. GH has been shown to potentiate the increase of both testosterone and androstenedione evoked by human chorionic gonadotropin (hCG) (30). It is unclear whether or not IGF-I mediates the GH action in the human testis, because both GH and IGF-I receptors have been found in the testis, and IGF-I is able to induce effects similar to those observed after GH administration (31). GH has also been found to enhance both basal and follicle-stimulating hormone (FSH)-stimulated aromatization of testosterone to estradiol (E_2) by human granulosa cells in vitro (32). Studies in animal models suggest that the induction and/or maintenance of estrogen receptors in the liver requires GH (33).

GH receptors are present in tissues involved in immunologic reactions (34), although clinical studies do not provide a clear picture of the effect of GH on immune function in humans. However, in mice, the administration of antisera to bovine GH results in decreased growth and large reductions in the weights of the thymus and spleen (35).

GH receptors and binding proteins are widely distributed within the central nervous system. GH is believed to play a role in neurotransmission, central behavior, growth, and development of the CNS (36).

Insulin-Like Growth Factors

Until about four decades ago, it was unclear whether promotion of skeletal elongation resulted directly from GH or from other factors stimulated by GH. In 1957 Salmon and Daughaday (37) established the existence of GH-dependent intermediary factors. In classic studies, they first showed that sulfate incorporation into cartilage chondroitin sulfate was reduced by hypophysectomy, and then demonstrated that the factors inducing sulfate uptake by cartilage were GH dependent, but not GH itself. Earlier, these factors were named somatomedins to acknowledge mediation of the skeletal growth-promoting effects of somatotropin. Subsequently, two factors were purified, and it was recognized that these polypeptides have structural similarity to proinsulin, and biologic actions similar to insulin as well. Therefore, they are now referred to as the insulin-like growth factors (IGF-I and IGF-II). The major site of production of circulating IGFs is the liver (38), but they are also produced locally in numerous organs and tissues. GH is an important regulator of both hepatic and local IGF-I production, but the local production of IGF-I is influenced by local factors as well.

Insulin-Like Growth Factors Binding Proteins (IGFBPs)

Both the endocrine and autocrine/paracrine actions of IGF-I are subject to positive and negative modulation by interstitial and plasma IGFBPs. In the circulation, both IGF-I and IGF-II are predominantly bound in a 150-kd insulin-like growth factor binding protein (IGFBP) complex. A subunit of this complex is one of six specific IGFBPs (IGFBP-1 to IGFBP-6) (21). The combination of IGFBPs with either IGF-I or IGF-II often acts to reduce the activity of the IGFs (32). However, there is evidence that a complex of IGF-I to at least one IGFBP (IGFBP-1 or -3) can enhance the activity of the growth factor in some systems (33). The levels of IGFBPs are themselves regulated by several factors, including GH, IGF-I, insulin, nutritional status, and physiologic states including puberty, pregnancy, and the stage of development.

IGFBP-3 is the predominant carrier of IGF-I in the circulation, and more than 90% of the IGFs in serum circulate as part of this binding protein complex. This complex is composed of an acid-stable subunit (IGFBP), an acid-labile subunit, and IGF-I or IGF-II linked to the IGFBP (39). There is strong evidence that production of IGFBP-3 from the liver is GH dependent (or dependent on IGF-I, which itself is GH dependent) (21). There is also evidence that GH increases IGFBP-3 indirectly via elevated IGF-I (25). The concentrations of IGFBP-3 are reduced when nutrients are restricted, and are restored by feeding (40).

In addition to different regulatory mechanisms, the IGFBPs are believed to have distinct functions. As the concentration of IGFBP-3 is the highest in the serum, it may play the principal role as a serum carrier protein for the IGFs. On the other hand, the concentrations of IGFBP-1 and IGFBP-2 are higher in lymph than in serum, and may play a role in transporting IGFs out of the vascular space (40). This concept is supported by the observation that IGFBP-1 can cross intact vascular endothelium (41).

Systemic Effects of IGF-I

An intravenous bolus of IGF-I in a dose that overcomes the binding capacity of IGFBPs causes hypoglycemia. The hypoglycemic effect of IGF-I due largely to the concentration of free IGF-I, whereas IGF-I attached to binding proteins (BPs) has less insulin-like action (42). Although the glucose-lowering effects of IGF-I and insulin are similar, the levels of free fatty acids decrease to a greater extent and remain lower for a longer duration with insulin as compared with IGF-I (42). This can be attributed to the abundance of insulin receptors as opposed to IGF-I receptors in human adipocytes (42). On the other hand, the IGF-I/insulin potency ratio is higher in muscle than in adipose tissue (42).

IGF-I administration leads to broad anabolic responses, including a decrease in creatinine and urea levels. IGF-I levels are decreased in insulin-dependent diabetes mellitus and this disease state is associated with growth retardation (43, 44). Control of diabetes mellitus with insulin therapy can improve growth (45). Scheiwiller et al. (46) suggested that this improvement in growth is due to an increase in IGF-I synthesis induced by insulin. They showed that (rh)IGF-I infusion in diabetic rats restores normal growth even in the presence of uncontrolled diabetes mellitus. Administration of IGF-I also stimulates growth in hypophysectomized rats, and mimics the effects of human GH (hGH) treatment (47, 48).

There is disagreement as to the relative importance of IGF-I reaching cartilage from the circulation and action as an endocrine factor, as compared with IGF-I synthesized by cartilage and acting as an autocrine/paracrine factor. Some evidence suggests that the autocrine/paracrine pathway of IGF-I action on growth cartilage is of less quantitative importance than the endocrine mode (49). Moreover, autocrine/paracrine action cannot explain the failure of GH added to isolated cartilage, even if obtained from growth plates, to stimulate parameters of growth and to reproduce the changes observed with IGF-I addition (49). In addition, the stimulation of cartilage growth by local administration of GH in vivo (50) is only a small fraction of that which can be achieved by systemic administration of GH with its attendant rise in serum IGF-I (51).

The specific pattern of organ growth observed with continuous, subcutaneous, or intravenous infusion of IGF-I suggests a relatively small effect of IGF-I on long-bone growth as compared with that of GH (42). There can be several explanations for this observation. First, IGF-I induced suppression of GH release may attenuate the expression and release of paracrine IGF-I in growth plates. Second, GH acts as a protein-anabolic hormone in part through mobilization of endogenous substrate. The lipolytic and gluconeogenic effects of GH provide a supply of free fatty acids and glucose, while IGF-I does not have this action. Third, IGF-I suppresses insulin release, in contrast to GH, which stimulates insulin release, and the lack of insulin may lead, in part, to growth retardation. Fourth, access of parenterally administered IGF-I to the local target sites is decreased, due to binding by IGFBPs (32). Fifth, the changes in IGFBP profile induced by IGF-I treatment are different from those observed with GH administration. In vivo, GH induces a rise in IGFBP-3 (52), but rat IGF-I (rIGF-I) lowers IGFBP-3 acutely (53). In cocultures of hepatic nonparenchymal and parenchymal cells, expression and secretion of IGFBP-3 are stimulated by addition of IGF-I but not by GH (54). As the IGFBPs are important regulators of IGF-I action (see below), differences in the IGFBP profile induced by IGF-I as compared with GH may also account for some of the differences between the growth promoting effects of IGF-I vs. GH treatment.

Local Actions of IGF-I

The IGFs act primarily as mitogens in some tissues, stimulate differentiation without proliferation in others, and in all responding tissues stimulate the production of cell products that are characteristic of that tissue.

Although IGFs were first described as growth factors for skeletal tissues, IGF-I or IGF-II in fact stimulate DNA synthesis and cell proliferation in cells of diverse embryologic origin.

The interaction of IGFs with other local growth factors is complex. Often, in the absence of other hormones or growth factors, the effects of IGF-I or IGF-II are relatively weak, and many of these actions can be demonstrated only in the presence of other growth factors or hormones. Thus, amplification of the effect of other agonists is a common theme of IGF-I action (55).

In general, transcripts for IGF-II are more abundant than those for IGF-I in the fetus, whereas IGF-I messenger RNA predominates postnatally (56). A striking exception to this developmental pattern is present in the brain, where IGF-II mRNAs predominate over those for IGF-I and appear to be regulated by GH (57).

IGFs are synthesized in the adrenals and the gonads in response to stimulation by their respective trophic hormones. Although inactive by themselves, IGFs potentiate the steroidogenic actions of ACTH and angiotensin II in the adrenals (58), of FSH in ovarian granulosa cells (59), and of LH on androgen production by theca-interstitial cells in the ovary (60) and Leydig cells in the testis (61).

The IGFs probably play an important role in the regulation of uterine and placental growth during pregnancy, as well as of early embryonic and fetal development (62). The endometrial content of IGF-I and IGF-I mRNA is high at implantation and during early embryogenesis in the sow (63). Autocrine and paracrine roles for the IGFs in uterine and placental tissues are postulated.

In muscle, IGFs stimulate the proliferation of myoblasts and differentiation into myotubes (40). The IGFs also appear to be involved in the proliferation and differentiation of lens epithelium. In the chick embryo, IGF-I serves as a differentiation factor for lens epithelium, an effect characterized by elongation of the cells and synthesis of the specific lens protein delta-crystallin (40).

The growth-promoting actions of GH on skeletal elongation are thought to be mediated in part by systemic production of IGF-I, and in part by the local production of IGF-I by prechondrocytes or neighboring cells in the epiphyseal growth plate (40). The importance of IGFs in the growth of established cancellous bone is less well understood. Although IGF-I plays a central role in epiphyseal growth, IGF-II may play the major role in maintenance of cancellous bone (40, 64).

Regulation of IGF-I Production

Regulation of IGF-I by Growth Hormone

GH regulates IGF-I at two main levels. At one level, GH is thought to regulate circulating concentrations of IGF-I through actions on the liver to stimulate IGF-I production and release. There is considerable evidence that the liver is the major source of plasma IGF-I (38). Estimated IGF-I production rates are sufficient to account for IGF-I turnover in the circulation. Moreover, hepatectomy reduces circulating IGF-I activity, whereas liver regeneration following partial hepatectomy restores circulating IGF-I activity (65). Thus, circulating IGF-I acts in an endocrine mode to mediate GH action on various tissues. This has been shown in animal models as well as in humans. Purified human IGF-I, administered subcutaneously as a constant infusion, has been shown to mimic the effects of GH in increasing growth (body weight gain, tibial epiphyseal width and [³H]thymidine incorporation into cartilage) in hypophysectomized rodents (66). Growth is also stimulated by IGF-I in humans. For instance, IGF-I administration is reported to be effective in stimulating growth in patients with Laron-type dwarfism who lack GH receptors (67). Moreover, IGF-I reduces circulating concentrations of uric acid and creatinine (42, 68). Arguably, this reflects shifts in nitrogen metabolism (42, 68).

It has also become evident that at another level, GH induces production and release of IGF-I in target tissues, and locally produced IGF-I can act in a paracrine or autocrine mode to promote organ-specific growth and nutritional homeostasis. Local stimulation of cartilage proliferation is observed when GH is infused directly into the tibial cartilage plate (69). Similarly, infusion of GH into one limb by way of a catheterized femoral artery, or administration directly into the growth plate, results both in cartilage development in the growth plate and in enhanced linear growth of the infused limb compared to the contralateral limb (70). Thus, all the key components for a local GH–IFG-I response mechanism are present in growth plate cartilage, including GH and IGF-I receptors (71). In cardiac and skeletal muscle, IGF-I acting as an endocrine factor may predominate in responses to GH, but the autocrine or paracrine mode may be involved in work hypertrophy and regeneration of muscle fibers (49).

The ability of IGFs to act in an autocrine and paracrine mode is also shared by other growth factors such as the transforming growth factors (TGFs) and platelet-derived growth factor (PDGF). Like these other factors, the IGFs should be considered as pleiotropic modulators of multiple aspects of cell physiology, involved not only in proliferation and calorie storage via mitogenic and anabolic actions, but also in the induction and maintenance of differentiation (72).

However, not all GH effects are mediated by IGF-I. For example, Ohlsson et al. (73) found that local infusion of GH stimulated the incorporation of [³H]thymidine into the germinal layer of the rat tibial epiphyseal plate in vivo, whereas IGF-I was inactive (73). The same selective action of GH has also been demonstrated on isolated rabbit prechondrocytes by Lindahl et al. (74). Accordingly, Lindahl et al. have hypothesized that GH action is focused on a precursor cell population, and when the cells have started to differentiate, IGF-I promotes clonal expansion of these cells (74). It is also possible that GH directly influences the growth of muscle and other tissues.

Local Regulation of IGF-I

IGFs were initially considered to be derived only from the liver, but now both their expression and local production have been demonstrated in numerous organs and tissues. Local regulation of IGFs is under the influence of GH as well as locally acting factors. Glucocorticoids appear to reduce the local abundance of IGF-I mRNA in several tissues in intact rats, and decrease the induction of IGF-I mRNA after treatment with GH in hypophysectomized animals (75). In contrast, thyroid hormone, estrogens and androgens affect the circulating IGF-I level indirectly, via effects on GH production (62). However, estrogens exert a direct regulatory action on the endometrium to control local IGF-I production in this tissue, independent of GH (76). Similarly, IGF-I production in the adrenals is stimulated by ACTH, angiotensin II, and fibroblast growth factor (FGF) (77), and in the gonads by gonadotropic hormones (78).

Local production of IGF-I is under the influence of GH in chondrocytes of various origins, including those of the growth plate (79). Locally acting IGF-I is also involved in bone growth. In adult skeletal muscle, immunostaining for IGF-I is not found in the muscle fibers (80). However, during regeneration after ischemic or toxic injury, immunostaining for IGF-I appears in activated satellite cells, and continues to be expressed when these cells develop into myoblasts and myotubes. With subsequent maturation of the regenerated muscle cells, the IGF-I staining eventually returns to normal low levels (80). The exact stimulus for this reappearance of local expression of IGF-I is unclear.

IGF-I appears to be produced by specific cell types in the kidney. Unilateral nephrectomy causes compensatory growth of the contralateral remaining kidney. A role for IGF-I in this growth process has been indicated by several studies (79). During compensatory renal growth, there is no increase in IGF-I in serum or in other organs, and there is no increase in hepatic IGF-I mRNA (81). IGF-I synthesis during compensatory growth after nephrectomy appears to be at least partly independent of GH (82), and may be regulated by systemic factors.

Local expression of IGF-I also plays a role in the reproductive system. In the ovary, the expression of IGF-I mRNA and levels of IGF-I both vary during the estrous cycle in rats, with increased levels between proestrus and estrus (83). Although the local production of IGFs is regulated predominantly by gonadotropic hormones, the effect of IGFs in responsive ovarian cells is also regulated by IGFBPs (40).

Des(1-3)IGF-I is a naturally occurring variant of IGF-I present in many tissues, which is biologically more potent than full-length IGF-I (84). This variant of IGF-I can be generated in serum by a trypsin-like acid protease.

The protease activity is significantly enhanced in states of GH deficiency, and replacement of GH normalizes this activity in serum (85). This represents another potential site of GH regulation of IGF-I.

Regulation of IGF-I by Insulin and Nutritional Status

Both the circulating levels of IGF-I protein and hepatic IGF-I abundance are reduced in situations of insulin-dependent diabetes mellitus (IDDM) and during nutritional deficiency. The low levels of IGF-I in these conditions are not entirely due to a decrease in GH secretion, based on evaluation of 24-hour profiles.

IGF-I levels are decreased in insulinopenic/type I diabetes mellitus in association with impaired skeletal elongation and diminished weight gain. Strasser-Vogel et al. (44) have reported a negative correlation between hemoglobin A1c (HbA1c) and the standard deviation scores (SDS) of IGF-I, and a positive association between HbA1c and IGFBP-1SDS or IGFBP-2SDS. Strong correlations were also observed between height SDS and IGF-ISDS and IGFBP-3SDS in prepubertal subjects who had IDDM for at least 2 years, but not in adolescents (44). This suggests that the lower plasma concentrations of serum IGF-I may play a role in the pathogenesis of growth impairment of poorly controlled prepubertal children with IDDM (44). Other studies have also reported lower height velocity in children with elevated HbA1c (43), and/or with elevated glucose levels found by home blood glucose monitoring (45). The decreased circulating IGF-I levels and defective anabolism are due in part to impaired GH action, since growth failure in insulinopenic states occurs despite increased circulating levels of GH. Tamborlane et al. (86) observed that an improvement in metabolic control in IDDM resulted in a 70% to 75% increase in IGF-I levels and a fall in GH levels; in two growing adolescents, growth velocity doubled during 13 to 15 months of insulin pump treatment (86). Levels of IGF-I are also significantly decreased in patients with diabetic ketoacidosis (87), whereas subjects with more typical metabolic control usually exhibit normal levels of IGF-I with significant increases in IGFBP-1 (88, 89). Possibly due to the rise in IGFBP-1, diabetes depresses the levels of free IGF-I more than the levels of total IGF-I, as estimated by radioimmunoassay (RIA) after separation from circulating IGFBPs in animal models (90); free IGF-I fell more rapidly and further below control levels in animals with progressive severity of diabetes, and free IGF-I was restored less than total IGF-I by insulin therapy in diabetic animals. Similar observations have been made in human subjects; Guler et al. (91) reported that rises in circulating free IGF-I were greater than changes in total IGF-I in patients receiving IGF-I infusions.

A blocked IGF-I response to exogenous GH has been found in IDDM (92). Thus, insulin is required for the GH-induced release of IGF-I. Insulin has been shown to influence IGF-I gene expression at the transcriptional level in vivo (93). Under more controlled conditions, IGF-I expression and gene transcription also been shown to be regulated by the provision of insulin in rat hepatocytes maintained in primary culture (94).

In addition to GH and other hormones, IGF-I is also dependent on nutritional status (95). In protein-energy malnourished children, levels of IGF-I are low (96). In girls with anorexia nervosa, levels of IGF-I are low despite high concentrations of GH (97). There appears to be a hierarchy of dietary components influencing GH, IGF-I, and their binding proteins. In healthy men of normal weight, a 5-day fast reduced the IGF-I levels by approximately half (98). Refeeding with a protein-deficient isocaloric diet restored the IGF-I levels to some extent, but a diet deficient in both protein and energy led to a further fall in the IGF-I levels (98). In obese adult women, 14 days of a hypocaloric diet enriched in fat or carbohydrate resulted in a 40% decrease in IGF-I levels, while a hypocaloric protein-enriched diet prevented the fall in IGF-I (99). In addition to the amount of protein ingested, the essential amino acid content of the dietary protein also appears to be important. Refeeding with an essential amino acid rich diet after fasting causes a larger increase in serum IGF-I than refeeding with a diet rich in nonessential amino acids (100). In another study, fasting followed by refeeding with normal protein but a low energy 11 kcal/kg diet failed to increase IGF-I levels, while refeeding with isocaloric but variable protein content diets revealed that in the presence of an adequate caloric intake, even low protein intake can increase IGF-I synthesis (101). Therefore, protein intake may be relatively more important than caloric intake, but there is a threshold of energy requirement below which even optimal protein intake fails to raise IGF-I.

The close relationship between the individual anabolic/catabolic state and the serum concentrations of IGF-I has also initiated interest in the use of IGF-I as a marker of nutritional status in severely ill patients, and as a guideline for nutritional support (42). The mechanism by which nutritional factors influence serum IGF-I in humans is not clear. Deprivation of food causes a state of GH resistance, as shown by the low concentration of IGF-I despite a normal to high level of GH in fasting humans (42). In fasting subjects, administration of GH is unable to restore IGF-I levels (102).

Studies in animal models suggest that the resistance to GH and the low serum concentrations of IGF-I that occur during fasting are due in part to a decrease in the GH receptors on hepatocytes (103). However, under conditions of protein restriction alone, serum IGF-I is decreased without a change in GH receptors, suggesting that a postreceptor defect exists (104). Adaptation of the GH–IGF-I axis to chronic and severe calorie and protein malnutrition was studied in young adult rats by Oster et al. (105). Caloric deprivation to 40% for 30 days resulted in a decrease in serum GH, growth hormone binding protein (GHBP), IGF-I, IGFBP-3, and liver IGF-I mRNA. Caloric restriction to 60% calories had no impact on IGFBP levels and only slightly lowered IGF-I levels, despite a 95% fall in GH levels. Protein deprivation lowered serum GH, IGF-I, IGFBP-3, and liver IGF-I mRNA, while GHBP levels were normal. The reduced total IGF-I under these dietary conditions could not be explained by an increase in IGFBP-3 protease activity, or a decrease in the association of IGF-I with IGFBP-3 and the acid labile subunit (105).

In cultured rat hepatocytes, amino acid availability modulates hepatic production of IGF-I independent of the contributions of regulatory hormones, which change along with circulating metabolic fuels in the malnourished state in vivo (106). Amino acids have been shown to regulate IGF-I gene expression at the transcriptional level in primary cultures of rat hepatocytes (107). Fasting for 48 hours has been shown to result in a reduction of IGF-I mRNA and an increase in IGFBP-1 mRNA in both spontaneous GH-deficient dwarf rats (SDRs) and normal rats (108). This suggests that a cause other than changes in GH levels is responsible for these fasting-induced changes.

Regulation of IGF-I During Catabolic States and Tissue Regeneration

In conditions such as malnutrition, surgery, severe infection, or burns, there is an increased release of "stress hormones" such as catecholamines, corticosteroids, and cytokines. This leads to a state of protein wasting and catabolism. However, in these states GH production is also increased. This may constitute a protective response of the body, as GH has protein anabolic actions. But the hypermetabolic states also involve some degree of GH resistance. This is suggested by the decreased circulating levels of IGF-I despite elevated GH levels in catabolic patients (109). Rapid changes in circulating IGFs and IGFBPs were observed in a study assessing alterations in the GH-IGF system in trauma patients (110). GH levels increased 25-fold on the first day of admission to the surgical intensive care unit (SICU), and were still elevated more than fivefold on the last day of the SICU stay. In contrast, trauma decreased the circulating levels of IGF-I by 50% to 60% and IGFBP-3 by 55% to 75%, while IGFBP-1 increased more than threefold. A subset of these patients was also studied within 24 hours of their discharge from the hospital (23 to 35 days after admission to SICU) and the IGF-I level was still reduced (30%), despite adequate nutritional intake and overall improvement in the patient's condition (110). In another study, the circulating levels of IGF-I in the catabolic flow phase of injury were measured in multiple trauma victims, before nutritional support was instituted and again 4 days after intravenous feeding (111). It was observed that feeding could restore IGF-I levels in nonobese, young patients, but obese and elderly subjects exhibited a decreased responsiveness to feeding (111).

Although the hepatic production and the systemic levels of IGF-I decrease in catabolic states, increased local synthesis of IGF-I is observed in many regenerating tissues during these states (112, 113). In the normal state, GH appears to regulate the synthesis of IGF-I in most tissues. This is suggested by the significantly lower levels of both IGF-I and IGF-I mRNA in a large number of tissues after hypophysectomy (114). However, it is likely that factors other than GH act as potent activators of local IGF-I production in injured regenerating tissue. The observation that IGF-I expression is increased in the regenerating tissues of both normal as well as GH-deficient hypophysectomized animals (113) supports this hypothesis. Precisely which factors regulate the local synthesis of IGF-I during tissue repair remains to be investigated.

Different tissues vary with regards to the specific growth factors synthesized at the local sites of injury. For example, local factors other than the IGFs may be responsible for regeneration of organs such as the liver. In a study assessing the relation of IGFs to tissue regeneration, partial hepatectomy, a potent stimulus for liver cell growth, was not accompanied with major changes in the tissue level of IGF-I or IGF-II (112). In another study, a decrease in hepatic and serum concentrations of IGF-I was observed during the course of hepatic regeneration (115). In contrast to liver repair, regeneration of muscle appears to be a potent stimulus of IGF-I mRNA levels. Studies suggest that IGF-I is locally produced and may take part in the regenerative process in muscle (112).

Conclusion

Alterations in the GH–IGF-I–IGFBP axis at several levels helps to maintain homeostasis in catabolic states. Increased production of GH by the pituitary acts directly in the periphery to restrain proteolysis and promote lipolysis, helping to spare nitrogen and facilitating use of alternate metabolic fuels. However, at the level of the liver, production of IGF-I is decreased, due in part to downregulation of hepatic GH receptors, and in part to postreceptor mechanisms. Levels of circulating "free" IGF-I may be decreased further because of an increase in hepatic release of IGFBP-1. Despite the decrease in circulating levels of IGF-I, there is increased expression of IGF-I at sites of tissue injury, aiding the regenerative response. Thus, the response to injury includes the increased pituitary secretion of GH, depressed production of endocrine IGF-I by the liver, and increased production of autocrine/paracrine IGF-I at local sites. These changes constitute an adaptive response, helping to promote local healing while conserving anabolic resources for vital tissues (Fig. 5.1).

Continued advances in understanding of the regulation of GH, IGFs, and IGFBPs should provide further insight into the regulation of both physio-

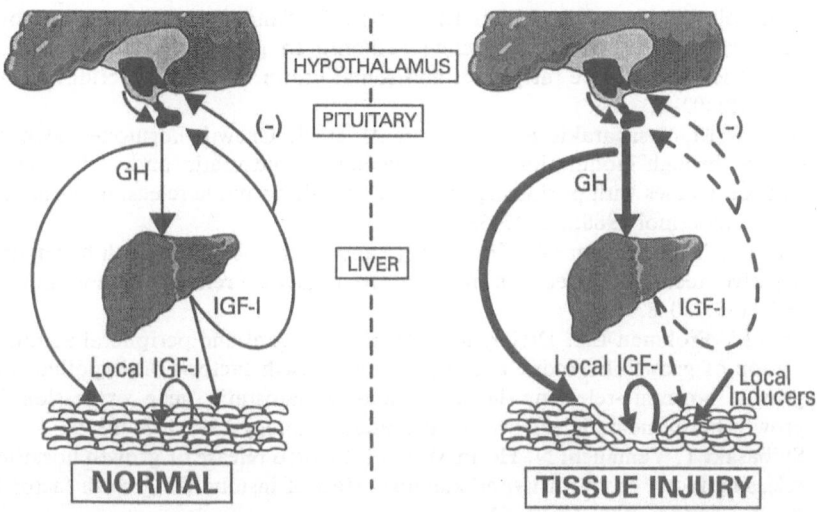

FIGURE 5.1. GH–IGF-I axis in the normal state and in catabolic states/tissue injury. The response to injury includes (a) increased pituitary secretion of GH due to decreased negative feedback, (b) decreased production of endocrine IGF-I by the liver, and (c) increased production of autocrine/paracrine IGF-I and other local growth factors at sites of injury, induced by GH and other as yet unidentified factors.

logic and pathophysiologic processes, and may lead to new therapies to enhance anabolism at both whole animal and local tissue levels.

Acknowledgments. The work was supported in part by a grant from Endocrine Fellows Foundation (A.Y.K.) and NIH grants DK-33475 and DK-48124 (L.S.P.). The authors thank Sharon DePeaza and Mary Lou Mojonnier for assistance in preparation of the manuscript.

References

1. Merimee TJ, Grant MB. Principles and practice of endocrinology and metabolism. Philadelphia: J.B. Lippincott, 1990:125.
2. Martin JB, Andet J, Saunders A. Effects of somatostatin and hypothalamic ventromedial lesions on growth hormone release induced by morphine. Endocrinology 1975;96:839.
3. Roth J, Glick SM, Yallow RS, Berson SA. Hypoglycemia: a powerful stimulus to secretion of GH. Science 1963;140:987.
4. Frantz AC, Rabkin MT. Effects of estrogen and sex difference on secretion of human GH. J Clin Endocrinol Metab 1965;25:1470.
5. Fraser RA, Harvey S. Ubiquitous distribution of growth hormone receptors and/or binding proteins in adenohypophyseal tissue. Endocrinology 1992;130:3593-600.

6. Pontiroli AE, Lanzi R, Monti LD, Pozza G, Sandoli E. Growth hormone autofeedback on growth hormone response to growth hormone-releasing hormone. Role of free fatty acids and somatostatin. J Clin Endocrinol Metab 1991;72:492–5.
7. Ross RJM, Ttsagarakis S, Grossman A, et al. Growth hormone feedback occurs through modulation of hypothalamic somatostatin under cholinergic control: studies with pyridostigmine and growth hormone releasing hormone. Clin Endocrinol 1988;27:727–33.
8. Lanzi R, Tannenbaum GS. Time course and mechanism of growth hormone's negative feedback effect on its own spontaneous release. Endocrinology 1992;130:780–8.
9. Sato M, Frohman LA. Differential effects of central and peripheral administration of growth hormone and insulin-like growth factor-I on hypothalamic growth hormone-releasing hormone and somatostatin gene expression in growth hormone-deficient dwarf rats. Endocrinology 1993;133:793–9.
10. Shibasaki T, Yamauchi N, Hotta M, et al. In vitro release of growth hormone releasing factor from rat hypothalamus: effect of insulin-like growth factor-I. Regul Peptides 1986;15:47–53.
11. Namba H, Morita S, Melmed S. Insulin-like growth factor-I action on growth hormone secretion and messenger ribonucleic acid levels: interaction with somatostatin. Endocrinology 1989;124:1974–99.
12. Blanchard MM, Goodyer CG, Charrier J. In vitro regulation of growth hormone release from ovine pituitary cells during fetal and neonatal development: effects of growth hormone-releasing factor, somatostatin, and insulin-like growth factor-I. Endocrinology 1988;122:2114–20.
13. Hoeffler JP, Hicks SA, Scanes CG. Existence of somatotrope subpopulations which are differentially responsive to insulin-like growth factor-I and somatostatin. Endocrinology 1987;120:1936–41.
14. Laron Z, Blum W, Chatelain P, et al. Classification of growth hormone insensitivity syndromes. J Pediatr 1993;122:241.
15. Frankel RJ, Jenkins JS. Hypothalamic-pituitary function in anorexia nervosa. Acta Endocrinol 1975;78:209–21.
16. Salerno F, Locatelli V, Muller EE. Growth hormone hyperresponsiveness to growth hormone-releasing hormone in patients with severe liver cirrhosis. Clin Endocrinol 1987;27:183–90.
17. Payne PR, Waterlow JC. Relative energy requirements for maintenance, growth and physical activity. Lancet 1971;2:210–1.
18. Panemangalore M, Clark AJ, Clark HE. Effects of dietary energy restriction and rehabilitation on growth and tissue composition in growing rats. J Nutr 1978;108:1297–305.
19. Muller EE. Clinical implications of growth hormone feedback mechanisms. Horm Res 1990;33(suppl 2):90–6.
20. Daughaday WH, Harvey S. Growth hormone release: pathophysiological dysfunction. In: Harvey S, Scanes CG, Daughaday WH, eds. Growth hormone. Boca Raton, FL: CRC Press, 1995:225–55.
21. MacGorman LR, Rizza R, Gerich J. Physiologic concentrations of growth hormone exert insulin-like and insulin antagonistic effects of both hepatic and extra hepatic tissues in man. J Clin Endocrinol Metab 1981;53:556–9.

22. Scanes CG. Growth hormone action: carbohydrate metabolism. In: Harvey S, Scanes CG, Daughaday WH, eds. Growth hormone. Boca Raton, FL: CRC Press, 1995:371-7.
23. Tai PK, Liao JF, Chen EH, Dietz J, Schwartz J, Carter-Su C. Differential regulation of two glucose transporters by chronic growth hormone treatment. J Biol Chem 1990;265:21828-34.
24. Scanes CG. Growth hormone action: protein metabolism. In: Harvey S, Scanes CG, Daughaday WH, eds. Growth hormone. Boca Raton, FL: CRC Press, 1995:379-87.
25. Solomon SS, Schwartz Y, Kawlinson T: Lipolysis in diabetic adipocytes: differences in response to growth hormone and adenosine. Endocrinology 1987;121:1056-60.
26. Vernon RG, Finley E, Flint DJ. Role of growth hormone in the adaptations of lipolysis in rat adipocytes during recovery from lactation. Biochem J 1987;242:931-4.
27. Vernon RG. Effect of growth hormone on fatty acid synthesis in sheep adipose tissue. Int J Biochem 1982;14:255-8.
28. Vernon RG, Finley E. Roles of insulin and growth hormone in the adaptation of fatty acid synthesis in white adipose tissue during the lactation cycle in sheep. Biochem J 1988;256:873-8.
29. Scanes CG. Growth hormone action: protein metabolism. In: Harvey S, Scanes CG, Daughaday WH, eds. Growth hormone. Boca Raton, FL: CRC Press, 1995;389-91.
30. Balducci R, Toscano V, Mangiantini A, Bianchi P, Guglielmi R, Boscherini B. The effect of growth hormone administration on testicular response during gonadotropin therapy in subjects with combined gonadotropin and growth hormone deficiencies. Acta Endocrinol 1993;128:19-23.
31. Chatelain PG, Sanchez P, Saez JM. Growth hormone and insulin-like growth factor-I treatment increase testicular luteinizing hormone receptors and steroidogenic responsiveness of growth hormone deficient mice. Endocrinology 1991;128:1857-62.
32. Mason HD, Martikainen H, Beard RW, Anyaoku V, Frank S. Direct gonadotrophic effects of growth hormone on oestradiol production by human granulosa cells in vitro. J Endocrinol 1990;126:R1-R4.
33. Norstedt G, Wrange O, Gustafsson JA. Multihormonal regulation of the estrogen receptor in rat liver. Endocrinology (Baltimore) 1981;108:1190-6.
34. Arrenbrecht S. Specific binding of growth hormone to thymocytes. Nature (Lond) 1974;252:255-7.
35. Pierpauli W, Sorkin E. Hormones and immunologic capacity. I. Effect of heterologous anti growth hormone (ASTH) antiserum on thymus and peripheral lymphatic tissue in mice. Induction of a wasting syndrome. J Immunol 1968;101:136-43.
36. Harvey S. Growth hormone action: neural function. In: Harvey S, Scanes CG, Daughaday WH, eds. Growth hormone. Boca Raton, FL: CRC Press, 1995:437-49.
37. Salmon WD, Jr., Daughaday WH. A hormonally controlled serum factor which stimulates sulfate incorporation by cartilage in vitro. J Lab Clin Med 1957;49:825-36.

38. Schalch DS, Heinrich UE, Draznin B, Johnson CJ, Miller LL. Role of the liver in regulating somatomedin activity: hormonal effects on the synthesis and release of insulin-like growth factor and its carrier protein by the isolated perfused rat liver. Endocrinology 1979;104:1143–51.
39. Hintz RL. Plasma forms of somatomedin and the binding protein phenomenon. Clin Endocrinol Metab 1984;13:31–42.
40. Underwood LE, Van Wyk JJ. Normal and aberrant growth. In Wilson, Foster, eds. Williams' textbook of endocrinology. Philadelphia: W.B. Saunders, 1992:1079–138.
41. Bar RS, Clemmons DR, Boes M, et al. Transcapillary permeability and subendothelial distribution of endothelial and amniotic fluid insulin-like growth factor binding proteins in the rat heart. Endocrinology 1990;127:1078–86.
42. Bang P, Kerstin H. Insulin-like growth factors as endocrine and paracrine hormones. In: Schofield PN, ed. The insulin-like growth factor — structure and biological functions. Oxford University Press, 1992:151–77.
43. Williams ML, Savage DCL. Glycosylated hemoglobin levels in children with diabetes mellitus. Arch Dis Child 1979;54:295–8.
44. Strasser-Vogel B, Blum WF, Past R, et al. Insulin-like growth factor (IGF)-I and -II and IGF-binding proteins-1, -2, and -3 in children and adolescents with diabetes mellitus: correlation with metabolic control and height attainment. J Clin Endocrinol Metab 1995;80:1207–13.
45. Baumer JH, Edelsten AD, Howlett BC. Impact of home blood glucose monitoring on childhood diabetes. Arch Dis Child 1982;57:195–9.
46. Scheiwiller E, Guler H, Merryweather J, et al. Growth restoration of insulin-deficient diabetic rats by recombinant human insulin-like growth factor I. Nature 1986;323:169–71.
47. Schoenle E, Zapf J, Humbel RE, Froesch ER. Insulin-like growth factor I stimulates growth in hypophysectomized rats. Nature 1982;296:252–3.
48. Schoenle E, Zapf J, Hauri C, Steiner T, Froesch ER. Comparison of in vivo effects of insulin-like growth factors I and II and of growth hormone in hypophysectomized rats. Acta Endocrinol 1985;108:167–74.
49. Daughaday WH. Evolving concepts of GH and IGF-I regulation of skeletal growth. Endocrine 1994;2:767–9.
50. Isaksson OGP, Lindahl A, Nilsson A, Isgaard J. Mechanism of the stimulatory effect of growth hormone on longitudinal bone growth [Review]. Endocrine Rev 1987;8:426–38.
51. Daughaday WH. A personal history of the origin of the somatomedin hypothesis and recent challenges to its validity. Perspect Biol Med 1989; 32:194–211.
52. Walton PE, Etherton TD. Effects of porcine growth hormone and insulin-like growth factor-I (IGF-I) on immunoreactive IGF-binding protein concentration in pigs. J Endocrinol 1989;120:153–60.
53. Laron Z, Klinger B, Blum WF, Silbergeld A, Ranke MB. IGF binding protein 3 in patients with Laron type dwarfism: effect of exogenous rIGF-I. Clin Endocrinol 1992;36:301–4.
54. Villafuerte BC, Koop BL, Pao C, Gu L, Birdsong GG, Phillips LS. Coculture of primary rat hepatocytes and non-parenchymal cells permits expression of insulin-like growth factor binding protein-3 in vitro. Endocrinology 1994; 134:2044–50.

55. Van Wyk JJ, Conti M, del Monte P. The role of somatomedins in growth and function of endocrine tissues. In: Sizonenko PC, Aubert ML, eds. The endocrinology of adolescence. New York: Raven 1990:127–40.
56. Lunk PK, Moats-Staats BM, Hynes MA. Somatomedin-C/insulin-like growth factor-I and insulin-like growth factor-II mRNAs in rat fetal and adult tissues. J Biol Chem 1986;261:14539–44.
57. Hynes MA, Brooks PJ, Van Wyk JJ. Insulin-like growth factor-II messenger ribonucleic acids are synthesized in the choroid plexus of the rat brain. Mol Endocrinol 1988;2:47–54.
58. Penhoat A, Jaillard C, Saez JM. Synergistic effects of corticotropin and insulin-like growth factor-I on corticotropin receptors and corticotropin responsiveness in cultured bovine adrenocortical cells. Biochem Biophys Res Commun 1989;165:355–9.
59. Adashi EY, Resnick CE, Hernandez ER, et al. Insulin-like growth factor-1 as an amplifier of follicle-stimulating hormone action: studies on mechanism(s) and site(s) of action in cultured rat granulosa cells. Endocrinology 1988; 122:1583–91.
60. Magoffin DA, Kurtz KM, Erickson GF. Insulin-like growth factor-I selectively stimulates cholesterol side-chain cleavage expression in ovarian theca-interstitial cells. Mol Endocrinol 1990;4:489–96.
61. Kasson BG, Hsueh AJW. Insulin-like growth factor-I augments gonadotropin-stimulated androgen biosynthesis by cultured rat testicular cells. Mol Cell Endocrinol 1987;52:27–34.
62. Fisher DA. Endocrinology of fetal development. In: Wilson, Foster (eds.). Williams' textbook of endocrinology. Philadelphia: W.B. Saunders, 1992: 1049–77.
63. Simmen FA, Simmon RCM, Letcher LR. IGFs in pregnancy: developmental expression in uterus and mammary gland and paracrine actions during embryonic and neonatal growth. In: LeRoith D, Raizada MK, eds. Molecular and cellular biology of insulin-like growth factors and their receptors. New York: Plenum, 1989:195–208.
64. McCarthy TL, Centrella M, Canalis E. Insulin-like growth factor (IGF) and bone. Conn Tissue Res 1989;20:277–82.
65. Uthne K, Uthne T. Influence of liver resection and regeneration on somatomedin (sulphation factor). Activity in sera from normal and hypophysectomized rats. Acta Endocrinol 1972;71:255–64.
66. Schoele E, Zapf J, Humbel RE, Froesch ER. Insulin-like growth factor-I stimulates growth in hypophysectomized rats. Nature (Lond) 1982;296:252–3.
67. Walker JL, Van Wyk JJ, Underwood LE. Stimulation of statural growth by recombinant insulin-like growth factor I in a child with growth hormone insensitivity syndrome (Laron type). J Pediatr 1992;121:641–6.
68. Scanes CG, Daughaday WH. Growth hormone: action. In: Harvey S, Scanes CG, Daughaday WH, eds. Growth hormone. Boca Raton, FL: CRC Press, 1995:351–69.
69. Isaksson OGP, Jansson J, Gause LAM. Growth hormone stimulates longitudinal bone growth directly. Science 1982;216:1237–9.
70. Russell SM, Spencer ER. Local injections of human or rat growth hormone or of purified human somatomedin-C stimulate unilateral tibial epiphyseal growth in hypophysectomized rats. Endocrinology 1985;116:2563–7.

71. Bentham J, Ohlsson C, Lindahl A, Isaksson O, Nilsson A. A double-staining technique for detection of growth hormone and insulin-like growth factor-I binding to rat tibial epiphyseal chondrocytes. J Endocrinol 1993;137:361-7.

72. Schoefield PN. Introduction. In Schofield PN, ed. The insulin-like growth factor — structure and biological functions. Oxford University Press, 1992: 1-4.

73. Ohlsson C, Nilsson A, Isaksson O, Lindahl A. Growth hormone induces multiplication of the slowly cycling germinal cells of the rat tibial growth plate. Proc Natl Acad Sci USA 1992;9826-30.

74. Lindahl A, Nilsson A, Isaksson OGP. Effects of growth hormone and insulin-like growth factor-I on colony formation of rabbit epiphyseal chondrocytes at different stages of nutrition. J Endocrinol 1987;115:263-71.

75. Luo H, Murphy LJ. Dexamethasone inhibits growth hormone induction of insulin-like growth factor-I (IGF-I) messenger ribonucleic acid (mRNA) in hypophysectomized rats and reduces IGF-I mRNA abundance in the intact rat. Endocrinology 1989;125:165-71.

76. Murphy LJ, Friesen HG. Differential effects of estrogen and growth hormone on uterine and hepatic insulin-like growth factor I gene expression in the ovariectomized hypophysectomized rat. Endocrinology 1988;122:325-32.

77. Penhoat A, Naville D, Jaillard C. Hormonal regulation of insulin-like growth factor I secretion by bovine adrenal cells. J Biol Chem 1989;264:6858-62.

78. Hammond JM, Hsu C, Klindt J, Tsang BK, Downey BR. Gonadotropins increase concentrations of immunoreactive insulin-like growth factor-1 in porcine follicular fluid in vivo. Biol Reprod 1988;38:304-8.

79. Jennische E, Isgaard J, Isaksson OGP. Local expression of insulin-like growth factors during tissue growth and regeneration. In Schofield PN, ed. The insulin-like growth factors: structure and biologic functions. Oxford University Press, 1992:221-39.

80. Jennische E, Olivecrona H. Transient expression of insulin-like growth factor 1 immunoreactivity in skeletal muscle cells during postnatal development in the rat. Acta Physiol Scand 1987;131:619-22.

81. Fagin JA, Melmed S. Relative increase in insulin-like growth factor I messenger ribonucleic acid levels in compensatory renal hypertrophy. Endocrinology 1987;120:718-24.

82. Stiles AD, Sosenko IRS, D'Ercole AJ, Smith BT. Relation of kidney tissue somatomedin-C/insulin-like growth factor I to postnephrectomy renal growth in the rat. Endocrinology 1985;117:2397-401.

83. Carlsson B, Carlsson I, Billig H. Estrus cycle-dependent co-variation of insulin-like growth factor-I (IGF-I) messenger ribonucleic acid and protein in the rat ovary. Mol Cell Endocrinol 1989;64:271-5.

84. Ballard FJ, Francis GL, Ross M, Bagley CL, May B, Wallace JC. Natural and synthetic forms of insulin-like growth factor-I (IGF-I) and the potent derivative, destripeptide IGF-I: biological activities and receptor binding. Biochem Biophys Res Commun 1987;149:398-404.

85. Yamamoto H, Murphy LJ. Enzymatic conversion of IGF-I to des(1-3)IGF-I in rat serum and tissues: a further potential site of growth hormone regulation of IGF-I action. J Endocrinol 1995;146:141-8.

86. Tamborlane WV, Hintz RL, Bergman M, Genel M, Felig P, Sherwin RS. Insulin-infusion-pump treatment of diabetes. Influence of improved metabolic control on plasma somatotmedin levels. N Engl J Med 1981;305:303-7.

87. Glaser EW, Goldstein S, Phillips LS. Nutrition and somatomedin. XVII. Circulating somatomedin-C during treatment of diabetic ketoacidosis. Diabetes 1987;36:1152–60.
88. Cotterill AM, Cowell CT, Baxter RC, McNeil D, Silinik M. Regulation of the growth hormone-independent growth factor-binding protein in children. J Clin Endocrinol Metab 1988;67:882–7.
89. Suikkari A, Koivisto VA, Rutanen E, Yki-Jarvinen H, Karonen S, Seppala M. Insulin regulates the serum levels of low molecular weight insulin-like growth factor-binding protein. J Clin Endocrinol Metab 1988;66:266–72.
90. Graubert MG, Goldstein S, Phillips LS. Nutrition and somatomedin XXVII. Total and "free" insulin-like growth factor 1 and IGF binding proteins in rats with streptozotocin-induced diabetes. Diabetes 1991;40:959–65.
91. Guler H, Zapf J, Froesch ER. Short-term metabolic effects of recombinant human insulin-like growth factor I in healthy adults. N Engl J Med 1987; 317:137–40.
92. Lanes R, Recker B, Fort P, Lifshitz F. Impaired somatomedin generation test in children with insulin-dependent diabetes mellitus. Diabetes 1985;34: 156–60.
93. Pao C-I, Farmer PK, Begovic S, Goldstein S, Wu G-J, Phillips LS. Expression of hepatic insulin-like growth factor-I and insulin-like growth factor-binding protein-1 genes is transcriptionally regulated in streptozotocin-diabetic rats. Mol Endocrinol 1992;6:969–77.
94. Phillips LS, Goldstein S, Pao C-I: Nutrition and somatomedin XXVI. Molecular regulation of insulin-like growth factor-1 by insulin in cultured rat hepatocytes. Diabetes 1991;40:1525–30.
95. Phillips LS, Vassilopoulou-Sellin R. Somatomedins. N Engl J Med 1980; 302:371–80;438–46.
96. Grant DB, Hambley J, Becker D, Pimstone BL. Reduced sulphation factor in undernourished children. Arch Dis Child 1973;48:596–600.
97. Hall K, Sara VR. Somatomedin levels in childhood, adolescence and adult life. In: Daughaday WH, eds. Clinics in endocrinology and metabolism. Philadelphia: W.B. Saunders, 1984:91–112.
98. Isley WL, Underwood LE, Clemmons DR. Dietary components that regulate serum somatomedin-C concentrations in humans. J Clin Invest 1983; 71:175–82.
99. Musey VC, Goldstein S, Farmer PK, Moore PB, Phillips LS. Differential regulation of IGF-I and IGF-binding protein-1 by dietary composition in humans. Am J Med Sci 1993;305:131–8.
100. Clemmons DR, Seek MM, Underwood LE. Supplemental essential amino acids augment the somatomedin-C/insulin-like growth factor-I response to refeeding after fasting. Metabolism 1985;34:391–5.
101. Isley WL, Underwood LE, Clemmons DR. Changes in plasma somatomedin-C in response to ingestion of diets with variable protein and energy content. JPEN 1984;3:407–11.
102. Merimee TJ, Zapf J, Froesch ER. Insulin-like growth factors in the fed and fasted states. J Clin Endocrinol Metab 1982;55:999–1002.
103. Postel-Vinay MC, Cohen-Tough E, Charrier J. Growth hormone receptors in rat liver membranes: effects of fasting and refeeding and correlation with plasma somatomedin activity. Mol Cell Endocrinol 1982;28:657–69.

104. Thissen JP, Triest S, Maes M, Underwood LE, Ketelslegers JM. The decreased plasma concentration of insulin-like growth factor-1 in protein-restricted rats is not due to decreased numbers of growth hormone receptors on isolated hepatocytes. J Endocrinol 1990;124:159–65.
105. Oster MH, Fielder PJ, Levin N, Cronin MJ. Adaptation of the growth hormone and insulin-like growth factor-I axis to chronic and severe calorie or protein malnutrition. J Clin Invest 1995;95:2258–65.
106. Harp JB, Goldstein S, Phillips LS. Nutrition and somatomedin XXIII. Molecular regulation of IGF-I by amino acid availability in cultured hepatocytes. Diabetes 1991;40:95–101.
107. Pao, C-I, Farmer PK, Begovic S, et al. Regulation of insulin-like growth factor-I (IGF-I) and IGF-binding protein-1 gene transcription by hormones and provision of amino acids in rat hepatocytes. Mol Endocrinol 1993; 7:1561–8.
108. Kobayashi S, Nogami H, Ikeda T. Growth hormone and nutrition interact to regulate expressions ofkidney IGF-I and IGFBP mRNAs. Kidney Int 1995; 48:65–71.
109. Bentham J, Rodriguez-Arnao J, Ross RJM. Acquired growth hormone resistance in patients with hypercatabolism [review]. Horm Res 1993;40:87–91.
110. Wojnar MM, Fan J, Frost RA, Gelato MC, Lang CH. Alterations in the insulin-like growth factor system in trauma patients. Am J Physiol 1995; 268:R970–7.
111. Jeevanadam M, Holaday NJ, Shamos RF, Petersen SR. Acute IGF-1 deficiency in multiple trauma victims. Clin Nutr 1992;11:352–7.
112. Norstedt G, Andersson G, Edwall D, Eriksson L, Hansson H, Jennische E, et al. Regulatory aspects of insulin-like growth factor expression in rodents. In: Isaksson O, Binder C, Hall K, Hokfelt B, eds. Growth hormone—basic and clinical aspects. New York: Elsevier Science, 1987:387.
113. Edwall D, Schaaling M, Jennische E, Norstedt G. Induction of insulin-like growth factor-I messenger ribonucleic acid during regeneration of rat skeletal muscle. Mol Cell Endocrinol 1989;63:1–14.
114. D'Ercole AJ, Stiles AD, Underwood LE. Tissue concentrations of somatomedin C: further evidence of multiple sites of synthesis and paracrine and autocrine mechanisms of actions. Proc Natl Acad Sci USA 1984;81:935–9.
115. Russel NE, D'Ercole AJ, Underwood LE. Somatomedin C/insulin like growth factor I during liver regeneration in the rat. Am J Physiol 1985;248:E618–23.

Part II

Role of Nutrients in
Wound Healing Responses

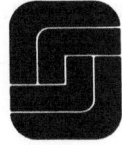

6

Use of Exogenous Amino Acids in Wound Healing

MICHAEL R. SCHÄFFER AND ADRIAN BARBUL

Host metabolism and physiology greatly influence the outcome of wound repair. Overall nutritional status has been shown to affect the healing process (1, 2). Human protein-calorie malnutrition (PCM) or experimentally induced PCM correlate with increased wound complications and decreased wound mechanical strength (3–5). Experimentally this is a reflection of decreased wound collagen synthesis (Fig. 6.1), while clinically there is an added component of reduced specific and nonspecific immune response. In humans the degree of PCM need only be mild and of short duration (1), as evidenced by the fact that patients with brief preoperative illness or reduced nutritional intake in the immediate postoperative or postinjury phase demonstrate impaired fibroplasia (6). The reverse is also true, namely that short-term and not necessarily full-target nutritional intervention can reverse or prevent the decreased deposition of connective tissue seen with protein-calorie malnutrition or with postoperative starvation (7, 8).

Under experimental conditions protein deprivation also leads to impaired wound healing, although the degree of deficiency needs to be quite extensive. Individual sulfur-containing amino acids have been shown to abrogate some of the healing defects in protein-deficient animals (9, 10), but the clinical relevance of these findings is not clear as pure protein deficiencies are rarely seen.

While deficiencies of many nutrients impair wound healing, there has been a recent surge of interest in the use of individual nutrients to promote normal healing, either in situations where there is need for enhanced healing or where healing failure has occurred (2). Often these nutrients are used in amounts well in excess of normal nutritional requirements and thus they are said to possess "pharmacologic" effects, to differentiate these uses from standard nutritional uses. In this regard several amino acids have been used most extensively. This chapter reviews the accumulated body of knowledge and makes some recommendations regarding clinical applications.

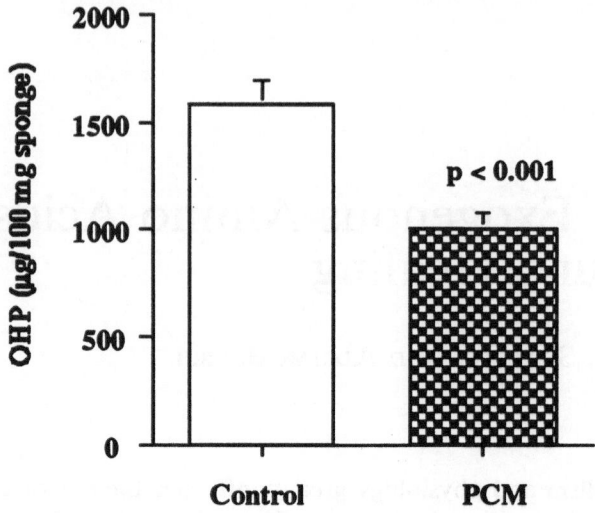

FIGURE 6.1. Effect of acute protein-calorie malnutrition (PCM) on wound collagen accumulation. Beginning 7 days prior to wounding, one group of rats was rendered malnourished by restricting its food intake to 50% of the level for the ad libitum–fed control group. Hydroxyproline (OHP) content in subcutaneously implanted polyvinyl alcohol sponges, an index of collagen deposition, was measured 10 days postwounding. Data show the means ± SEM of 10 animals.

Arginine

Arginine, a dibasic amino acid, is considered to be a dietary conditionally dispensable amino acid (11). Arginine is synthesized endogenously from ornithine via citrulline as a result of interorgan reactions. The quantities produced, sufficient to maintain muscle and connective tissue mass, may be less than that required for optimal protein biosynthesis and therefore optimal growth. In times of immaturity and severe stress, such as sepsis, trauma, and nitrogen overload, endogenous synthesis arginine is insufficient to meet the increased demands that increased protein turnover requires. Therefore, in such situations arginine is an indispensable amino acid for optimal growth and maintenance of positive nitrogen balance (12–14).

Arginine is a normal constituent of numerous body proteins and is associated with a variety of essential reactions of intermediary metabolism. The intestinal absorption of arginine involves a transport system shared with lysine, ornithine, and cysteine. This system is energy and sodium dependent and has substrate specificity. Arginine, ornithine, and lysine also share a common uptake and transport system in the brain involving leukocytes, erythrocytes, and fibroblasts (15).

Arginine serves as a vehicle for the transport, storage, and excretion of nitrogen. The transamidation between arginine and glycine results in guanidioacetic acid, which is further methylated to form the high-energy phosphagen creatine phosphate. The reversible release of fumaric acid by dismutation of argininosuccinic acid further links arginine metabolism with cellular energetics via the tricarboxylic acid cycle. Arginine and its metabolite ornithine are also utilized for polyamine biosynthesis, an important requirement for cellular division. The urea cycle represents the major metabolic pathway for ammonia detoxification, and arginine plays a key regulatory role within this cycle (16).

Recently, L-arginine has been shown to be the unique substrate for the production of the biologic effector molecule nitric oxide (NO). This important pathway has been shown to be present in many tissues and cells including endothelium, brain, inflammatory cells (lymphocytes, macrophages, neutrophils, mast cells), platelets, and hepatocytes (17).

The feeding of arginine deficient diets to young adult rats subjected to dosal skin incisions and subcutaneous implantation of polyvinyl alcohol sponges resulted in decreased wound mechanical strength and wound collagen accumulation (Fig. 6.2) (14). Furthermore, arginine deficiency resulted in increased postoperative weight loss and mortality when compared with controls fed a normal laboratory chow. Subsequently, chow-fed animals were given a 1% arginine supplement and this resulted in increased wound mechanical strength and collagen deposition (Fig. 6.2) (14). Improvement of wound healing was also reported after intravenous hyperalimentation with high arginine levels (65 mg/kg body weight/hr) when compared to controls (36 mg arginine/kg body weight/hr) (18). Mature and old rats fed a diet supplemented with both arginine (2.4%) and glycine (1.0%) demonstrated improved nitrogen retention, increased wound collagen deposition, and higher ratios of type III/type I collagen (19). Type III collagen is the dominant collagen isoform during the early phases of healing (20, 21) and is found in significantly higher concentrations in granulation tissue than in normal skin (22). Although type I collagen constitutes most of the collagen in mature wounds, there is chemical evidence that types I and III are linked and can be present in the same fibril (23). The effect of arginine on wound repair in rats is dependent on the presence of an intact hypothalamic-pituitary axis. Hypophysectomized rats, whether or not treated with growth hormone, do not demonstrate any beneficial effects on wound healing from arginine supplementation (24).

Two studies in healthy human volunteers looked at the effect of arginine supplementation on wound collagen accumulation. Young healthy human volunteers (25 to 35 years) were found to have significantly increased wound collagen accumulation and enhanced lymphocyte immune response following oral supplementation with either 30 g of arginine aspartate (17 g of free arginine) or 30 g of arginine hydrochloric acid (HCl) (24.8 g of free arginine) daily for 14 days (Fig. 6.3) (25). In a subsequent experiment of healthy aged humans (67 to 82 years) daily supplements of 30 g arginine

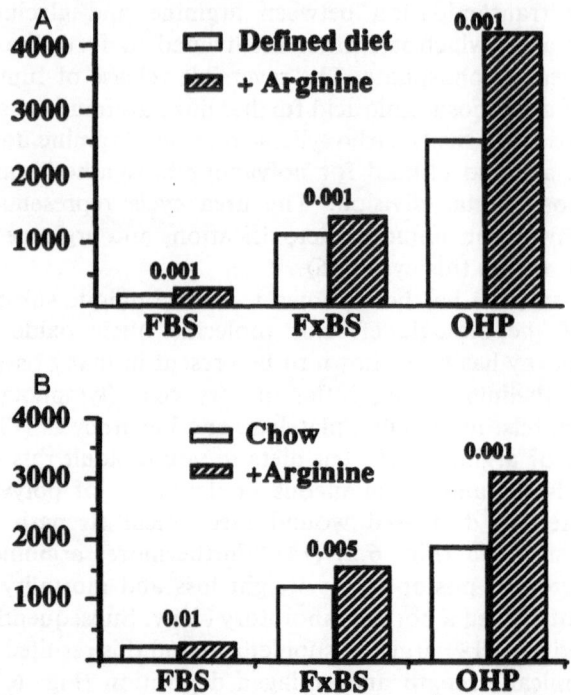

FIGURE 6.2. Effect of arginine-free diet (defined diet) (A) and arginine-supplemented chow (B) on wound healing in rats. FBS, fresh breaking strength of scar, g ± SEM; FxBS, formalin-fixed breaking strength, g ± SEM; OHP, hydroxyproline content of subcutaneously implanted polyvinyl alcohol sponges, μg/100 mg sponge dry weight ± SEM.

aspartate resulted in enhanced collagen and total protein deposition in subcutaneously implanted polytetrafluoroethylene catheters (Fig. 6.4). No effect on the rate of epithelialization of superficial skin defects, however, was noted, suggesting that the main effect of arginine on wound healing is mediated by increased collagen formation (26).

The mechanism of action by which arginine promotes wound healing is not clear. Arginine levels are essentially undetectable in wound fluid. Arginine can be metabolized to ornithine and urea by arginase and to NO and citrulline by NO synthase. Sustained substrate utilization for these metabolic pathways may account for undetectable arginine levels in the wound (27). Ornithine is a precursor of proline, a potentially limiting substrate for collagen production (28, 29). Ornithine supplementation of animal diet has been shown to have stimulatory effects on wound breaking strength (30). Thus, some of the effects of arginine on wound repair may be mediated through ornithine synthesis (29). Systemic treatment of Balb/C mice with competitive inhibitors of NO synthase, including methyl isothiouronium and aminoguanidine, has been found to decrease wound collagen

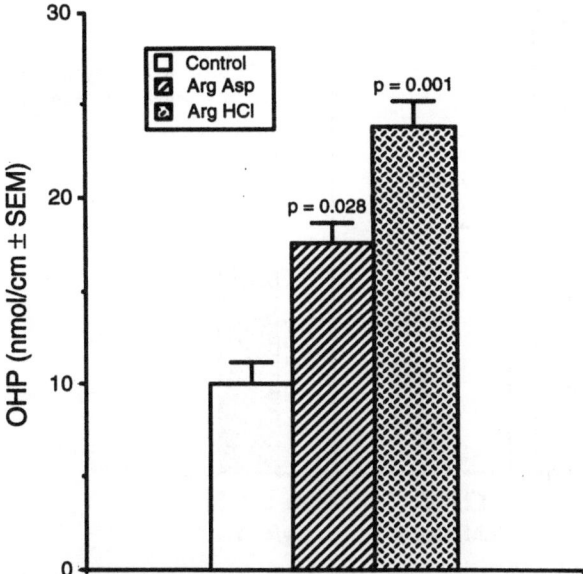

FIGURE 6.3. Effect of 2 weeks of arginine supplementation on hydroxyproline (OHP) accumulation in subcutaneously implanted polytetrafluoroethylene catheters in young human volunteers. Each group of 12 volunteers received a placebo syrup (control), 30 g arginine aspartate (Arg, Asp), or 30 g arginine HCl (Arg HCl) for 2 weeks.

deposition and wound mechanical strength (31). Also, impaired wound healing caused by acute protein-calorie malnutrition was accompanied by decreased wound NO synthesis. Diminished wound collagen accumulation was paralleled by decreased type III, but not type I, collagen gene expression (32).

In the treatment of severely burned patients a low-fat enteral diet supplemented with 0.4% arginine, 0.25% cysteine, and 0.5% omega-3 fatty acids has been found to reduce wound infection when compared with other standard enteral formations (33, 34). In another prospective trial, surgical patients undergoing surgery for upper gastrointestinal malignancies were randomized to receive either a supplemented (arginine 12.5 g/L, RNA 1.25 g/L, and omega-3 fatty acids 1.7 g/L) diet or a standard enteral diet postoperatively (35). Wound complications were decreased and length of hospital stays were found to be reduced in the supplemental group.

Ornithine α-Ketoglutarate

Ornithine α-ketoglutarate (OKG) is formed of two molecules of ornithine and one molecule of α-ketoglutarate. When given parenterally or enterally

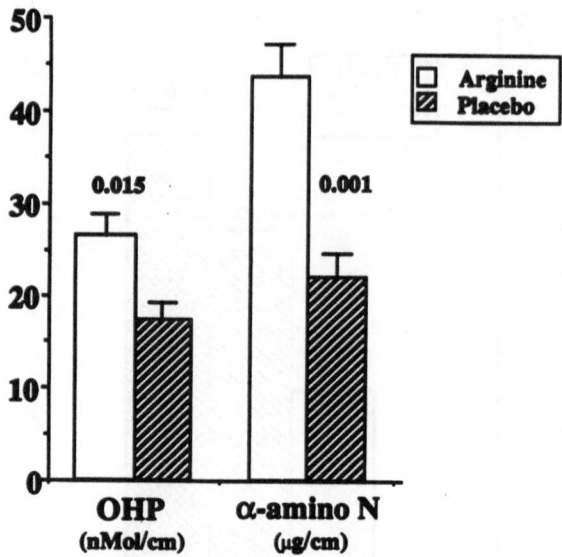

FIGURE 6.4. Effect of arginine on wound healing parameters in healthy elderly human volunteers. Accumulation of hydroxyprolin (OHP) and total α-amino nitrogen (N) in subcutaneously implanted polytetrafluoroethylene catheters was measured at the end of 2 weeks. Controls ($n = 15$) received a placebo syrup; the arginine group ($n = 30$) received 30 g of arginine aspartate in double-blind fashion.

to animals or humans, OKG decreases muscle protein catabolism and enhances liver anabolism in trauma, sepsis, and burn injury (36). In addition, in patients having undergone reconstructive surgery, daily supplements of 10 to 15 g OKG resulted in significantly enhanced healing rates and decreased wound complications (36). The mechanism of action of OKG is thought to be due to its stimulatory effect on anabolic hormone secretion and to the synthesis of active metabolites, including ornithine, glutamine, arginine, polyamines, and ketoacids. The interaction between ornithine and α-ketoglutarate seems to be critical for at least some of the effects of OKG, since individual applications did not show similar results (37).

Glutamine

Glutamine is the most abundant amino acid in the body, accounting for approximately 20% of the total circulating free amino acid pool and for more than 60% of the free intracellular amino acid pool (38). It is an important vehicle for nitrogen transfer between tissues (39). In addition, glutamine is a regulator of protein synthesis (40) and an essential precursor for nucleotide biosynthesis in all cells (41). It serves as an energy fuel for the gut mucosa (42) and other rapidly dividing cells such as fibroblasts, lymphocytes, and epithelial cells (43, 44). Trauma, severe illness, and sepsis are followed by a rapid fall of muscle and plasma glutamine levels (45, 46). Intracellular loss is thought to be due to impaired sodium-dependent glutamine transport (47, 48). The decrease in glutamine concentration correlates, in general, with the severity of the underlying pathologic condition, and a greater than 50% decrease in muscle glutamine levels is associated with increased mortality (46). Glutamine-enriched parenteral nutrition has been shown to improve postoperative nitrogen balance in humans (49, 50).

In acutely undernourished rats (animals were fed a 3.5% agar diet for 6 days preoperatively, resulting in a 10% decrease of body weight and mild hypoalbuminemia), glutamine-enriched (1.2%) parenteral nutrition has been reported to increase mucosal protein content. However, no improvement of healing of colonic anastomosis was seen (51). The effect of glutamine as a single amino acid on human would healing is unknown.

Branched-Chain Amino Acids

The branched-chain amino acids (BCAAs), leucine, iso-leucine, and valine, have been shown to promote protein synthesis and inhibit protein breakdown in posttraumatic situations (52–54). BCAAs have been shown also to increase nitrogen retention during trauma and sepsis (55, 56). It has been hypothesized that trauma patients may have an enhanced consumption of BCAAs as they may be metabolized as caloric substrates as an alternative energy fuel; the secondary depletion of the intracellular BCAA pool may thus reduce their availability for protein synthesis (57, 58). Exogenous BCAA supply may not only restore intracellular levels (59), but may also increase muscle sensitivity to insulin, resulting in enhanced protein synthesis (60). Clinical trials examining the effect of BCAA supplementation on protein synthesis in severely injured patients have obtained conflicting results (61, 62). This points out the need for further clinical studies to identify those patients that would most benefit from enhanced BCAA intake.

The effects of BCAAs on posttraumatic nitrogen metabolism led to several experimental studies examining the possible effects of BCAAs on wound healing. However, no improvement in wound healing has been noted using high supplements of these amino acids. Total parenteral nutrition utilizing amino acid mixtures containing 45% BCAA showed no stimulating effect on the healing of musculo-aponeurotic wounds in rats with acute PCM when compared with conventional mixtures (8% BCAA) (63). Another study failed to show any effect on the healing of colonic anastomoses in jaundiced rats given a BCAA-enriched formula (43% BCAA) when compared with two standard solutions containing 21%

BCAA (64). Rats subjected to a 40% burn and tibial osteotomy were found to have impaired bone healing 3 weeks postinjury when treated with an enriched BCCA solution (45%) (65). Overall it appears that although BCAA may improve host nitrogen metabolism postinjury, no beneficial effect on wound healing has been noted.

Topical Amino Acid Application

In a prospective controlled trial, topical irrigation with an amino acid solution has been shown to result in faster healing of chronic leg ulcers when compared with treatment with normal saline (66). Osmolarity had no significant effect on the outcome of healing. Local hyperalimentation, i.e., application of glucose and amino acid mixtures, has been found to improve, both experimentally and clinically, the healing of open wounds of traumatic origin and second- and third-degree burns (67–69). A mixture of amino acids and glucose, electrolytes, and vitamins increases the number of collagen-producing cells and causes a changeover of metabolism from anaerobic toward a more oxidative pathway in subcutaneously implanted viscose cellulose sponges (67). Histologic examination of human wounds treated with amino acid solutions showed enhanced capillary growth and increased numbers of fibroblasts (69).

Amino Acid Metabolism

This topic is discussed in greater detail by Jorge Albina and Michael Caldwell in this volume. The wound environment, as represented by wound fluid, mirrors cell metabolic activity and contains a complex mixture of active and nonactive extracellular factors. Wound amino acid concentrations represent the net effect of change of wound water content, equilibration with plasma amino acid levels, proteolysis within the wound, synthesis and degradation of individual amino acids, and release of intracellular stores of amino acid levels. Wound amino acid levels increase from day 1 to day 10 postwounding and reach concentrations close to those recommended for optimal cell proliferation, except for arginine, cysteine, glutamine, isoleucine, and phenylalanine (70, 71). Also, the stimulatory effect of growth factors on fibroblast replication has been shown to be dependent on the concentration of certain amino acids (71).

Relative deficiencies of amino acids may occur during excessive ammonia concentrations, growth, pregnancy, trauma, or protein-calorie malnutrition (72). Intestinal absorption of arginine involves an energy and sodium-dependent transport system shared with lysine, ornithine, and cysteine. This active process, however, may be compromised in situations of increased amino acid demands, such as sepsis, and may limit the ability of enteral feeding alone to supply nutritional requirements (73). Wounds containing a marked dead space or large regenerative area exhibit chronic lack of oxygen and other nutrients. Local imbalance of wound amino acid metabolism, combined with impaired intestinal absorption and systemic metabolic disorders, provides the biologic rationale for exogenous supplementation of amino acids to support the healing process in compromised patients. Nutritional requirements, however, may differ for individual patients, due to the kind and size of wound, underlying diseases, and acute systemic metabolic complications.

Summary

Exogenous amino acids have been shown to improve wound healing; notably individual amino acids, in particular arginine, exhibit a pharmacologic effect and promote normal wound repair in rodents and humans. The exact mechanism of action is not known. Recent studies, however, suggest that arginine metabolic products, including ornithine and nitric oxide, play a key role in mediating the stimulatory effect of arginine on wound healing. Clinically it is important to maintain as normal an intake of calories and amino acids as possible and to start such intake as close to the time of injury/surgery as possible. The specialized use of individual amino acid awaits further definition.

References

1. Haydock DA, Hill GL. Impaired wound healing in surgical patients with varying degrees of malnutrition. J Parenter Enteral Nutr 1986;10:550–4.
2. Barbul A, Purtill WA. Nutrition in wound healing. Clin Dermatol 1994; 12:133–40.
3. Irvin TT. Effects of malnutrition and hyperalimentation on wound healing. Surg Gynecol Obstet 1978;146:33–7.
4. Casey J, Flinn WR, Yao JS, Fahey V, Pawlowski J, Bergan JJ. Correlation of immune and nutritional status with wound complications in patients undergoing vascular operations. Surgery 1983;93:822–7.
5. Dickhaut SC, DeLee JC, Page CP. Nutritional status: importance in predicting wound healing after amputation. J Bone Joint Surg 1984;66:71–5.
6. Goodson WH, Lopez-Sarmiento A, Jensen JA, West J, Gramja-Mena L, Chavez-Estrella J. The influence of a brief preoperative illness on postoperative healing. Ann Surg 1987;205:250–5.
7. Haydock DA, Hill GL. Improved wound healing response in surgical patients receiving intravenous nutrition. Br J Surg 1987;74:320–3.
8. Schroeder D, Gillanders L, Mahr K, Hill GL. Effects of immediate postoperative enteral nutrition on body composition, muscle function and wound healing. J Parenter Enteral Nutr 1991;15:376–83.

9. Williamson MB, Fromm JH. The incorporation of sulphor amino acids into protein of regenerating wound tissue. J Biol Chem 1955;212:705-12.

10. Localio SA, Morgan ME, Hinton JW. The biological chemistry of wound healing. The effect of methionine on the healing of wounds in protein depleted animals. Surg Gynecol Obstet 1948;86:582-90.

11. Rose WC. The nutritive significance of the amino acids and certain related compounds. Science 1937;86:298-300.

12. Rose WC. Amino acid requirements of man. Fed Proc 1949;8:546-52.

13. Nakagawa I, Takahashi T, Suzuki T, Kobayashi K. Amino acid requirements of children: minimal needs of tryptophan, arginine, histidine based on nitrogen balance method. J Nutr 1963;80:305-10.

14. Seifter E, Rettura G, Barbul A, Levenson SM. Arginine: an essential amino acid for injured rats. Surgery 1978;84:224-30.

15. Barbul A. Arginine: biochemistry, physiology and therapeutic implications. J Parenter Enteral Nutr 1986;10:227-38.

16. Fahey JL. Toxicity and blood ammonia rise resuling from intravenous amino acid administration in man: the protective effect of L-arginine. J Clin Invest 1957;36:1647-55.

17. Moncada S, Higgs EA, eds. Nitric oxide from arginine: a bioregulatory system. New York: Elsevier, 1990.

18. Barbul A, Fishel RS, Shimazu S, Wasserkrug HL, Yoshimura NN, Tao RC, et al. Intravenous hyperalimentation with high arginine levels improves wound healing and immune function. J Surg Res 1985;38:328-34.

19. Chyun J, Griminger P. Improvement of nitrogen retention by arginine and glycine supplementation and its relation to collagen synthesis in traumatized mature and aged rats. J Nutr 1984;114:1697-704.

20. Gay S, Viljanto J, Raekallio J, Penttinen R. Collagen types in early phases of wound healing in children. Acta Chir Scand 1978;144:205-11.

21. Clore JN, Cohen IK, Diegelmann RF. Quantitation of the collagen types I and III during wound healing in the rat skin (40548). Proc Soc Exp Biol Med 1979;161:337-40.

22. Bailey AJ, Sims TJ, LeLous M, Bazin S. Collagen polymorphism in experimental granulation tissue. Biochem Biophys Res Commun 1975;66:1160-5.

23. Henkel W, Glanville RW. Covalent crosslinking between molecules of type-I and type-III collagen. The involvement of the N-terminal, nonhelical regions of the alpha 1 (I) and alpha 1 (III) chains in the formation of intermolecular crosslinks. Eur J Biochem 1982;122:205-13.

24. Barbul A, Rettura G, Levenson SM, Seifter E. Wound healing and thymotropic effects of arginine: a pituitary mechanism of action. Am J Clin Nutr 1983;37:786-94.

25. Barbul A, Lazarou SA, Efron DT, Wasserkrug HL, Efron G. Arginine enhances wound healing and lymphocyte immune responses in humans. Surgery 1990;108:331-7.

26. Kirk SJ, Hurson M, Regan MC, Holt DR. Wasserkrug HL, Barbul A. Arginine stimulates wound healing and immune function in elderly human beings. Surgery 1993;114:155-60.

27. Albina JE, Mills CD, Barbul A, et al. Arginine metabolism in wounds. Am J Physiol 1987;254:E459-67.

28. Rojkind M, DeLeon D. Collagen biosynthesis in cirrhotic rat liver slices: a regulatory mechanism. Biochim Biophys Acta 1970;217:512-22.

29. Albina JE, Abate JA, Mastrofrancesco B. Role of ornithine as a proline precursor in healing wound. J Surg Res 1993;55:97–102.
30. Rettura G, Stratford F, Levenson SM, Barbul A, Seifter E. Improved wound healing: anti-catabolic and thymotropic actions of supplemental ornithine (Abstract). Mid-Atlantic Regional Meeting of the American Society 17th Washington, DC, 1983.
31. Schäffer M, Tantry U, Gross SS, Wasserkrug HL, Barbul A. Nitric oxide regulates wound healing (abstract). 29th Annual Meeting of the American Association for Academic Surgery, Dearborn, MI, 1995.
32. Schäffer M, Tantry U, Ahrendt G, Wasserkrug HL, Barbul A. Acute protein-calorie malnutrition (PCM) impairs wound healing: role of decreased wound nitric oxide (NO) synthesis (abstract). Annual Meeting of the Baltimore Academy of Surgery, Baltimore, MD, 1995.
33. Alexander JW, Gottschlich MM. Nutritional immunomodulation in burn patients. Crit Care Med 1990;18:S149–53.
34. Gottschlich MM, Jenkins M, Warden GD, et al. Differential effects of three enteral dietary regimens on selected outcome variables in burn patients. J Parenter Enteral Nutr 1990;14:225–36.
35. Daly JM, Lieberman MD, Goldfine J, et al. Enteral nutrition with supplemental arginine, RNA, and omega-3 fatty acids in patients after operation: immuno-logic, metabolic, and clinical outcome. Surgery 1992;112:56–67.
36. Cynober L. Ornithine α-ketoglutarate in nutritional support. Nutrition 1991;7:313–22.
37. Cynober L, Coudray-Lucas C, De Banddt JP, et al. Action of ornithine α-ketoglutarate, ornithine hydrochloride and calcium α-ketoglutarate on plasma amino acid and hormonal patterns in health subjects. J Am Coll Nutr 1990;9:2–12.
38. Bergstrom L, Furst P, Noree LO, Vinnars F. Intracellular free amino acid concentrations in human muscle tissue. J Appl Physiol 1974;36:693–7.
39. Souba WW. Interorgan ammonia metabolism in health and disease: a surgeon's view. J Parenter Enteral Nutr 1987;11:569–79.
40. Jepson MM, Bates PC, Broadbent P, Pell JM, Millward DJ. Relationship between glutamine concentration and protein synthesis in rat skeletal muscle. Am J Physiol 1988;18:E166–72.
41. Frisell WR. Synthesis and catabolism of nucleotides. In: Frisell WR, ed. Human biochemistry. New York: Macmillan, 1982:292–304.
42. Souba W, Smith R, Wilmore D. Glutamine metabolism by the intestinal tract. J Parenter Enteral Nutr 1985;9:608–17.
43. Zetterberg A, Engstrom W. Glutamine and the regulation of DNA replication and cell multiplication in fibroblasts. J Cell Physiol 1981;108:365–73.
44. Ardawi MS, Newsholme EA. Glutamine metabolism in lymphocytes of the rat. Biochem J 1983;212:835–42.
45. Askanazi J, Carpentier JA, Michelsen CB, et al. Muscle and plasma amino acids following injury: influence of intercurrent infection. Ann Surg 1980;192:78–85.
46. Roth E, Funovics J, Muhlbacher F. Metabolic disorders in severe abdominal sepsis: glutamine deficiency in skeletal muscle. Clin Nutr 1982;1:25–32.
47. Rennie MJ, Hundal HS, Babil P, McLennan PA, Taylor PM, Watt PW. Characteristics of a glutamine carrier in skeletal muscle have important conse-quences for nitogen loss in injury, infection and chronic disease. Lancet 1986;2(8514):1008–12.

48. Ahmed A, Taylor PM, Rennie MJ. Characteristics of glutamine transport in sarcolemmal vesicles from rat skeletal muscle. Am J Physiol 1990;259:E284–91.
49. Hammargvist F, Wernerman J, Ali R, von der Decken A, Vinnars E. Addition of glutamine to total parenteral nutrition after elective abdominal surgery spares free glutamine in muscle, counteracts the fall in muscle protein synthesis, and improves nitrogen balance. Ann Surg 1989;209:455–61.
50. Stehle P, Zander J, Mertes N, et al. Effect of parenteral glutamine peptide supplements on muscle glutamine loss and nitrogen balance after major surgery. Lancet 1989;1(8632):231–3.
51. McCauley R, Platell C, Hall J, McCulloch R. Effects of glutamine infusion on colonic anastomotic strength in the rat. J Parenter Enteral Nutr 1991;15:437–9.
52. Hedden MP, Buse MG. General stimulation of muscle protein synthesis by branched-chain amino acids in vitro. Proc Soc Exp Bio Med 1979;160:410–5.
53. Buse MG, Reid M. Leucine. A possible regulator of protein turnover in muscle. J Clin Invest 1975;56:1250–61.
54. Freund HR, Lapidot A, Fischer JE. The use of branched-chain amino acids in the injured septic patients. In: Walser M, Williamson JR, eds. Metabolism and clinical implications of branch chain amino acids and keto acids. New York: Elsevier, 1981;18:527–32.
55. Cerra FB, Shronts EP, Konstantinides NN, et al. Enteral feeding in sepsis: a prospective, randomized double-blind trial. Surgery 1985;98:632–9.
56. Sax HC, Talamini MA, Fischer JE. Clinical use of branched chain amino acids in liver disease, sepsis, trauma, and burns. Arch Surg 1986;121:358–66.
57. Elia M, Farell R, Ilie V, Smith R, Williamson DH. The removal of infused leucine after injury, starvation and other conditions in man. Clin Sci 1980;59:275–83.
58. Desai SP, Bistrain BR, Moldawere LL, Miller MM, Blackburn GL. Plasma amino acid concentrations during branched-chain amino acid infusion in stressed patients. J Trauma 1982;22:747–52.
59. Moss G, Maylor ED. Postoperative enteral hyperalimentation results in earlier elevation of serum branched-chain amino acid levels. Am J Surg 1994;168:33–5.
60. Garlick PJ. Grant I. Amino acid infusions increase the sensitivity of muscle protein synthesis in vivo to insulin. Biochem J 1988;254:579–84.
61. Yu YM, Wagner DA, Walesreswski JC, Burke JF, Young VR. A kinetic study of leucine metabolism in severely burned patients. Ann Surg 1988;207:421–9.
62. Brennan MF, Cerra F, Daly JM, et al. Report of a research workshop: branched-chain amino acids in stress and injury. J Parenter Enteral Nutr 1986;10:446–52.
63. McCauley R, Platell C, Hall J, McCulloch R. Influence of branched chain amino acid infusions on wound healing. Aust N Z Surg 1990;60:471–3.
64. Delemarre JB, van de Velde CJ, de Brauw LM, Vree R, Giesberts M, Hermans J. Internal biliary drainage, parenteral nutrition, and variation in the total parenteral nutrition feeding solutions: influence on the healing of colon anastomosis in jaundiced rats. J Parenter Enteral Nutr 1990;14:629–33.
65. Dudrick SJ, Matheny RG, O'Donnell JJ, Dudrick PS, Yoshimura NN. Effect of enriched branched chain amino acid solutions in traumatized rats. J Parenter Enteral Nutr 1984;8:86.
66. Bulstrode CJK, Goode AW, Scott PJ. A prospective controlled trial of topical irrigation in the treatment of delayed cutaneous healing in human leg ulcers. Clin Sci 1988;75:637–40.

67. Niinikoski J, Kivisaari J, Viljanto J. Local hyperalimentation of experimental granulation tissue. Acta Chir Scand 1977;143:201–6.
68. Kaufmann T, Levin M, Hurwitz DJ. The effect of topical hyperalimentation on wound healing rate and granulation tissue formation of experimental deep second degree burns in guinea-pigs. Burns Incl Therm Inj 1984;10:252–6.
69. Viljanto J, Raekallio J. Local hyperalimentation of open wounds. Br J Surg 1976;63:427–30.
70. Caldwell MD, Mastrofrancesco B, Schaerer J, Bereiter D. The temporal change in amino acid concentration within the wound fluid—a putative rationale. In: Barbul A, Caldwell MD, Eaglestein WH, et al., eds. Progress in clinical and biological research: clinical and experimental approaches to dermal and epidermal repair. New York: Wiley-Liss, 1991;365:205–22.
71. Gartner MH, Shaerer JD, Bereiter DF, Mills CD, Caldwell MD. Wound fluid amino acid concentrations regulate the effect of epidermal growth factor on fibroblast replication. Surgery 1994;110:448–56.
72. Zieve L. Conditional deficiencies of ornithine or arginine. J Am Coll Nutr 1985;5:167–76.
73. Sodeyama M, Gardiner KR, Regan MC, Kirk SJ, Efron G, Barbul A. Sepsis impairs gut amino acid absorption. Am J Surg 1993;165:150–4.

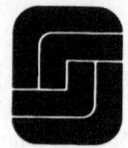

7

Vitamin A–Growth Factor Interactions in Wound Healing

Anders E. Ulland and Michael D. Caldwell

Vitamin A and Wound Healing

Early work by Ehrlich and Hunt (1) demonstrated that vitamin A improved the impairment of wound healing induced by cortisone treatment. Their studies were based on the hypothesis that the inhibition of wound healing caused by cortisone was mediated through the lysosome. Cortisone was known to stabilize lysosomal membranes, while vitamin A had the opposite effect (2). In these experiments they showed that cortisone treatment reduced incisional tensile strength in rats. Rats treated with both cortisone and vitamin A had tensile strength unchanged from that of controls. Vitamin A alone did not increase tensile strength. In a subsequent study (3), these investigators tested topical vitamin A on open wounds in cortisone-treated and control rabbits. Vitamin A treatment of nonimpaired wounds showed no increase in the rate of healing. Rabbits that received cortisone and topical vitamin A had healing rates that were similar to controls. The improved rate of healing was the result of improved epithelialization. Vitamin A appeared to have no effect on cortisone-impaired wound contraction. They also examined the effects of cortisone and vitamin A on inflammation and collagen synthesis (4). In these rodent experiments, they demonstrated that vitamin A stimulated fibroplasia and collagen accumulation and restored polymorphonuclear leukocyte infiltration, all of which had been depressed by cortisone treatment.

The impairment of wound healing by other mechanisms has also been shown to be improved by treatment with vitamin A. Wound healing impaired by streptozocin-induced diabetes, traumatic stress, and radiation are all improved with supplemental vitamin A (5–7). Weinzweig et al. (8) demonstrated that supplemental dietary vitamin A mitigated the impairment of wound healing seen in tumor-bearing mice. Some studies have suggested that vitamin A can improve normal wound healing as well. A study of wound healing accelerators by Herrmann and Woodward (9) demonstrated that local and systemic vitamin A treatment increased the rate of collagen accumulation in polyvinyl alcohol sponges and increased incisional breaking strength relative to normal. In a double-blind, placebo-controlled, prospective, randomized study of 16 human males, Hevia et al. (10) examined the effect of topical retinoic acid on healing after a chemical skin peel. They found that pretreatment with topical retinoic acid for 14 days prior to tochloroacetic acid peel accelerated healing of the peeled areas. Topical retinoic acid pretreatment of photoaged skin in humans also accelerated healing of punch biopsies (11).

These experiments, and others, established vitamin A as an important factor in improving wound healing that has been impaired by a variety of causes, and possibly in normal healing as well. Several other important points emerged from these studies. First, both systemic and local application of vitamin A appear to be effective in improving impaired healing. Second, the effects of vitamin A on healing are not species specific, but have been observed in rats, mice, rabbits, and humans. Third, the effects appear to be most pronounced and consistent in situations of impaired healing. Fourth, the observation that vitamin A increases epithelialization but not contraction in cortisone-treated wounds (3) suggests that vitamin A antagonizes some, but not all, aspects of impaired healing. Thus, the mechanism of vitamin A's effect on healing appears to be somewhat selective.

These important observations led to extensive interest in and investigation of the mechanism of action of vitamin A's effects on wound healing. Despite this effort, the mechanisms of vitamin A action have remained somewhat elusive. Ehrlich's original hypothesis of lysosomal mediation of these effects was consistent with available data, but no direct evidence supported it. Even so, it proved to be a useful paradigm for continued study of the mechanisms involved in vitamin A–improved wound healing.

Retinoic Acid Receptor

The discovery that the retinoic acid receptor (RAR) belongs to the steroid-thyroid hormone receptor superfamily of transcriptional activators (12, 13) was a tremendous advance in understanding how vitamin A might exert its effects. The steroid-thyroid hormone receptor superfamily is the largest known family of transcription factors in eukaryotes. It includes receptors for the steroids progesterone and estrogen, glucocorticoids, mineralcorticoids, and androgens. Also included are the thyroid hormone and vitamin D receptors, as well as the receptors for retinoic acid and 9-*cis* retinoic acid (RXR). A variety of isoforms of RAR exist that may be expressed in distinct cell types and developmental stages, thereby offering a potential broad diversity of physiologic roles for the retinoids. At least three distinct genes have been identified that encode high-affinity RARs, termed α, β, and γ. Each of these isoforms is able to bind to specific elements of DNA, termed retinoic acid response elements (RAREs), and activate transcription of target genes in response to nanomolar concentrations of retinoic acid.

The general structure and functional domains of steroid receptors are reviewed by Tsai and O'Malley (14). The defining feature of this family of receptors is the highly conserved DNA-binding domain, termed the C region. In the RAR it consists of 69 amino acids with nine invariantly placed cysteine residues, eight of which make up two zinc fingers. These are responsible for DNA recognition and dimerization. Directly downstream from the DNA binding domain (DBD) is a variable hinge region (D region) that may allow bending of the protein or conformational alterations. The E region or ligand binding region, is large (about 250 amino acids) and functionally complex. The most important function of the E region appears to be ligand binding. It is also a major site of protein-protein interactions and dimerization. No specific function is as yet described for the F region. The N-terminal A/B region is variable in sequence and length, contains a transactivation function, and may be important for enabling different RAR isoforms to recognize the same response elements.

In the case of the RAR there appears to exist a large number of cell-type specific proteins (termed coregulators) capable of interacting with the RAR to enhance binding to various retinoic acid response elements (15). Binding to DNA by the RAR, therefore, can take place both in the absence of coregulators (intrinsic binding) or in their presence (enhanced binding). Intrinsic binding to DNA does not appear to depend on the ligand-binding domain, whereas enhanced binding depends on it completely. These properties of RAR binding offer even more complexity to the control and regulation of retinoic acid responsive genes.

Earlier work on the steroid receptors demonstrated that the progesterone, glucocorticoid, and mineralcorticoid receptors could all recognize identical response elements. In a similar manner, Umesono et al. (16) showed that the RAR can bind to the thyroid response element. Further work by Graupner et al. (17) demonstrated that the thyroid hormone receptor, in the absence of thyroid hormone, can inhibit transcription activated by the RAR by binding to two distinct thyroid hormone response elements. With these findings in mind, it seems likely that the RARs could participate in the complex regulation of the overlapping gene networks belonging to this extensive family of nuclear receptors. Furthermore, the varying isoforms of the RAR, and complex DNA binding modulated by cell-type specific coregulators, offer a complex array of potential physiologic roles for RAR and may begin to explain some of the seemingly conflicting data regarding vitamin A effects both in vivo and in vitro.

Fibroblast Proliferation, Collagen Metabolism, and Phenotypic Transformation

Because wound breaking strength is directly dependent on collagen content, the observations of increased breaking strength and increased collagen accumulation are roughly equivalent. Increased reparative collagen has been consistently observed in the studies of vitamin A action on impaired wound healing. It seems useful, therefore, to examine the effect of vitamin A on fibroblast replication and collagen synthesis. Numerous studies of fibroblast in culture indicate that like steroids, retinoids usually suppress fibroblast replication and collagen synthesis, suggesting that the vitamin A–stimulated increase in reparative collagen is not the result of a direct effect of vitamin A on fibroblasts. For example, Hein et al. (18) demonstrated a dose-dependent inhibition of the growth rate of human adult and fetal fibroblasts with vitamin A, 13-*cis* retinoic acid, and etritiniate. This study also demonstrated inhibition of collagen production induced in a dose-dependent manner in the same cells. Oikarinin et al. (19) used all-*trans* retinoic acid and 13-*cis* retinoic acid at a concentration of 10^{-5} M in normal and keloid human fibroblasts in culture. Both forms of retinoic acid induced significant decreases in procollagen production as measured by ^{3}H-hydroxyproline production. They also showed a 51% reduction in procollagen messenger RNA (mRNA) levels in normal human fibroblast, and an even more pronounced reduction of procollagen mRNA and product in keloid fibroblast cultures.

In addition to inhibiting fibroblast proliferation and collagen production, retinoic acid appears to inhibit transformation of certain cell types to fibroblast-like phenotypes in fibrotic diseases. The process of hepatic fibrosis in rats appears to be mediated in part through the transformation of the rat Ito cell from an adipocyte-like phenotype to a collagen-producing, fibroblast-like phenotype (20). Retinoic acid treatment inhibits rat Ito cell proliferation and interstitial collagen production in culture as well as in vivo. Inhibition of collagen mRNA was observed in these cells in cultures, but could not be demonstrated in vivo. These data suggested that retinoic acid modulation of collagen metabolism of rat Ito cells in vitro may occur via a different mechanism from in vivo inhibition of collagen production.

In contrast to these findings, other investigators found that vitamin A may increase collagen production by fibroblasts. Demetriou et al. (21), for example, demonstrated that while vitamin A and retinoic acid decreased Balb 3t3 mouse fibroblast replication in culture, collagen accumulation was enhanced. They also observed morphologic differentiation induced by retinoid treatment. In a similar way, Kim et al. (22) demonstrated a differential effect of retinoic acid on radiation-damaged versus normal skin in mice. Topical retinoic acid applied to the skin of ultraviolet B irradiated hairless mice increased types I and III collagen mRNA in the skin. Retinoic acid had no effect on age-matched, nonirradiated controls. These investigators also found an increase in transforming growth factor-β_1 (TGF-β_1) protein immunostaining in the epidermis of these animals. Corresponding changes in TFG-β_1 mRNA could not be demonstrated. The time course of TFG-β_1 increase paralleled that of the increase collagen mRNA. Since TFG-β_1 is known to promote collagen and matrix synthesis in general, they proposed that retinoic acid improved healing in radiation-damaged skin via an initial stimulation of TFG-β_1, which then stimulates dermal fibroblasts to synthesize collagen.

A variety of factors have been postulated to account for these seemingly conflicting data. The age of the cells in culture, culture conditions, and the source of the cells have all been suggested to affect the response to retinoids. To begin to address these factors, Varani and Mitra (32) studied the effect of all-*trans* retinoic acid on growth-inhibited human dermal fibroblasts in culture. They showed that retinoic acid can stimulate fibroblast proliferation in growth-inhibited cultures, but has no effect on rapidly proliferating cells. Furthermore, the concentration range within which retinoic acid promoted proliferation was very narrow. They also examined the effect of retinoic acid on thrombospondin and laminin production, two components of extracellular matrix. Retinoic acid stimulated production of these two components under both conditions (growth inhibited and proliferating), but the effect was see within the same narrow concentration range that stimulated proliferation.

Collagenase Metabolism

Because wound breaking strength depends on collagen content, and collagen content, in turn, must depend on the relative balance of synthesis and degradation, it is possible that regulation of the collagen degradation pathway may influence vitamin A effects on wound healing as well. No studies that directly addressed the effects of retinoids on collagenase activity in healing wounds in vivo have been done. But a large body of work has been devoted to the study of collagenase production in disease conditions such as rheumatoid arthritis and epidermolysis bullosa. In these diseases, overproduction of collagenase by synoviocytes and fibroblasts, respectively, is thought to play a major role in producing the pathologic, destructive lesions that characterize these conditions. Brinkerhoff et al. (24) studied the effects of all-*trans* and 12-*cis* retinoic acid on collagenase production in monolayers of human synovial tissue. With both all-*trans* and 13-*cis* retinoic acid treatment, collagenase production was inhibited. Retinoic acid also inhibits interleukin-1–stimulated collagenase gene expression in human synovial cells (25). In their experiments, Lafyatis et al. (25) found that the ligand-bound RAR complex inhibits, and interleukin-1 stimulates, collagenase gene expression through the 5′ phorbol-ester response element (TRE) of the collagenase gene. The DNA-binding protein activator protein-1 (AP-1) enhances transcription of the collagenase gene by binding to the TRE. Activator protein-1 is a complex composed of the *jun* and *fos* oncoproteins. *Fos* is necessary for AP-1 function. Retinoic acid inhibits IL-1–stimulated *fos,* thereby inhibiting the collagenase gene activation. This finding raises the possibility that other *fos*-dependent gene interactions may be modulated by retinoic acid and the RAR as well.

This effect of retinoic acid inhibition of collagenase is not limited to mesenchymal cells such as the synoviocyte. Skin fibroblasts derived from both healthy human volunteers and patients with dystrophic epidermyosis bullosa responded to retinoic acid treatment in culture with reduced collagenase production also (26). Furthermore, retinoic acid inhibited gelatinase activity. Gelatinase is the second enzyme in the collagen degradation pathway.

The Inflammatory Response

The majority of studies of vitamin A effects on collagenase production in various systems indicate that in general vitamin A is inhibitory. But the effects on collagen production and fibroblast proliferation are variable. In this regard, the effects of vitamin A are likely dependent on a number of factors including age and state of differentiation of the cells or tissue, culture (or in vivo) conditions, and the influence of other factors in the local environment. With this in mind, it seems unlikely that the consistent effects of improved wound healing that have been observed in a wide variety of conditions could be attributed to a direct effect of vitamin A on fibroblast collagen metabolism. This implies that vitamin A may be influencing collagen metabolism and ultimately wound healing through indirect mechanisms.

One such possible indirect mechanism that has received considerable attention has been the ability of vitamin A to restore the early inflammatory response. Ehrlich and Hunt, in addition to the findings discussed above, demonstrated that vitamin A restored depressed polymorphonuclear leukocyte infiltration into the wound site that was depressed by cortisone treatment. They could not evaluate the effects on monocytic cells because of small numbers (4). Seifter et al. (5) fed supplemental vitamin A to rats made diabetic by streptozocin and showed that diabetes induced a peripheral leukopenia and monocytopenia. The rats fed supplemental vitamin A had less leukopenia, and the peripheral monocytopenia was returned to normal. Barbul et al. (27) studied the effect of vitamin A on various white cell populations in normal rats and rats injured by unilateral femoral fracture. Supplemental dietary vitamin A induced a temporary peripheral leukocytosis (45–50% greater WBC) compared with the unsupplemented (chow fed) controls prior to fracture. After injury these differences persisted for one day only, after which time no significant difference was observed in peripheral total WBC between the groups. The differential WBC was further characterized by lymphocytosis, monocytosis, and a relative neutropenia in the vitamin A-supplemented rats prior to fracture. These differences persisted for one day after injury. On days 2 and 3 after fracture the percentage of lymphocytes and neutrophils was not different between the groups. However, the vitamin A–supplemented rats maintained a 50% greater percentage of circulating monocytes compared with their chow-fed controls on days 1 through 5 after fracture. These findings were reflected at the wound site as well. Polyvinyl alcohol sponges implanted next to the fracture site showed increased migration of white blood cells into the wound area in the vitamin A supplemented rats. This increased cellular infiltrate included significantly larger numbers of monocytes and macrophages (27).

Macrophage Function

The critical role of macrophages in normal wound healing had been firmly established. In the classic experiments by Leibovich and Ross (28), systemic hydrocortisone given to guinea pigs induced a circulating monocytopenia as well as reduced numbers of wound macrophages. Debridement within the wound was reduced in these animals, but fibrosis appeared unaffected. However, when local subcutaneous injection of antimacrophage serum was given in conjunction with systemic hydrocortisone, wound macrophages were eliminated from the wound. This resulted in delayed wound debridement and fibroblast infiltration, as well as reduced fibrosis (28). Hunt et al. (29) showed that macrophages aspirated from subcutaneous rabbit wounds and transplanted autogenously into the cornea released substances that stimulate angiogenesis, fibroplasia, and collagen synthesis. If these wound macrophages are exposed to steroids prior to corneal transplantation, these effects are prevented (29).

Considering, then, the central role the macrophage and its factors plays in normal wound healing and the apparent ability of vitamin A to restore depressed circulating and local macrophage numbers, the hypothesis that the beneficial effects of vitamin A on impaired wound healing are mediated via the macrophage is very appealing. However appealing it may be, it still is little more than a description of events and begs the question, How does vitamin A stimulate macrophage function? Retinoids are known to have complex effects on immune cell function. For example, retinoic acid treatment of human promyelocytic leukemia cells induces their differentiation into granulocytes. Lower concentrations of retinoic acid induce these cells to express both TGF-β mRNA and TGF-B protein (30). Thus, it is possible that retinoids may influence differentiation via an autocrine action of TGF-β. One study that examined directly the effects of retinoids on macrophage function demonstrated a mixed effect on guinea pig peritoneal macrophage function in culture. Retinoids were shown to increase concentrations of the bacteriocidal and tumoricidal enzyme arginase. On the other hand, Fc receptor–mediated binding and phagocytosis were inhibited by vitamin A. Regulation of cytokine production by macrophages may play a central role in mediating vitamin A effects. Interleukin-1 and -3 are stimulated in a dose-related fashion by retinoic acid in human peripheral monocytes and murine WEHI-3 cells, respectively (31). In another experiment suggesting mediation of retinoid effects via the macrophage Szabo et al. demonstrated that retinoic acid could modulate TGF-β production in both THP-1, human myelomonocytic cells, and in human peripheral blood monocytes.

Growth Factor Interactions

EGF Peptide and Receptor, PDGF-α, and RAR

Many interactions of vitamin A and growth factors have been described but mostly with regard to embryogenesis and tumorigenesis. However, several studies with potential applications in healing deserve mention. In 1980 Harper and Savage (32) demonstrated that vitamin A potentiated the mitogenic effects of epidermal growth factor (EGF) in human skin fibroblasts (32). Retinoic acid alone had no effect on growth. Epidermal growth factor alone stimulated growth by 69%. When EGF and retinoic acid were added in combination, cell growth increased 159% to 224%. Subsequent study of this interaction has suggested this potentiation of EGF mitogenicity by retinoic acid may be due to upregulation of EGF receptors, possibly through EGF receptor gene promotion. Interestingly, other investigators have demonstrated inhibition of EGF receptor gene expression (33). Two other gene-encoding receptors, platelet-derived growth factor-α (PDGF-α) receptor (34) and retinoic acid receptor-β_2 (35), exhibit retinoid responsiveness as well.

Transforming Growth Factor-β

Of the multitude of growth factors and peptides that participate in events associated with inflammation and tissue repair, TGF-β seems to be the key mediator of vitamin A effects. Transforming growth factor-β is a potent chemoattractant for macrophages and fibroblasts (36) and may potentiate recruitment and differentiation of the cellular components needed for effective repair (37). In general, TGF-β strongly inhibits epithelial cell growth (38), but promotes production of extracellular matrix components such as collagen and fibronectin (39). Several investigators have demonstrated accelerated healing of impaired wounds by TGF-β treatment (40–42). The mechanistic interrelationships among the steroid/retinoid receptors and TGF-β are complex and extensive (reviewed in 43). Pioneering work of Glick et al. (44) demonstrated for the first time the widespread regulation of TGF-β expression by retinoic acid in vivo. Using polyclonal antibodies to TGF-β_1, TGF-β_2, and TGF-β_3, these investigators examined the effect of retinoic acid on the expression of these three TGF-β isoforms in the rat epithelia of the epidermis, intestine, respiratory tract, and vagina. Retinoic acid induced the expression of all isoforms in the epidermis, and TGF-β_2 and TGF-β_3 in respiratory epithelium as well as in intestinal mucosa and lamaina propria. Vitamin A–deficient rats had basal diminution of TGF-β_2 expression except in the vaginal epithelium, where all three isoforms were increased. Subsequent retinoic acid treatment reduced expression of all three in the vagina (44). Danielpour et al. (45) studied the effects of various hormone and growth factors on TGF-β_1 and TGF-β expression. They showed that retinoic acid increased in TGF-β_2 and NRK-49F normal rat kidney fibroblasts and human lung carcinoma cells, and decreased the level of TGF-β_1 peptide in both cell lines. Also, epidermal growth factor (EGF) blocked the induction of TGF-β_2 mRNA and peptide induced by retinoic acid in the NRK-49F cells. These studies and others illustrate an important feature of TGF-β regulation. The expression of TGF-β depends on the particular milieu of growth factors and hormones acting on the cells, the cell type, and its state of differentiation. In our lab, we have examined the effect of corticosterone and retinoic acid on TGF-β_1 concentrations in rats' wound fluid recovered from polyvinyl alcohol sponges implanted subcutaneously under an incisional wound. Corticosterone treatment resulted in diminished TGF-β_1 peptide concentrations from day 1 through day 15 postwounding. Concomitant treatment with retinoic acid restored TGF-β_1 concentration to normal by day 10 postwounding. This time course correlated with the improvement of incisional breaking strength observed in this model (45). These data suggest that the in vivo effects of retinoic acid may be mediated by TGF-β_1 in this steroid-impaired wound healing model.

To understand the molecular mechanisms operative in the interaction of retinoids and TGF-β, Salbert et al. (46) examined the ability of RARs to inhibit TGF-β_1 promotion via AP-1 binding sites. Transforming growth factor-β promotion is controlled by three AP-1 binding sites on two promoters. They showed repression of TGF-β_1 promoter activity by RAR-α, RAR-β, and RXR-α. Furthermore, RXR-α inhibited three different AP-1 controlled promoters (TGF-β_1, collagenase, and c-*fos*). Based on the demonstration that RXR inhibits *jun* and *fos* DNA binding (which is necessary for AP-1 function), they suggested that these inhibitory effects may involve a mechanism of direct protein-protein interaction between RXR and AP-1. These findings are consistent with the work of Lafyatis et al. (25). Clearly more work needs to be done to determine which cells make and respond to TGF-β in response to retinoids, and under what conditions they do so. Nevertheless, based on these data, the proposition put forward by Roberts and Sporn that the effects of retinoids on growth and differentiation of target cells and tissues are often mediated locally by TGF-β is well grounded.

Summary

Vitamin A treatment can improve impaired wound healing by increasing collagen accumulation, even though in many circumstances it appears to inhibit fibroblast proliferation and collagen production. This can be explained by the wide range of responses to retinoids by cells both in vitro and in vivo. Responses to retinoids appear to vary according to the age of the cells, culture conditions, concentration of retinoid, and the local environment, and appear to be mediated via regulation of other growth factors and hormones. This mediation is likely carried out through the retinoic acid receptor, which belongs to the steroid-thyroid hormone receptor superfamily, the largest known family of transcription factors in eukaryotes. Complex interactions among the steroids and retinoids confer a great degree of variety on the regulation of retinoid responsive genes. Of the many growth factors that interact with the retinoids, TGF-β appears to be the key mediator of retinoid action in wound healing.

References

1. Ehrlich H, Hunt T. Effects of corticosterone and vitamin A on wound healing. Ann Surg 1968;167:324–8.
2. Weissmann. The effects of corticosteroids upon connective tissue and lysosomes. Recent Prog Horm Res 1964;20:215.
3. Hunt T, Erlich H, et al. Effect of vitamin A on reversing the inhibitory effect of cortisone on healing of open wounds in animals and man. Surgery 1969; 170:633–41.
4. Ehrlich H, Tarver H, et al. Effect of vitamin A and glucocorticoids upon inflammation and collagen synthesis. Ann Surg 1973;177:222–7.
5. Seifter E, Rettura G, et al. Impaired wound healing in streptozotocin diabetes: prevention by supplemental vitamin A. Ann Surg 1981;914:42–50.
6. Seifter E, Crowley B, et al. Influence of vitamin A on wound healing in rats with femoral fracture. Ann Surg 1975;181:836–41.
7. Levenson S, Rettura G, et al. Supplemental vitamin A prevents the acutes radiation-induced defect in wound healing. Ann Surg 1984;200:494–512.
8. Weinzweig J, Levenson S, et al. Supplemental vitamin A prevents the tumor-induced defect in wound healing. Ann Surg 1989;211:269–76.
9. Herrmann J, Woodward S. An experimental study of wound healing accelerators. Am Surg 1972;38:26–34.
10. Hevia O, Nemeth A, et al. Tretinoin accelerates healing after trichloroacetic acid chemical peel. Arch Dermatol 1991;127:678–82.
11. Popp C, Kligman A, et al. Pretreatment of photoaged forearm skin with topical tretinoin accelerates healing of full-thickness wounds. Br J Dermatol 1995; 132:46–53.
12. Petkovich M, Nigel N, et al. A human retinoic acid receptor which belongs to the family of nuclear receptors. Nature 1987;330:444–50.
13. Giguere V, Ong E, et al. Identification of a receptor for the morphogen retinoic acid. Nature 1987;330:624–35.
14. Tsai M, O'Malley B. Molecular mechanisms of action of steroid/thyroid receptor superfamily members. Annu Rev Biochem 1994;63:451–86.
15. Glass C, DiRenzo J, et al. Regulation of gene expression by retinoic acid receptors. DNA Cell Biol 1991;10:623–38.

16. Umesono K, Giguere V, et al. Retinoic acid and thyroid hormone induce gene expression through a common responsive element. Nature 1988;336:262–5.
17. Graupner G, Wills K, et al. Dual regulatory role for thyroid-hormone receptors allows control of retinoic acid receptor activity. Nature 1989;340:653–6.
18. Hein R, Mensing H, et al. Effect of vitamin A and its derivatives on collagen production and chemotactic response of fibroblasts. Br J Dermatol 1980; 107:2113–4.
19. Oikarinin A, Tan E, et al. Modulation of procollagen gene expression by retinoids. J Clin Invest 1985;75:1545–53.
20. Davis B, Kramer R, et al. Retinoic acid modulates rat Ito cell proliferation, collagen, and transforming growth factor β production. J Clin Invest 1990;86:2062–70.
21. Demetriou A, Levenson S, et al. Vitamin A and retinoic acid: induced fibroblast differentiation in vitro. Surgery 1985;98:931–4.
22. Kim H, Bogdan N, et al. Effect of topical retinoic acids on the level of collagen mRNA during the repair of UVB-induced dermal damage in the hairless mouse and the possible role of the TGF-β as a mediator. J Invest Dermatol 1992; 98:359–63.
23. Varani J, Mitra R. All-trans retinoic acid stimulates growth and extracellular matrix production in growth-inhibited cultured human skin fibroblasts. J Invest Dermatol 1990;4:717–23.
24. Brinkerhoff C, McMillan R, et al. Inhibition by retinoic acid of collagenase production in rheumatoi synovial cells. N Engl J Med 1980;303:432–6.
25. Lafyatis R, SJ K, et al. Interleukin-1 stimulates the all-trans-retinoic acid inhibits collagenase gene expression through its 5' activator protein-1-binding site. Mol Endocrinol 1990;4:973–80.
26. Bauer E, Seltzer J, et al. Inhibition of collagen degradative enzymes by retinoic acid in vitro. Am Acad Dermatol 1982.
27. Barbul A, Thysen B, et al. White cell involvement in the inflammatory, wound healing, and immune reactions of vitamin A. J Parenter Enteral Nutr 1978; 2:129–40.
28. Leibovich S, Ross R. The role the macrophage in wound repair. Am J Pathol 1975;78:71–91.
29. Hunt T, Knighton D, et al. Studies on inflammation and wound healing: angiogenesis and collagen synthesis stimulated by resident and activated wound macrophages. Surgery 1984;96:48–54.
30. Falk L, DeBenedetti F, et al. Induction of transforming growth factor-beta$_1$ receptor expression and TGF-β_1 protein production in retinoic acid-treated IL-60 cells: possible TGF-β1-mediated autocrine inhibition. Blood 1991; 77:1248–55.
31. Treschel U, Evequoz V, et al. Stimulation of interleukin 1 and 3 production by retinoic acid in vitro. Biochem J 1985;230:339–44.
32. Harper R, Savage C Jr. Vitamin A potentiates the mitogenic effect of epidermal growth factor in cultures of normal adult human skin fibroblast. Endocrinology 1980;107:2113–4.
33. Zheng Z, Goldsmith L. Modulation of epidermal growth factor receptors by retinoic acid in ME180 cells. Cancer Res 1990;50:1201–5.
34. Wang C, Kelly J, et al. Retinoic acid promotes transcription of the platelet-derived growth factor alpha-receptor gene. Mol Cell Biol 1990;10:6781–4.
35. Harnish D, Jiang H, et al. Retinoic acid receptor β2 mRNA is elevated by

retinoic acid in vivo in susceptible regions of mid-gestation mouse embryos. Dev Dynam 1992;194:239–46.
36. Wahl S, Hunt T, Andy U, et al. Transforming growth factor type beta induces monocyte chemotaxis and growth factor production. Proc Natl Acad Sci USA 1987;84:5788–92.
37. Assoian R, Fleurdelys B, et al. Expression and secretion of type beta transforming growth factor by activated macrophages. Proc Natl Acad Sci USA 1987;84:6020–4.
38. Moses H, Yang H, et al. TGF-β stimulation and inhibition of cell proliferation: new mechanistic insights. Cell 1990;63:245–7.
39. Sporn M, Roberts A, et al. Polypeptide transforming growth factors isolated from bovine sources and used for wound healing in vivo. Science 1983; 219:1329–31.
40. Beck L, Deguzman L, et al. TGF-β_1 accelerates wound healing: reversal of steroid-impaired healing in rats and rabbits. Growth Factors 1991;5:295–304.
41. Pierce G, Mustoe T, et al. Transforming growth factor β reverses the glucocorticoid-induced wound-healing deficit in rats: possible regulation in macrophages by platelet-derived growth factor. Proc Natl Acad Sci USA 1989;86:2229–33.
42. Slavin J, Nash J, et al. Effect of transforming growth factor beta and basic fibroblast growth factor on steroid-impaired healing intestinal wounds. Br J Surg 1992;79:69–72.
43. Roberts A, Sporn M. Mechanistic interrelationships between two superfamilies: the steroid/retinoid receptors and transforming growth factor-β. Cancer Surv 1992;14:205–20.
44. Glick A, McCune B, et al. Complex regulation of TGF-β expression by retinoic acid in the vitamin A deficient rat. Development 1991;111:1081–6.
45. Danielpour D, Kim K, et al. Differential regulation of the expression of transforming growth factor-βs 1 and 2 by retinoic acid, epidermal growth factor, and dexamethasone in NRK-49F and A 549 cells. J Cell Physiol 1991;148:235–44.
46. Salbert G, Fanjul A, et al. Retinoic acid receptors and retinoid X receptor-alpha down-regulate the transforming growth factor-beta 1 promoter by antagonizing AP-1 activity. Mol Endocrinol 1993;7:1347–56.

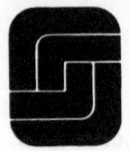

8

Interactions Between Nutrients and Growth Factors in Cellular Anabolism and Tissue Repair

THOMAS R. ZIEGLER, ALAN B. PUCKETT, DANIEL P. GRIFFITH, AND JOHN L. GALLOWAY

Appropriate administration of nutrient substrates appears to be important for optimal wound healing and growth factor–induced tissue anabolism in animals and in man. Endogenously derived and dietary amino acids are utilized as key substrates for new protein and collagen synthesis. Energy sources (amino acids, carbohydrate, fat) support the wound healing process directly, and indirectly by providing fuel for neutrophils, macrophages, lymphocytes, and other cells. Generalized protein-energy malnutrition (marasmus-like), protein depletion (kwashiorkor-like), or specific micronutrient deficiency (e.g., zinc, vitamin C, and vitamin A) may delay or impair normal tissue regeneration and healing in vivo. Nutritional repletion in these settings often improves wound healing and tissue function and tissue repair. Recent work suggests that "pharmacologic" doses of specific amino acids or novel nutrient substrates (e.g., glutamine, arginine, ornithine-α-ketoglutarate) may enhance tissue restoration during catabolic states in humans.

Endogenous peptide growth factors, including growth hormone (GH), insulin-like growth factor-I (IGF-I), epidermal growth factor (EGF), keratinocyte growth factor (KGF), and platelet-derived growth factor (PDGF), appear to mediate many of the key processes required for normal tissue growth and repair. In addition, several growth factors (e.g., insulin, GH, and IGF-I) promote tissue amino acid uptake, enhance protein synthesis, and/or decrease protein degradation, and thus facilitate anabolic processes by healing tissues. Exogenous administration of recombinant growth factors such as GH, IGF-I, and PDGF enhances wound healing and tissue repair in animal and human studies. Other studies have demonstrated marked whole body and tissue-specific anabolic effects of certain growth factors when combined with nutritional support. Many of these studies have focused on wounds, skeletal muscle, and intestine as target tissues for growth factor action.

A large proportion of the data on nutrition-growth factor interactions involves studies on the nutritional regulation of the GH–IGF-I axis. Generalized malnutrition or protein depletion diminishes serum IGF-I levels, alters circulating IGF binding proteins, and reduces tissue IGF-I messenger RNA (mRNA) levels. Depletion of certain micronutrients (e.g., magnesium, thiamine, and zinc) also decreases plasma IGF-I levels and reduces tissue IGF-I production in animal models. Additional studies suggest that specific nutrients may upregulate tissue production or secretions of certain hormones, as evidenced by the increase in plasma insulin, GH, and IGF-I with enteral arginine supplementation. For example, administration of large doses of the amino acid glutamine in combination with GH, IGF-I, or EGF induces additive or synergistic effects on intestinal growth and adaptation in short bowel syndrome or in states of gut atrophy.

Nutrients and growth factors may interact to facilitate specific processes critical to wound and tissue repair. Both IGF-I and glutamine administration enhance blood flow in tissues such as gut and muscle, while exogenously administered nutrient antioxidants including vitamin E, cysteine, zinc, and selenium diminish oxidative tissue damage in catabolic states. Effects such as these may facilitate cell growth and repair induced by specific nutrients and growth factors. Thus, several lines of evidence support the concept that nutrient metabolism and growth factor physiology are interactive. The molecular basis for the specific interaction among general nutritional status, single nutrients, and growth factor action pathways is being increasingly investigated. This chapter reviews some of the interactions between nutritional status and growth factors in cellular anabolism and tissue repair.

General Nutritional Status and Specific Nutrients in Protein Anabolism and Tissue Repair

Effects of Protein-Energy Malnutrition and Nutritional Repletion

It has long been recognized that adequate nutritional status is an important determinant of somatic growth, tissue function, tissue regeneration, and repair (1–8). For example, both endogenously derived and dietary amino acids are utilized as key substrates for new protein and collagen synthesis. Amino acids, carbohydrate, and fat support cellular reactions in tissues and the wound healing process directly as energy sources for cells. Nutrients also play an indirect role in wound healing and tissue repair by providing fuel for neutrophils, macrophages, lymphocytes, and other cells that are critical for these processes. The quantity and quality of dietary fat intake is known to regulate cell membrane composition, and possibly cell function (5). It has been shown that either generalized protein-energy malnutrition or deficiency of specific micronutrients (e.g., zinc, vitamin C, and vitamin A) delays or impairs normal tissue regeneration and healing in vivo (6). In addition, macro- or micronutrient repletion after nutritional depletion often results in protein accrual and anabolic effects such as improved wound healing (1–6). The underlying mechanisms involved in nutrient-mediated effects in individual cell types remain poorly understood (7).

Either protein malnutrition or combined protein-energy malnutrition is associated with poor growth throughout infancy, childhood, and adolescence in animals and in humans (8). In addition, generalized malnutrition reduces whole body and tissue mass, and inhibits tissue repair and wound healing throughout the life cycle (4, 8–13). In 1972 Daly et al. (4) showed that protein depletion in rats significantly impaired bursting strength of colonic anastomoses (an index of intestinal healing) by 17% after 1 week and 26% after 6 weeks of protein restriction. Other studies in animal models demonstrated that prolonged administration of protein-free diets significantly impaired colonic anastomoses (9) and healing of abdominal wall wounds (10). After a 24- to 96-hour period of fasting in otherwise healthy rats, both noncollagen and, especially, collagen production in bone and cartilage rapidly declined (11). Refeeding resulted in a rapid return of noncollagen protein and a slower recovery of collagenous proteins (11).

In rats subjected to a 72-hour fast, marked small intestinal atrophy (decreased intestinal wet weight, DNA, and protein content) occurred in association with loss of body weight (13). The atrophic response in gut tissue was rapidly reversed with 24 to 72 hours of enteral refeeding, and body mass also rapidly increased (13). The loss and repletion of intestinal mass with fasting and refeeding is proportionally greater than changes in whole body mass, suggesting that certain tissues may be differentially sensitive to alterations in general nutritional status (12, 13). Additional studies in animals demonstrate that enteral feeding after catabolic stress, such as burn injury or abdominal operation, is associated with decreased body weight loss, increased tissue protein anabolism, and improved wound healing responses (6, 14, 15).

Clinical studies also suggest that nutrition plays an important role in protein anabolism, organ regeneration, and wound healing in humans; however, data on this issue are in many cases conflicting (1, 2, 6, 16). In 1936 Studley (1) demonstrated that increased postoperative morbidity and mortality occurred in surgical patients with preoperative body weight loss of >20%. However, Moore (2) noted that wounds heal reasonably well in most patients with concomitant weight loss and malnutrition. Nonetheless, in the face of either (a) chronic moderate to severe protein or protein-energy malnutrition or (b) rapid weight loss and protein catabolism (as occurs during critical illness), marked erosion of lean body mass occurs in humans

(2, 5, 16). Loss of body protein is associated with changes suggesting deleterious effects on structural and functional protein-rich tissues. These alterations include immunosuppression (17), increased hospital infections (18), delayed wound healing and tissue repair (19, 20), skeletal muscle weakness (21), and reduced muscle bioenergetic capacity (22).

While it seems clear that general nutritional repletion after starvation or semistarvation facilitates growth, tissue anabolism, and wound repair in humans (1), clinical data on the effects of nutritional repletion on anabolic processes during catabolic states remain limited. However, several studies in hospitalized patients do suggest that increased protein and energy intake is beneficial in human wound healing (23–25) and other clinical outcomes (26, 27). Accumulation of hydroxyproline (a measure of collagen content) in standardized subcutaneous wounds was significantly decreased in patients with protein-energy malnutrition compared with well-nourished individuals undergoing general surgical procedures (0.48 ± 0.3 μg/cm versus 0.34 ± 0.23 μg/cm; $p < .05$) (23). However, a marked increase in hydroxyproline content occurred after 7 to 11 days of total parenteral nutrition support (to 0.88 ± 0.62 μg/cm) (23). Another study indicated that early postoperative tube feedings in patients undergoing intestinal operations were associated with improved wound healing responses compared with patients receiving routine hypocaloric fluids and gradual progression to enteral diet (24). Adequate preoperative enteral food intake was associated with improved wound healing in adult patients compared with those with a history of poor dietary intake in the immediate 7 days prior to operation (25). Alexander et al. (26) demonstrated that increasing enteral dietary protein intake (from 16% of total calories to 23% of calories) significantly improved survival in children with moderate- to large-sized burns. Müller et al. (27) found that preoperative parenteral nutrition improved overall morbidity and mortality, but not wound healing in postoperative patients. In contrast to these findings, the VA Cooperative Trial (28), conducted during the 1980s and published in 1991, found that only severely malnourished patients (≈ 5% of the subjects studied) appeared to benefit from preoperative parenteral feeding in terms of noninfectious complications. No overall effects of parenteral nutritional support on wound healing were observed. However, subjects deemed to absolutely require parenteral feeding were not randomized in this trial; thus, the design may have been biased against an effect of nutritional support.

Despite limited and somewhat conflicting data on clinical outcome, the current standard of care in patients with catabolic illness, significant wounds, and/or organ dysfunction is to prevent significant malnutrition with specialized feeding as appropriate and to nutritionally replete patients with moderate to severe forms of protein-energy malnutrition (29). However, it is now appreciated that current forms of nutrition support are relatively inefficient in stimulating protein synthesis or inhibiting protein breakdown rates during critical illness, and are usually unable to induce positive nitrogen balance (16). Numerous studies have investigated the role of growth factors in enhancing the efficiency of nutritional repletion in catabolic states (30), and these are discussed in more detail below.

The actual contribution of underlying nutritional status and nutritional repletion in patient morbidity and tissue recovery is difficult to determine in malnourished patients with an associated illness. Nutritional depletion may be a result of the underlying condition, rather than a direct cause or contributor to morbidity. As an example, the interactions between whole body nutritional status, immune cell function, and infection rates have been well documented (7, 17). Infection accelerates body protein loss (7), while protein-calorie malnutrition itself decreases host resistance to bacterial, fungal, and viral infection (17). Nonetheless, general nutritional status and specific nutrients are believed to play key roles in wound healing and tissue anabolism (Table 8.1).

Effects of Specific Nutrients

Vitamins and Minerals

Studies both in animal models and in humans suggest that deficiencies of specific nutrients, including amino acids, electrolytes, vitamins, and trace elements, impair growth and inhibit normal tissue regeneration and repair in vivo. Micronutrients are critical cofactors involved in cell structure and function. For example, inadequate zinc, vitamin C, and vitamin A nutriture have been classically associated with poor wound healing (6). Isolated riboflavin deficiency in rats impairs skin wound healing (31). Dietary deficiencies of the electrolytes potassium and magnesium each individually induce poor somatic growth, inhibit protein synthesis, and reduce protein accrual in animal models or in in vitro cell culture systems (32). Correction of micronutrient deficiencies by dietary supplementation often results in improved protein synthesis, enhanced growth, and improved wound healing in these settings.

Zinc is a critical trace element in cell proliferation and cell differentiation

TABLE 8.1. Some roles of nutrients in wound healing and tissue growth and regeneration.

Amino acids, CHO, fat serve as energy sources
  For new cell renewal (direct support)
  For PMNs, macrophages, lymphocytes, other immune cells
Dietary fat regulates cell membrane composition
Endogenous and exogenous amino acids are substrates for synthesis of collagen and other
  key proteins involved in tissue repair
Micronutrients (vitamins and trace elements) are critical cofactors involved in cell structure,
  tissue functions, and cellular reactions
Nutrient antioxidants diminish oxidative tissue damage and may facilitiate tissue repair

reactions and in normal cellular immune function (6, 33–36). Zinc deficiency causes growth failure and inhibits poor protein synthesis in animal models (33). In addition, zinc depletion is associated with immune cell dysfunction, poor wound healing, depressed gut mucosal turnover, diarrhea, and hypogonadism that can be reversed with zinc repletion (34, 35). Zinc deficiency occurs commonly in catabolic, hospitalized patients, especially those with diarrhea or other gastrointestinal losses (6, 30, 36, 37). Serum and tissue zinc concentrations are also reduced due to poor zinc intake, urinary losses, and zinc redistribution in tissue compartments in these settings (35–37). Several studies in human subjects indicate that zinc supplementation improves wound healing responses (35–38). However, it appears that zinc is beneficial in tissue repair only when concomitant depletion of zinc exists (38). As discussed in detail below, zinc nutrition has significant interactions with the GH–IGF-I system in vivo (32).

Vitamin C is a critical micronutrient involved in collagen synthesis, chemotaxis, and macrophage function (36). Vitamin C is essential for appropriate hydroxylation of lysine and proline residues in the synthesis of procollagen and for cross-linking of extracellular collagen (39). Scurvy, or vitamin C deficiency, is associated with poor accumulation of extracellular matrix and collagen into wounds and microhemorrhages, which inhibits angiogenesis, and thus healing (6). Although available data are somewhat conflicting, vitamin C depletion is not uncommon in hospitalized patients, and vitamin C supplementation enhances wound healing in such subjects (6, 36). Administration of supplemental vitamin A also enhances wound healing in animal models and in some clinical settings, particularly when given during administration of corticosteroids, which are known inhibitors of tissue repair (6, 36, 40, 41). While the mechanisms of vitamin A action in tissue repair remain unclear, vitamin A may influence healing via fibroblast differentiation (42) or collagen formation (43). In addition to the nutrients noted above, other vitamins and minerals, including thiamine, copper, manganese, and pantothenic acid, are important cofactors in collagen production and other important cellular aspects of tissue repair (6, 36).

Specific Amino Acids

The amino acids arginine and glutamine are both classified as nonessential amino acids during health; however, they appear to become conditionally essential during certain catabolic states (44, 45). Consistent improvement in wound healing indices has been noted with enteral arginine administration in rats and in humans (44, 46–49). In a study focusing on the effects of oral arginine on experimental wound healing, Barbul et al. (47) studied healthy adults with subcutaneously implanted polytetrafluoroethylene (PTFE) tubing inserted into the deltoid region. The subjects were randomized into three groups, and given 30 g arginine HCL (24.8 g free arginine), 30 g arginine aspartate (17 g free arginine), or placebo, daily for 2 weeks with an ad libitum diet. Mitogenic responses of peripheral blood lymphocytes to PHA and concanavalin A (ConA) were assessed at baseline and after 2 weeks. The hydroxyproline content in the PTFE tubes was assessed after 2 weeks as an index of collagen formation and wound healing (47). Both arginine-supplemented groups demonstrated significantly enhanced hydroxyproline concentrations in the experimental wounds, and a greater response occurred with oral arginine HCL. Both arginine regimens significantly increased lymphocyte blastogenic responses versus the controls (47).

A similar randomized, double-blind protocol was performed by Kirk et al. (48) in healthy elderly adults. The experimental subjects (mean age 72 years) were given 30 g arginine aspartate for 14 days; age-matched control patients received placebo. Subcutaneously placed deltoid PTFE tubes were assessed for nitrogen, DNA, and hydroxyproline content. Also 2 × 2 cm split-thickness wounds were created on the upper thigh for evaluation of skin re-epithelialization. Peripheral blood mitogenic responses were also assessed before and after the 14 days of treatment. In these elderly, healthy subjects, oral arginine supplementation significantly enhanced wound catheter hydroxyproline content (an index of collagen deposition) and protein content (48).

In a randomized, blinded, prospective trial, Daly et al. (49) evaluated immune and metabolic effects of L-arginine (25 g/day) or isonitrogenous L-glycine added to enteral feeding solutions given via needle-catheter jejunostomy for 7 days postoperatively in 30 elderly patients with GI malignancies (49). Immune parameters were measured preoperatively, and on days 1, 4, and 7 postoperatively. The L-arginine–supplemented group demonstrated significantly increased plasma arginine levels by day 7 (from a preoperative value of 87 μM to 213 μM postoperatively). In addition, enteral arginine administration significantly increased plasma ornithine levels (approximately fourfold) and tended to improve nitrogen balance. Supplemental arginine significantly enhanced mean T-lymphocyte responses to mitogens versus control group responses on postoperative days 4 and 7 (49). Serum levels of IGF-I were $\approx 50\%$ higher in the arginine group by day 7 (49), reflecting arginine's known effect as a GH secretagogue (50). The interaction between arginine administration and GH and IGF-I secretion is discussed below. Arginine's role in wound healing is considered in more detail elsewhere in this volume.

Glutamine (Gln), which has classically been considered a nonessential amino acid, has received increasing attention by the research community as a potentially beneficial amino acid under certain conditions (45). Data are now available to support the concept that Gln is conditionally essential in various catabolic states (51, 52). Gln is the most abundant free amino acid in plasma, skeletal muscle, and in the human body as a whole (45). Gln exhibits dynamic interorgan metabolism, particularly between skeletal muscle and the splanchnic bed and kidney, and plays an important physiologic role in several key metabolic processes that are involved in tissue synthesis, repair, and regeneration (Table 8.2). The small intestine extracts 25% to 30% of circulating Gln in the postabsorptive state; thus, intestinal tissues (and other rapidly replicating cells) are perhaps the major utilizer of circulating Gln (53). Gln concentrations in plasma, and especially skeletal muscle pools, may decrease markedly during various catabolic states, including sepsis, burns, or trauma (35, 53). In animal models and postoperative humans, a relationship exists between Gln concentrations and rates of muscle protein synthesis and breakdown (45).

Dietary Gln requirements increase markedly during catabolic states because cellular requirements of the primary Gln-utilizing tissues (such as intestinal and immune cells, kidney, and wounds) are increased (45, 53). A relative Gln deficiency may develop if increased Gln requirements are not met by adequate dietary provision of Gln. Reduced Gln concentrations in intracellular and plasma pools appears to be coupled with altered structure and function of the key tissues that synthesize and/or utilize Gln (45, 51, 53). Net catabolism of skeletal muscle and muscle Gln efflux may increase during stress to provide increased quantities of Gln for certain tissues and wounds.

Numerous animal and human studies indicate that dietary supplementation of Gln during catabolic states improves structure and function of organs and tissues, in association with reduced morbidity and mortality (Table 8.3). For example, in animal studies, the beneficial effects of Gln-enriched nutrition have been compared with isonitrogenous, isocaloric control diets containing little or no Gln (45, 51). Benefits of dietary Gln include increased whole body protein anabolism, attenuation of intestinal and pancreative atrophy during parenteral feeding, increased gut mucosal repair after burn injury, trauma, sepsis, chemotherapy and/or irradiation, improved gut nutrient absorption and barrier function after trauma and sepsis, increased immune cell number and function after injury, and increased animal survival (45, 51-53).

In human studies, little data on the clinical effects of enteral diets enriched in Gln have been published to date, although a number of trials are in progress. However, Gln enriched parenteral nutrition given to catabolic hospitalized patients improves nitrogen retention and protein synthesis

TABLE 8.2. Some important metabolic functions of glutamine.

Essential substrate for nucleotide synthesis
Constituent amino acid in synthesis of body proteins
Regulator of protein synthetic and breakdown rates
Important metabolic fuel source for rapidly replicating cells
  (e.g., enterocytes and immune cells)
Major substrate for gluconeogenesis
Prominent amino acid in interorgan nitrogen and carbon transport
Substrate for renal ammoniagenesis
Stimulation of glycogen synthesis

TABLE 8.3. Beneficial effects reported with enteral and/or parenteral glutamine supplementation in animal models and in clinical trials of hospitalized patients.

Improved nitrogen retention (animals and humans)
Reduced skeletal muscle protein breakdown during catabolic stress (animals)
Maintained skeletal muscle glutamine concentrations (animals and humans)
Increased protein synthesis (animals and humans)
Enhanced intestinal mucosal cellularity, decreased pancreatic atrophy, and reduced hepatic
    steatosis during elemental enteral feeding (animals)
Improved gut mucosal repair, decreased bacteremia, and improved survival after
    irradiation, chemotherapy, or sepsis (animals)
Reduced ulceration and enhanced mucosal repair in experimental colitis (animals)
Increased intestinal adaptation in experimental short bowel syndrome (animals)
Enhanced growth and nutrient absorption in transplanted small intestine and enhanced gut
    water and electrolyte absorption across inflamed small bowel (animals)
Maintained or improved intestinal and systemic immune functions during parenteral feeding
    (animals and humans)
Attenuated extracellular fluid expansion after bone marrow transplantation (humans)
Maintained intestinal villus height and gut barrier function during parenteral nutrition
    (humans)
Imcreased D-xylose absorption in critical illness (humans)
Improved intestinal nutrient absorption in severe short bowel syndrome, combined with a
    modified diet and growth hormone (humans)
Reduced microbial colonization and clinical infection, enhanced lymphocyte recovery, and
    shortened hospital length of stay after bone marrow transplantation (humans)

(54–56), and maintains plasma Gln concentrations in muscle and plasma (54, 55). Intravenous Gln administration exerts gut-trophic effects in clinical settings, including increased villus height with decreased intestinal permeability in patients requiring total parenteral nutrition (57) and enhanced absorption of D-xylose in critical illness, indicating improved small bowel mucosa functional capacity (58). Two randomized, double-blind, controlled studies in catabolic adult bone marrow transplant (BMT) patients demonstrated that Gln-supplemented parenteral nutrition shortened hospital length of stay (56, 59). In the first trial, nitrogen balance was significantly improved by ≈ 2.8 g/day with Gln treatment (Gln, 1.4 ± 0.5 g/day versus control, 4.2 ± 1.2 g/day), with a significant reduction in the 3-methylhistidine (3-MH)/creatinine excretion ratio, suggesting that dietary L-Gln diminished the rate of whole body protein breakdown (56). In addition, post-BMT infectious morbidity was diminished with Gln supplementation (Table 8.2). The incidence of clinical infection, both total and site-specific microbial colonization, and the length of hospital stay were significantly reduced versus the controls (56). Additional blinded studies in a subgroup of this patient population demonstrated that Gln-enriched parenteral feeding attenuated the expansion of extracellular and total body water observed in controls receiving standard, Gln-free parenteral feeding following BMT (60). The latter finding suggests that dietary Gln may affect cell membrane function or other factors related to alterations in both water compartments during catabolic stress. Additional studies in this patient population and in postoperative patients suggest that circulating lympho-cyte recovery is enhanced with L-Gln supplementation (61, 62).

Animal and in vitro studies support a key role for Gln in wound healing processes (63). Dietary Gln supplementation was able to modulate both acute and chronic inflammation in rats, in association with diminished inflammatory granulation and tissue edema after experimental injury (64). This anti-inflammatory effect has also been observed with oral administra-tion of other amino acids, including L-tryptophan, cysteine, and alanine in experimentally induced inflammation models (65). Of interest, standard parenteral feedings do not contain Gln and few enteral products are currently enriched in this amino acid. The apparent interactions between Gln and the GH–IGF-I system are covered in detail below.

Antioxidant Nutrients

Oxygen free radicals are known to be mediators of tissue damage during catabolic states (66, 67). The body utilizes antioxidant substances, made endogenously or provided in the diet as free radical scavengers, to attenuate oxidant-mediated peroxidation of lipid membranes and disruption of cell proteins in extracellular fluid and in tissues (68–71). Several dietary nutrients, including zinc, selenium, vitamins A, C, and E, and glutamine, appear to function as antioxidants or are involved directly or indirectly in the generation of critical antioxidants such as glutathione (GSH) (52, 66–71). Maintenance of GSH concentrations in tissues and in the circulation serves to inhibit lipid peroxidation of cell membranes; thus, GSH (a glutamate-cysteine-glycine tripeptide) is a key antioxidant in the body (68). The metabolism of nutrient antioxidants are interrelated. For example, tissue protection by ascorbate and glutathione against microsomal lipid peroxidation is dependent on vitamin E (72). Enzymes involved in GSH generation, such as glutathione peroxidase, are dependent on adequate supplies of the trace metal cofactors such as zinc and selenium (68, 70, 71).

It is known that catabolic illnesses associated with tissue damage, organ failure, and oxidant injury (e.g., sepsis, trauma, burn injury, pancreatitis, and surgical operations) are associated with marked depletion of both nutrient antioxidants and GSH in blood and tissues (73–75). It follows that depletion of key nutrients involved in scavaging oxygen radicals may increase tissue damage caused by oxidant-mediated processes and also may impair wound healing via this mechanism (52, 66–71, 76, 77). Several studies indicate beneficial effects on tissue GSH production with Gln administration in animal models of tissue injury and inflammation (67, 78, 79). Emerging clinical trials suggest that administration of single antioxi-dants, such as vitamins C and E, or antioxidant nutrient "cocktails" reduces indices of oxidant damage and tissue injury in selected groups of catabolic patients, including those with pancreatitis or burn injury and after opera-tion (80–85). In addition, several studies suggest that beneficial clinical effects occur with administration of enteral diets enriched in combinations of antioxidant and "immunomodulating" nutrients, including arginine, glutamine, fish oil, selenium, zinc, and vitamin C (86–91). Although there is as yet little evidence for interactions between growth factor hormones and antioxidant nutrient action pathways, it is likely that diminution of oxidative tissue damage by certain nutrients serves to facilitate growth factor–induced tissue growth and repair. In addition, as discussed below, several individual micronutrients appear to be critical for normal functioning of the GH–IGF-I axis.

Mechanisms of Cellular Nutrition

The metabolic and molecular mechanisms that underlie cellular responses to nutritional status or specific nutrients are not well understood (92). However, amino acids taken in the diet or derived endogenously (primarily from skeletal muscle protein breakdown) are utilized as substrates for new structural and circulating proteins. Energy sources (amino acids, carbohydrate, fat) directly support cells involved in tissue reparative processes directly, and also indirectly by providing fuel for neutrophils, macrophages, lymphocytes, and other cells critical to wound healing and tissue regeneration (Table 8.1).

As outlined by Bettger and McKeehan (92), it is clear that (a) specific nutrients are required for cell survival, proliferation, and differentiation; (b) cells require available energy sources; and (c) critical nutrients and nutrient sources for energy production contribute to the chemical milieu constituting the external environment of cells. The concentration of nutrients in the cellular microenvironment appears to be an important determinant of cell function, as graded reductions in nutrients such as glutamine (93), magnesium (94), and zinc (95) result in significantly reduced cell proliferation. Cellular nutrient requirements also clearly differ both qualitatively and quantitatively in different cell types and under different conditions. It is known that deficiency in certain nutrients, including amino acids, glucose, or lipids, arrests certain cells within the G_1 portion of the cell cycle (96); however, the exact role of nutrition in the progression of cells through the cell cycle is poorly understood at the molecular level (92). Cellular nutrient deficiency eventually leads to cell death by either passive degeneration (cell necrosis) or programmed cell death (apoptosis) (97). However, the effects of specific nutrient deficiencies on cell death has not been well investigated (92).

Nutrients may serve as substrates or products to determine the rate of biochemical reactions or may serve as reaction catalysts or allosteric effector molecules (92). Certain nutrients are compartmentalized within cells, and the intracellular nutrient concentration may then determine certain biochemical reactions and processes. For example, it has been suggested that the intracellular concentration of the amino acid glutamine (the most abundant intracellular amino acid involved in protein synthesis) in the skeletal muscle intracellular pool is a key regulator of muscle protein synthesis rates (98). Finally, certain nutrients may regulate the control of gene expression in specific cell types. In vitro studies indicate that mRNA levels of IGF-I are significantly decreased in rat hepatocytes maintained in medium depleted of the essential amino acid tryptophan, while significant recovery of cellular IGF-I mRNA occurs after tryptophan supplementation (99). This example demonstrates that specific nutrients may be critical for endogenous growth factor production.

Role of Growth Factor Hormones in Tissue Anabolism and Wound Repair

Endogenous hormones and peptide growth factors play essential roles in normal cellular growth and function. Growth factors mediate anabolic effects in tissues via endocrine, paracrine, or autocrine mechanisms (100). Available animal and limited human studies indicate that the sequence of events involved in wound healing processes, including inflammation, cell migration to the wound, angiogenesis and collagen, and wound protein synthesis, may be favorably modulated by exogenous administration of selected growth factors (101). Details on the effects of specific growth factors and their mechanisms of action are covered in more detail elsewhere in this volume. This chapter focuses primarily on studies concerning the GH–IGF-I axis in tissue anabolism, particularly when combined with nutritional support in catabolic states.

Insulin

Insulin is the major anabolic hormonal growth factor in the body and is critical for cellular amino acid and glucose uptake and metabolism (92). A number of studies have demonstrated reduced nitrogen loss with insulin administration in nondiabetic injured patients (102–104). Marked reductions in body protein breakdown rates and urea generation occurred with administration of high doses of regular insulin (200 to 600 units/day or 2 to 20 units/hr, respectively) with hypertonic dextrose in burn or trauma patients (102, 103). Addition of insulin at a dose of 25 units/L to parenteral nutrition in stable malnourished patients significantly improved lean body mass compared with effects with parenteral nutrition alone, as determined by body composition analysis (104).

PDGF, EGF, KGF, and FGF

PDGF mediates chemotaxis and fibroblast proliferation after platelet aggregation in wounds (105), and appears to accelerate healing rates when given topically in patients with diabetic foot ulcers (106) and in the elderly with decubitus ulcers (107). EGF enhances epidermal repair in animal burn injury models (108) and appears to modestly stimulate wound healing in burn-injured patents (109). Exogenous administration of EGF, normally secreted in saliva and gastric/duodenal secretions into the gut lumen, has trophic effects on the intestinal mucosa in rat models of intestinal atrophy, mucosal injury, and in mucosal adaptation after bowel resection (110–112). KGF is made by fibroblasts and is a key mediator of epithelial cell differentiation and proliferation in many tissues (101, 113). KGF expression has been shown to be significantly increased in wounds, and thus may be involved in normal wound healing processes (101). Fibroblast growth factor (FGF) stimulates angiogenesis and has been shown to increase wound granulation tissue (101, 114), but no significant effects on wound healing in humans have been published to date.

GH, IGF-I, and IGF Binding Proteins in Wound Healing

GH undoubtedly plays a role in normal anabolic responses because GH deficiency is characterized by erosion of lean body mass in otherwise healthy individuals (115). Endogenous production of IGF-I is thought to mediate many of the anabolic effects of GH on body tissues (100). IGF-I synthesis quantitatively occurs primarily by liver, but this growth factor is also made in most other cells and tissues of the body, including in fibroblasts, wounds, and wound fluid (101, 116, 117). IGF-I synthesis in tissues is dependent on GH and to a lesser extent insulin secretion, but is also markedly sensitive to nutritional status (13, 118). IGF-I circulates in plasma largely bound to one of several IGF binding proteins (IGFBP), with IGFBP-3 being by far the most abundant (118). Six IGFBPs have been characterized to date and they are synthesized in multiple tissues throughout the body, including fibroblasts and epithelial cells. IGFBPs appear to variously potentiate or inhibit IGF-I action, and may influence plasma and tissue IGF-I half-life and/or tissue distribution. However, the regulation and biologic actions of the IGFBPs are still incompletely understood (118).

Human skin has been shown to express GH receptor, IGF-I receptor, and IGF-I mRNA and protein, suggesting that the GH–IGF-I axis is important in normal skin growth and repair after injury (119). Studies in animals demonstrate that parenteral administration of recombinant GH enhances formation of wound granulation tissue (120), increases the mechanical strength of skin graft wounds (121), and stimulates healing and breaking strength of intestinal anastomoses (122, 123). Parenteral IGF-I significantly enhanced tissue healing indices when administered alone in rats given corticosteroids to inhibit wound healing responses (124). IGF-I also enhanced re-epithelialization when administered topically in an ex vivo system using human skin biopsies (125). The IGFBPs appear to be able to upregulate IGF-I–induced wound healing responses. For example, combining topical IGF-I with IGFBP-1 significantly enhanced healing of dermal wounds and skin ulcers in rodents (126, 127). Topical IGFBP-3 complexed to IGF-I is significantly more effective than IGF-I alone in reversing corticosteroid-impaired wound healing (128). Several studies also indicate that combining IGF-I with other growth factors, such as PDGF, may be synergistic in wound healing (101, 129). Unfortunately, the role of dietary nutrient intake or underlying nutritional status in investigations of growth factors and wound healing has often not been well characterized or controlled.

Interactions Between Specific Nutrients, Nutritional Status, and Peptide Growth Factors

General Concepts

Proliferation and function of many cell types has been shown to be dependent on both an appropriate hormonal milieu and an adequate supply of nutrients (92). It has been proposed that hormones influence the external concentrations of specific nutrients in the cellular environment by alternating such points of control as cell membrane permeability, local nutrient metabolism, and/or nutrient compartmentalization inside the cell (92). Thus, EGF reduced the requirement for magnesium and calcium in multiplication of human fibroblasts in culture (130). Various other growth factor hormones regulate nutrient uptake in specific cell types. For example, insulin and IGF-I are well known to increase tissue uptake and metabolism of glucose in adipocytes and skeletal muscle cells (92, 118). In addition, both the quantity and quality of food intake are known to regulate gastrointestinal hormones, including somatostatin, gastrin, EGF, and IGF-I that are important in gut growth and repair (131). Milk of various species, including man, is a nutrient source rich in a variety of gut-trophic growth factors including GH, IGF-I, insulin, prolactin, and EGF (132). These may interact with receptors in gut mucosa to stimulate regeneration and function of enterocytes or may be absorbed for systemic effects on the whole body (133). In fact, the gut is a target tissue for nutrient-stimulated growth factors, such as IGF-I, which are derived from the circulation (endocrine route), the gut lumen (via milk, saliva, and pancreatic-biliary secretions), and mucosal cells themselves (autocrine/paracrine route) (Table 8.4).

Although the mechanisms for nutrient-induced growth factor production remain elusive, Bettger and McKeehan (92) propose that nutritional status can have four major effects on growth factor production: (a) generalized

TABLE 8.4. Sources of nutrient-stimulated IFG-I for gut mucosal growth and regeneration.

Circulation (interaction with basolateral region)
Mucosal cells (autocrine/paracrine effects)
Gut lumen (interaction with apical region)
Saliva
Milk
Pancreatic-biliary secretions
Mucosal secretions/sloughed enterocytes

overnutrition or undernutrition may stimulate or depress synthesis of growth factor hormones in tissues; (b) stimulation of synthesis may be due to the presence or absence of a specific nutrient that corrects an imbalance of that nutrient in the cellular environment; (c) particular growth factors may require specific nutrient sets for optimal synthesis; and (d) particular growth factors may require particular specific nutrients for their synthesis. For example, in rats a 3-day total fast reduced jejunal IGF-I mRNA levels to 18% of fed controls, but with enteral refeeding gut IGF-I mRNA levels were rapidly normalized (13) (Fig. 8.1). Similar up- and downregulation of IGF-I production are seen in liver cells in response to fasting and refeeding and with the depletion or repletion of specific amino acids (99, 118).

Interactions Between Nutritional Status and Specific Nutrients and the GH/IGF-I Action Pathway

Effects of Generalized Malnutrition and Nutritional Repletion

It is well documented that nutritional status markedly effects the GH–IGF-I axis in humans (134–136). For example, it was demonstrated in the 1970s that the bioactivity of somatomedin C (IGF-I) was significantly reduced in children with primarily protein depletion (kwashiorkor) and in those with combined protein-energy malnutrition (137, 138). In humans and animal models, serum levels of total IGF-I are reduced in general proportion to the severity of malnutrition, and rise over time in response to refeeding (13, 134–136). In contrast, circulating GH levels are often elevated during starvation and other states of malnutrition, indicative of a GH-resistance state (136, 139–141). For example, fasting increases GH pulse amplitude and pulse frequency (140), while after 2 days of fasting endogenous GH production increased 2.4-fold (141).

A total fast in otherwise healthy adults causes a significant decrease in plasma IGF-I levels after 2 to 3 days (in association with markedly negative nitrogen balance (142). In one study, IGF-I levels in plasma continued to decrease steadily over a 9-day period of fasting, and were increased to only 50% of baseline with 3 days of refeeding (142). In obese individuals or

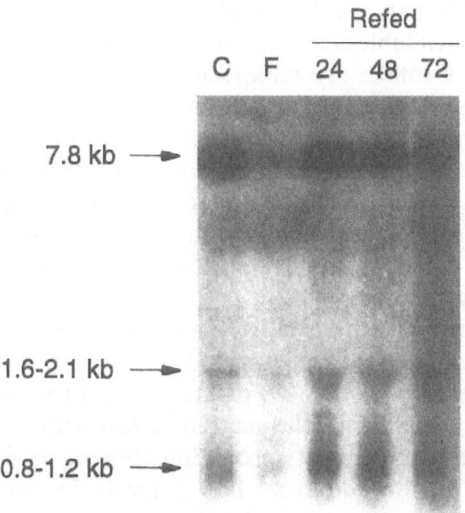

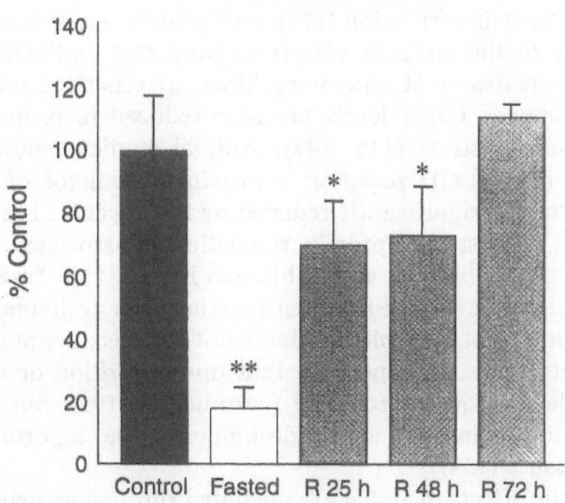

FIGURE 8.1. Rat jejunal IGF-I mRNA expression with fasting and enteral refeeding. A Northern blot of total jejunal RNA derived from control fed (C), 72-hour fasted (F), and 24-hour, 48-hour, and 72-hour refed conditions is shown on the left. Quantitative data for the 7.8-kb IGF-I transcript is shown on the right. *$p < .05$ vs. 72-hour refed; **$p < .01$ vs. all other groups. (Based on ref. 13.)

patients with hyperphagia, IGF-I levels are either normal or only modestly increased (136). Available data in animals and humans suggest that both energy and protein intake are important for IGF-I production. Adequate protein and energy intake is required to normalize plasma IGF-I levels after a period of fasting (143). With adequate protein intake, the rise in IGF-I levels after a 5-day fast was generally proportional to the level of calories provided (144). Further, it appears that provision of nonprotein calories primarily in the form of carbohydrates has a more potent effect on raising IGF-I levels after a period of undernutrition than isocaloric diets with fat as the primary energy source (145).

The level of protein intake also markedly effects IGF-I mRNA and protein production in liver, as well as IGF-I levels in human plasma (136). Enteral protein refeeding with 80% of the dietary protein as essential amino acids significantly increased plasma IGF-I levels (and nitrogen balance) compared with results with diets providing 80% of protein as nonessential amino acids (146). In addition, IGF-I levels in hospitalized patients generally correlate with general nutritional status, protein intake, and nitrogen balance (134–136). Available data suggest that the impact of protein nutritional status on IGF-I production is more marked than the effects of caloric intake (134, 135). In rats, IGF-I clearance from plasma is increased with protein restriction (136), and protein restriction is associated with resistance to the anabolic effects of both GH and IGF-I infusions. Undoubtedly, the degree of underlying illness affects these relationships in hospital patients, as IGF-I levels are also reduced in proportion to the degree of catabolic stress (115, 147). Animal studies demonstrated that mRNA levels for the GH receptor, a proximal mediator of GH-induced IGF-I production, is significantly reduced by fasting (134, 148). Additional studies in rats suggest that protein restriction is associated with normal hepatic GH-receptor binding with a blunted hepatic IGF-I response at the protein and mRNA level (149). Taken together, the available data suggest that malnutrition (protein depletion) induces GH resistance at both receptor and postreceptor sites. It is possible that undernutrition deprives cells of essential nutrients required for IGF-I production (99), but also reduces cellular exposure to insulin, a peptide known to be important for IGF-I synthesis in tissues (134).

The metabolic effects of IGF-I are mediated through its heterotetrameric receptor, a tyrosine kinase that shares structural and functional homology with the insulin receptor (13). IGF-I, insulin, and IGF-II all may bind to the IGF-I receptor in descending order of affinity (150). Fasting for 48 hours was shown to increase IGF-I binding and IGF-I receptor mRNA in several nonintestinal tissues in rats (151). We found a nonsignificant rise in rat jejunal IGF-I receptor number and mRNA in response to a 3-day fast (13). However, with 24 to 74 hours of enteral refeeding, IGF-I receptor expression in small bowel rose significantly (60–80%) at the same time that plasma IGF-I and jejunal IGF-I mRNA levels were increased (Fig. 8.2). This finding suggests that the small intestinal population of IGF-I receptors (and

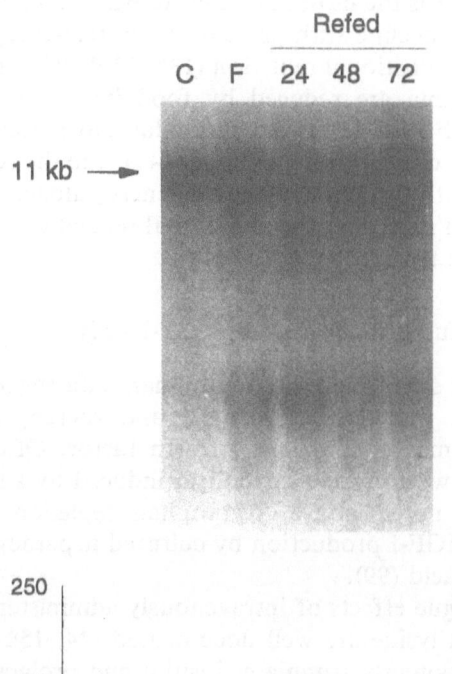

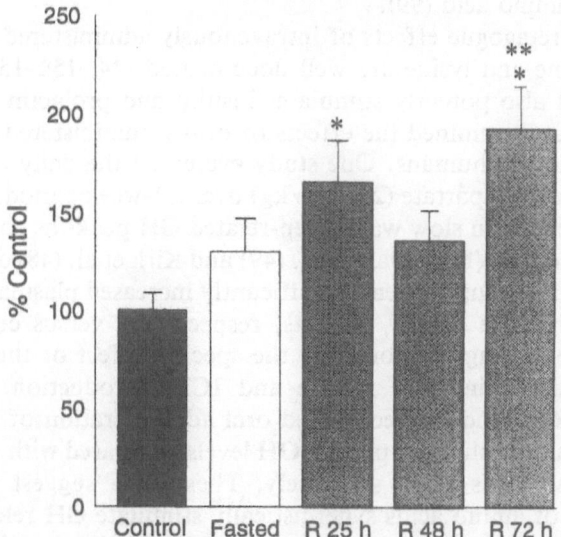

FIGURE 8.2. IGF-I receptor mRNA expression in jejunum during fasting and refeeding. A Northern blot demonstrating the 11.0-kb rat IGF-I-R transcript from control (C), 72-hour fasted (F), and 24-hour, 48-hour, and 72-hour refed conditions is shown on the left. Quantitative data from multiple experiments are shown on the right. *$p < .01$ vs. control; **$p < .05$ vs. fasted. (Based on ref. 13.)

thus the capacity for IGF-I action) is maintained during fasting-induced intestinal atrophy and increased during nutrient-induced intestinal growth with refeeding (13).

Nutritional status also appears to regulate IGFBPs in plasma and in tissues (118). IGFBP-3 is the most abundant IGFBP in human plasma and, like IGF-I, exhibits a decline with protein- or protein-energy malnutrition and an increase with nutritional repletion (135, 136). In contrast, IGFBP-1 and -2 levels in plasma are reduced by food intake and increase with starvation (135). IGFBP-2 levels in particular have been shown to be inversely regulated by dietary protein intake (141), and the IGFBP-2 mRNA is increased in liver with fasting, depletion of energy alone, or protein alone (135). Little is known regarding the nutritional regulation of IGFBP-4, -5, and -6 in plasma and tissues.

Effects of Specific Nutrients on the GH–IGF-I Axis

A number of animal studies and limited human data suggest that specific nutrients upregulate the GH–IGF-I axis, and thereby increase IGF-I production and plasma levels of this growth factor. Often these results occur in association with protein anabolism induced by administration of these nutrients. As noted above, tryptophan repletion was shown to specifically increase IGF-I production by cultured hepatocytes deprived of this essential amino acid (99).

The GH secretagogue effects of intravenously administered amino acids such as arginine and lysine are well documented (44, 152–154). Arginine administration also potently stimulates insulin and prolactin release (44). Few studies have examined the effects of orally administered amino acids on GH secretion in humans. One study evaluated the daily oral adminis-tration of arginine aspartate (250 mg/kg) over a 1-week period. All subjects had a 60% increase in slow wave sleep-related GH peaks as compared with their control periods (155). Daly et al. (49) and Kirk et al. (48) demonstrated that oral L-arginine supplements significantly increased plasma IGF-I levels in postoperative and elderly patients, respectively, versus controls given glycine. These findings demonstrate the specific effect of the amino acid arginine in stimulating GH release and IGF-I production. Isidori and colleagues (156) found that combined oral administration of arginine and lysine significantly enhanced plasma GH levels compared with similar doses of these amino acids given separately. These data suggest that specific combinations of amino acids synergistically stimulate GH release.

Zinc depletion is common in catabolic and hospitalized patients due to a combination of urinary, gastrointestinal, and wound losses, coupled with insufficient intake. Zinc deficiency is associated with poor wound healing, reduced protein synthesis, immunosuppression, diarrhea, dermatitis, and diminished gonadal steroid concentrations (34, 35). Zinc nutritional status has been shown to markedly influence the GH–IGF-I axis (157–162) (Table 8.5). In rats prefed a low-zinc, low-protein diet, plasma levels of IGF-I fell significantly, but increased in response to the amount of zinc or zinc and protein in the diet. However, no increase in IGF-I occurred when only dietary protein was increased (157). Growing lambs fed a zinc-deficient diet

TABLE 8.5. Zinc nutrition and growth factor regulation.

Zinc depletion is comon in catabolic and hospitalized patients
Zinc deficiency is associated with poor wound healing, reduced protein synthesis,
  immunosuppression, diarrhea, dermatitis, and diminished gonadal steroid concentrations
Zinc depletion is associated with reduced plasma concentrations of GH and GHBP, and
  diminished hepatic GH binding capacity
Zinc deficiency is associated with diminished hepatic IGF-I mRNA levels and reduced
  plasma IGF-I concentrations
Zinc repletion in zinc deficient animals normalizes the GH–IGF-I axis at the protein and
  mRNA level

GHBP, GH binding protein.

demonstrated significantly reduced plasma insulin, GH, and IGF-I levels, and insulin levels rose significantly more in response to feeding with zinc repletion (158). Of interest, topical zinc treatment in full-thickness wounds in pigs improved wound healing in association with a 50% increase in IGF-I mRNA levels in the wound granulation tissue (160). In rats, experimental zinc deficiency significantly reduced body weight, serum IGF-I and GH concentrations, hepatic GH receptor abundance, and serum GHBP levels (an index of GH receptor number) versus pair-fed controls (161). Liver IGF-I mRNA levels were also specifically reduced by zinc depletion (161). These data suggest that the reduction in IGF-I levels with zinc deficiency is due, in part, to reduced GH concentrations in plasma and reduced GH receptors in tissues. Zinc repletion in zinc-deficient animals normalizes the GH–IGF-I axis at both the protein and mRNA levels. Zinc deficiency also impairs intestinal growth and adaptation in response to massive small bowel resection (163), a process believed to be mediated, in part, by local generation of IGF-I (164). The relationship between zinc status and the GH–IGF-I and insulin axes is outlined in Table 8.5.

Another example of an interaction between specific nutrients and growth factors is the reduction in plasma and tissue IGF-I concentrations with potassium or magnesium depletion (32, 165, 166). When rats were given magnesium-deficient diets for 12 days, serum magnesium fell markedly, growth and protein synthesis rates diminished, and serum IGF-I levels fell by 44% versus pair-fed animals. Magnesium repletion reversed these alterations (32, 165). Similarly, potassium depletion in rats led to growth retardation, a fall in protein synthesis, and a significant fall in serum IGF-I and insulin levels. These effects are reversed with potassium repletion (32, 166). These findings are consistent with those of Rudman et al. (167), who demonstrated that deficiency of phosphorus, potassium, sodium, or nitrogen each individually impairs nitrogen and mineral retention in adults receiving parenteral feeding. Finally, recent data suggest that experimental thiamine deficiency in rats reduces IGF-I levels in plasma and tissues by 40% (168). Thiamine repletion enhanced the IGF-I response to GH administration in this model (168).

These examples demonstrate that specific nutrients are able to modulate major somatic growth factor systems in vivo (Table 8.6). Therefore, adequate intake of these nutrients appears to be critical to ensure optimal anabolic responses mediated by the GH–IGF-I and/or insulin action pathways, including wound healing, protein retention, and intestinal growth and repair.

Anabolic Effects of GH and IGF-I Combined with Specialized Nutrition During Catabolic States

Growth Hormone

Pituitary GH administration in clinically stable non–GH-deficient patients has long been known to enhance retention of nitrogen, phosphorus, potassium, sodium, magnesium, and calcium (16, 115). GH also causes lipolysis, diminishes urea production, and increases plasma insulin levels (115). A number of early studies in severely catabolic burn patients given pituitary GH (5–10 mg/day s.c. or i.m.) demonstrated improved nitrogen and mineral retention, increased appetite, and improved wound healing with this agent (169, 170). Recombinant GH as an adjunct to nutritional support has been extensively studied in clinical stable patients during the postoperative period (171–174) and in malnourished patients with end-stage renal disease (175, 176), chronic obstructive lung disease (177), acquired immunodeficiency syndrome (178), or gastrointestinal diseases including inflammatory bowel disease, intestinal fistulas, chronic pancreatitis, and short bowel syndrome (179–181).

In general, these studies in noncritically ill patients demonstrated markedly improved nutrient utilization efficiency with recombinant GH therapy. In one study positive nitrogen and mineral balance was achieved in patients

TABLE 8.6. Specific nutrients known to modulate the GH–IGF-I axis.*

Amino acids
Arginine
Glutamine
Lysine
Tryptophan
Trace metals
Zinc
Vitamins
Thiamine
Electrolytes
Potassium
Magnesium

*Downregulation with depletion of these nutrients and upregulation with nutrient repletion.

receiving parenteral nutrition that provided adequate protein and micronutrients but only 60% of calorie needs (181) (Fig. 8.3). This demonstrates that exogenous GH enhances the efficacy of nutritional support, compared with responses in individuals receiving identical isonitrogenous, isocaloric diets.

In clinically stable patients, GH at doses ranging from 0.06 to 0.20 mg/kg/day improved whole body protein synthesis rates (171), reduced muscle amino acid efflux (171, 173), diminished urea generation (171–176, 179–181), and enhanced whole body retention of nitrogen, potassium, phosphorus, and sodium (171–182). Of interest, the anabolic effects of GH were consistently observed over a wide range of nutrient intakes and clinical conditions. Significantly increased plasma insulin and IGF-I levels were observed in patients receiving GH, and these anabolic peptides undoubtedly facilitate the GH-induced protein-anabolic effects.

Limited data are available on skeletal muscle function with GH therapy in stable patients. In two studies, GH administration significantly improved skeletal muscle strength as shown by maintained hand grip strength in the postoperative period (171) and improved respiratory muscle strength (177). However, in another study in stable chronic obstructive pulmonary disease (COPD) patients, anabolic responses occurred, but these were not associated with improved indices of respiratory muscle strength (182).

A recent double-blind randomized study from Spain demonstrated that GH may improve clinically important end points in stable patients (172). In this study, hypocaloric parenteral nutrition (≈ 900 kcal/day) with adequate protein was given with either s.c. GH (8 IU/day or ≈ 2.5 mg/day) or saline placebo for 7 days after cholecystectomy. The patients were clinically and demographically matched at entry, and underwent similar operative courses (93 controls and 87 GH treated). With GH, a significant reduction in postoperative nitrogen and potassium excretion was noted, despite hypocaloric feedings (172). Blood levels of GH, insulin, and IGF-I rose significantly, and blood glucose slightly during GH treatment (NS). In control patients, serum albumin, prealbumin, transferrin, retinol binding protein, and immunoglobulins A, G, and M fell significantly by the fifth postoperative day. In contrast, levels of circulating proteins and immunoglobulins were maintained at levels significantly above controls with GH therapy (172).

Patients receiving GH in this study were significantly less likely to become hypoanergic or anergic to skin test antigens after operation than controls. The number of normergic patients in the control group fell from 60% to 43%, and the number of hypoanergic patients rose from 28% to 45% after operation (172). In contrast, in GH-treated patients the number of normergic patients rose from 68% to 93% after operation, while the number of hypoergic patients fell from 29% to 7%. Importantly, GH treatment was associated with significantly lower wound infections (control 17% versus GH 3%), and a shorter hospitalization time (12.5 days versus 9.6 days) compared with the control group (172).

Several studies evaluating short-term (3 days to 6 weeks) recombinant GH

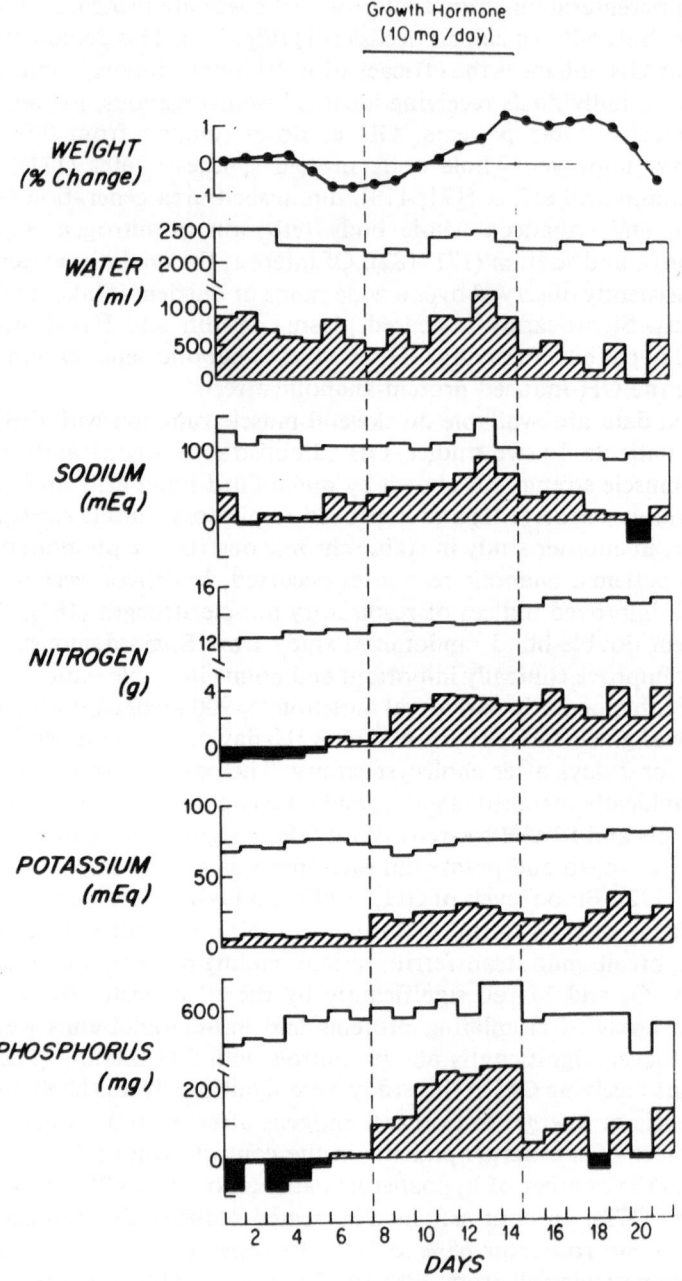

FIGURE 8.3. Improved nutrient utilization efficiency with growth hormone (GH) therapy (181). Body weight and elemental balances of sodium, nitrogen (N), potassium (K), and phosphorus (P) were determined in clinically stable adults with gastrointestinal disease receiving total parenteral nutrition. Patients were studied

treatment in critically ill patients receiving specialized nutrition have been reported (183–191). In general, these studies document significantly improved net protein anabolism; enhanced nitrogen, potassium, and phosphorus retention; reduced urea generation; and stimulated wound healing with GH therapy at doses ranging from 0.1 to 0.2 mg/kg/day. However, minimal anabolic effects were seen in three studies using lower GH doses for short periods following sepsis, trauma, or burn injury (192–194). These data suggest that some critically ill patients are resistant to the anabolic effects of GH, especially as plasma levels of IGF-I (believed to be the major mediator of GH-induced anabolism) were significantly elevated (192, 194).

The metabolic and clinical effects of up to 6 weeks of recombinant GH therapy (10 mg/day; dose range 0.096 to 0.172 mg/kg/day) were studied in severely catabolic adult patients receiving conventional enteral/parenteral nutrition support following severe burn injury ($\approx 60\%$ body surface area) or trauma (184). Body protein, potassium, and phosphorus losses decreased markedly and rapidly with GH treatment in all patients, and these anabolic effects persisted throughout GH therapy. Serum IGF-I levels rose approximately fivefold, and serum calcium rose slightly during GH therapy. Potassium, sodium, and phosphorus levels also rose in serum, despite significant retention of these with GH therapy. This finding suggests that the minerals were incorporated into protein-rich tissue in these critically ill patients (182).

Additional studies in other groups of critically ill and septic patients have documented increased whole body and limb protein synthetic rates, improved nitrogen balance, increased plasma amino acid levels, and increased fat oxidation rates with short-term GH administration compared with clinically similar patients receiving placebo injections and comparable diets (185–187). The improvement of nitrogen balance with GH in these studies has ranged from ≈ 2 to 5 g/day versus results with comparable feeding without GH. This change represents a relative improvement in protein-rich tissue of between 0.35 and 0.875 kg/week with GH therapy (180).

In a blinded, controlled trial in adult burn patients, 2 weeks of GH therapy (10 mg/day) was shown to attenuate expansion of the extracellular

←──────────────────────────────────────

during an initial control period, a GH treatment period and a post-GH control period, during which constant hypocaloric (60% of requirements) parenteral feedings with adequate protein were administered. During hypocaloric feeding, body weight fell and nutrient balances were near equilibrium (sodium and K) or negative (N and P). With GH therapy, body weight increased in association with positive sodium and water balances. GH induced a rapid increase in N balance, despite hypocaloric feeding. Protein anabolism occurred in association with positive K and especially P balance. After GH discontinuation, K and P balances returned toward baseline, while N balance remained positive. The upper line for each nutrient represents intake, the hatched area above the zero line represents positive nutrient balance, and the black area denotes negative nutrient balance.

water (ECW) compartment and to minimize loss of intracellular water (ICW), effects opposite those in control patients, who demonstrated the usual expansion of ECW and contraction of ICW common in the critically ill (190). This study suggests that GH may affect cell membrane stability or permeability. A recent study in trauma patients appeared to confirm these effects of GH on water metabolism (194).

Although several authors report anecdotal improvements in respiratory muscle strength, weaning from the ventilator, and other indices of physical rehabilitation during GH therapy in critical illness, such end points have not been well characterized in the small patient groups reported on to date. Thus, whether or not skeletal muscle function is improved by GH in ICU patients is unclear at present. Negative data have recently been published suggesting that GH is not effective in facilitating ventilator weaning in elderly COPD patients (183). Significantly improved wound healing of skin graft donor sites with GH administration in burn patients was confirmed in two blinded, randomized trials (188, 189). In addition, markedly decreased hospital length of stay occurred in the pediatric burn patients given GH therapy (189).

The mechanisms of GH anabolic effects when combined with nutritional support are multifactorial. For example, consistent and marked elevations in blood IGF-I occur with GH in these clinical settings and undoubtedly play a role in tissue anabolic responses. Of interest, this IGF-I response is attenuated as injury severity increases in ICU patients (191). The IGF-I response is also directly related to nutritional status (115, 118). Thus, certain severely ill patients, for example those receiving low caloric or protein intakes, or patients with cirrhosis or multiple organ failure, may not generate adequate IGF-I responses to induce significant anabolic effects. The stimulation of insulin release, production of endogenous fuel as free fatty acids via enhanced lipolysis, and regulation of circulating or tissue IGF binding proteins with GH treatment represent additional mechanisms of GH anabolic action (115). Although short-term GH treatment has been well tolerated in the studies published to date in catabolic patients, GH therapy may cause hyperglycemia and insulin resistance, hypercalcemia, mild fluid and sodium retention, and arthralgias in some individuals, and as a growth factor, may theoretically stimulate neoplastic growth (115). Some of the beneficial metabolic and clinical effects observed with GH therapy in catabolic states to date are shown in Table 8.7.

Insulin-Like Growth Factor (IGF-I)

A number of studies have evaluated the protein-anabolic effects of IGF-I (or somatomedin C) in humans without GH deficiency (195–201).

When administered intravenously in acute studies in healthy humans, IGF-I increased peripheral glucose disposal and suppressed hepatic glucose production (195). Free fatty acid (FFA) levels fell significantly with IGF-I

TABLE 8.7. Metabolic and functional effects of growth hormone in patients receiving specialized nutrition.

Metabolic effects
  Insulin resistance
  Improved nitrogen retention and stimulated protein synthesis
  Reduced amino acid efflux from muscle and urea generation
  Enhanced potassium, magnesium, sodium, and phosphorus retention
  Maintained skeletal muscle intracellular glutamine concentrations
  Enhanced lipolysis
  Increased metabolic rate
  Increased serum IGF-I, IGFBP-3, and insulin concentrations
Clinical and functional effects
  Improved wound healing in burn patients
  Variable effects on skeletal and respiratory muscle strength
  Shortened length of hospital stay (postoperative and burn patients)

infusion, indicating reduced lipolysis, while total branched-chain amino acid levels fell by $\approx 50\%$, indicating a possible protein-anabolic effect (195). Clemmons et al. (196) documented that parenteral IGF-I could reverse the protein catabolic effects of hypocaloric (20 kcal/kg/day) oral diets in healthy adults (196). Subjects were fed the hypocaloric diets for 8 days prior to a 6-day infusion of either recombinant IGF-I (12 μg/kg/hr over 16 hr/day) or GH (50 μg/kg/day s.c.). IGF-I significantly attenuated nitrogen losses, similar to the protein-anabolic effect observed with GH. In a subsequent study, these authors compared the protein anabolic effects of combined 6-day GH plus IGF-I infusion versus IGF-I infusion alone (197). Combined GH plus IGF-I therapy resulted in a significantly improved nitrogen balance over the baseline diet period compared with results with IGF-I alone. Both therapies significantly reduced urea appearance; however, combination therapy with GH and IGF-I was more potent in lowering blood urea nitrogen and in reducing urea and potassium excretion compared to IGF-I treatment alone (197). In another study, healthy adult subjects were given hypocaloric, adequate protein intravenous nutrition for 10 days prior to a 6-day infusion of saline or IGF-I at a dose of 25 μg/kg/hr (198). Subjects receiving IGF-I demonstrated improved nitrogen balance and reduced amino acid efflux from skeletal muscle, without changes in fat oxidation (198).

The results of IGF-I use in catabolic patients have recently been reported (199–201). In one trial, recombinant IGF-I (10 μg/kg/hr) or saline was infused for 14 days after severe head trauma in 24 adult patients. In controls, daily nitrogen balance was negative (-2.9 g/day), and worsened to -5.0 g/day during the second week after injury. Nitrogen was significantly conserved during the first week postinjury with IGF-I ($+1.3$ g/day), and IGF-I serum concentrations rose significantly from 78 to 466 ng/ml. However, IGF-I levels subsequently fell to 220 ng/ml by day 14, despite continued IGF-I infusion, and the nitrogen-retaining effect of IGF-I was lost (199). In a more recent short-term study, recombinant IGF-I infused over a several hour period significantly reduced protein oxidation rates in burn patients (200). Finally, IGF-I (80 μg/kg/day s.c.) or placebo was given for 5 days to patients after gastric surgery in a double-blind, randomized trial in Germany (201). IGF-I was well tolerated, but had no effect on postoperative nitrogen balance or 3-methylhistidine excretion, despite significantly increased plasma IGF-I levels with hormonal therapy (201). Thus, IGF-I therapy appears to be less efficacious than GH in promoting protein-anabolism in catabolic patients receiving otherwise adequate nutritional support.

Trophic Effects of Growth Factors During Malnutrition

Several studies in rats indicate that administration of peptide growth factors overcomes the catabolic effects of malnutrition during wound healing and intestinal growth. In one study, rats subjected to protein malnutrition exhibited a marked reduction in skin wound tensile strength after open laparotomy (202; Table 8.8). Wound tensile strength was further diminished when malnourished animals were given corticosteroids. However, perioperative administration of GH abolished the inhibitory effects of protein malnutrition combined with corticosteroids on wound healing, and values in this group were similar to controls (Table 8.8). In rats kept undernourished from birth to 24 days of age, marked atrophy of the small intestinal mucosa and loss of body weight was reversed in the undernourished group given s.c. EGF during the final 7 days of malnutrition (203). These data are consistent with studies demonstrating that positive nitrogen balance can be achieved in hospitalized patients given recombinant GH even with hypocaloric feeling (172, 181). Thus, exogenous growth factors are able to improve nutrient utilization for anabolism in both the whole body and in specific target tissues such as intestine and wounds.

TABLE 8.8. Improved skin wound healing with GH in protein-malnourished rats treated with corticosteroids.

Group	Wound breaking strength (mm Hg)
Controls	136 ± 13
Protein-malnourished	110 ± 23*
Protein-malnourished + corticosteroids	77 ± 7*†
Protein-malnourished + corticosteroids + GH	124 ± 20†¶

GH, perioperative growth hormone treatment.
*$p < .025$ vs. controls; †$p < .05$ vs. protein malnourished; ¶$p < .05$ vs. protein malnourished and corticosteroids.

Interactive Effects of Glutamine and Growth Factors In Vivo

Several studies suggest that the anabolic and tissue-specific trophic effects of dietary Gln are enhanced by exogenous EGF or GH administration in a synergistic or additive fashion. These and other data support the concept that the metabolism of Gln and certain peptide growth factors may be physiologically interactive. As noted previously, both EGF and dietary Gln administration each individually are trophic to gut mucosa in experimental animals (30, 52, 110–112). Jacobs et al. (204) studied the effects of dietary Gln with or without EGF s.c. in rats given standard Gln-free parenteral nutrition for 4 days, which rapidly results in gut mucosal atrophy when enteral food is given. When Gln was added to the parenteral nutrient solution, colonic mucosal thickness, DNA content, and protein content were moderately increased compared with controls given isonitrogenous, isocaloric parenteral diets (NS; Fig. 8.4). EGF treatment with Gln-free feeding had little effect on mucosal cellularity. However, the combination of Gln and EGF resulted in a marked additive effect on colonic mucosal mass and DNA content (204; Fig. 8.4). In other studies, jejunal glutamine transport was shown to be significantly upregulated in rats given exogenous EGF, probably due to an induction of Gln transporter proteins by this growth factor (205). In an in vitro study, glutamine was found to be essential for EGF-stimulated cell proliferation and DNA, RNA, and protein synthesis in IEC-6 cells, a rat small intestinal crypt cell line (206). Taken together, these reports indicate that Gln is a key nutrient that interacts with EGF to support intestinal cell growth, and that EGF is able to regulate gut Gln metabolism.

Enteral administration of L-Gln to healthy adults stimulates GH release (207, 208). Administration of recombinant GH to postoperative patients significantly decreases skeletal muscle Gln efflux (171, 173) and attenuates the usual fall in muscle intracellular Gln concentrations (209). In hypophysectomized rats, GH administration upregulates hepatic specific activity and mRNA levels for Gln synthetase, the rate-limiting enzyme involved in endogenous Gln synthesis (210). In experimental short bowel syndrome in rats, the combination of Gln-enriched enteral diet and IGF-I s.c. administration synergistically increased ileal protein content (Fig. 8.5), ileal wet weight, and plasma IGF-I and Gln levels compared with treatment with Gln or IGF-I alone (211). Of interest, dietary Gln has been shown to significantly increase splanchnic blood flow in rats, and this effect may facilitate delivery of nutrients and growth factors to the intestinal mucosa (212). The available studies suggest that Gln metabolism and the GH–IGF-I action pathways are interactive in animal tissues.

Based on the above data, one strategy to enhance tissue anabolism in humans is to combine anabolic hormones such as GH with key nutrient substrates such as Gln. In a series of studies, Byrne et al. (180) recently investigated the combined effects of Gln (0.45 g/kg/day by the intravenous

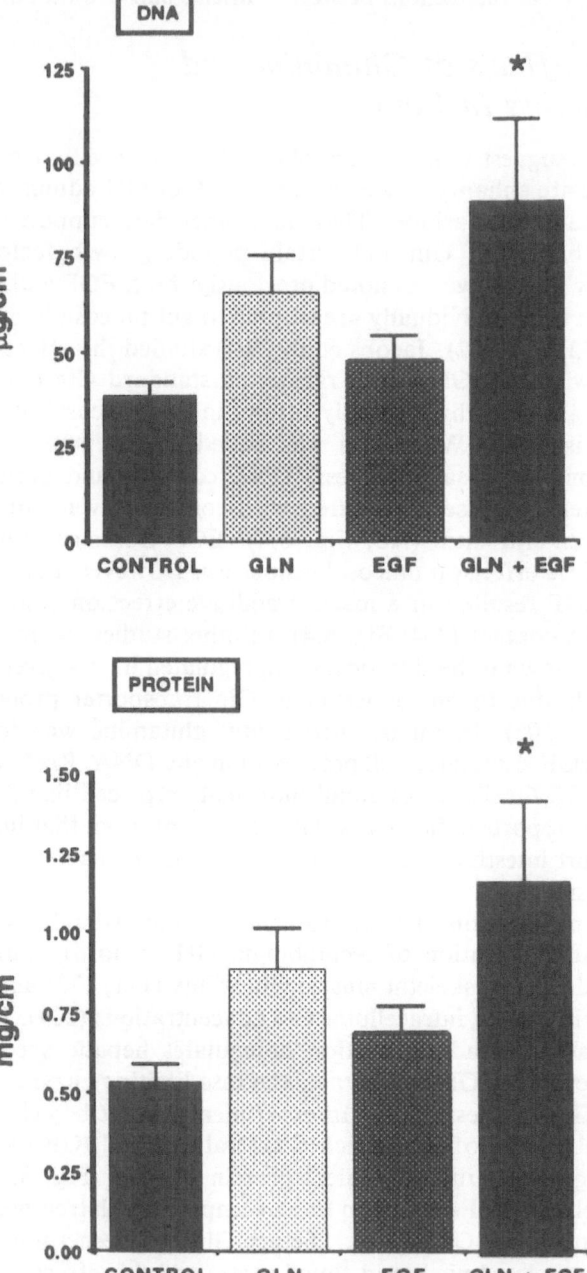

FIGURE 8.4. Colonic mucosal DNA content (top) and protein content (bottom) in rats maintained on parenteral nutrition (PN) for 4 days. Control rats received standard Gln-free PN and saline injection; Gln-treated rats (Gln) received isonitrogenous, isocaloric diets with 2% Gln and saline injections; EGF-treated animals (EGF) received daily s.c. injections of recombinant EGF (0.1 μg/g body weight twice daily) for 3 days; the final group received both Gln-enriched diet and EGF (gln + EGF). A marked additive effect of combined treatment on colon cellularity was noted.

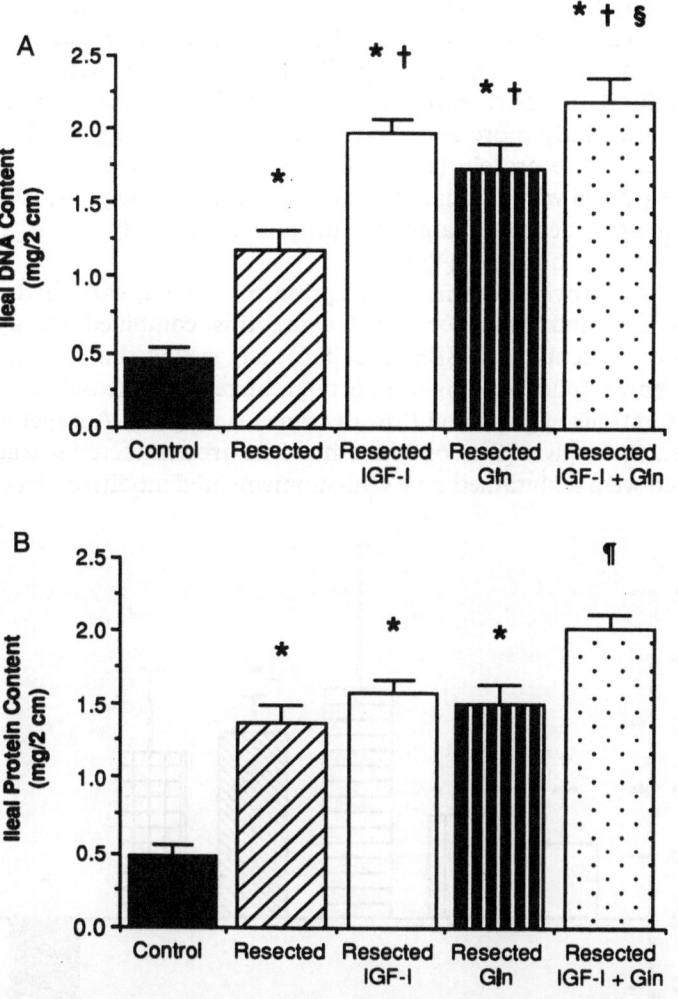

FIGURE 8.5. A: Ileal DNA content after 7 days of diet-hormone infusion. The five experimental groups are from left to right: (1) transected/non-Gln-supplemented diet/vehicle infused (control); (2) resected/non-Gln-supplemented diet/vehicle-infused (resected); (3) resected/non-Gln-supplemented diet/IGF-I-infused (resected/ IGF-I); (4) resected/Gln-supplemented diet/vehicle-infused (resected/Gln); and (5) resected/Gln-supplemented diet/IGF-I-infused (resected/IGF-I + Gln). *$p <$ .01 vs. control; †$p <$ .01 vs. resected; §$p <$ .05 vs. resected/Gln. B: Ileal protein content per centimeter. The combination of IGF-I plus Gln-enriched diet synergistically increased ileal protein content during intestinal adaptation. *$p <$ .01 vs. control; ¶$p <$ .01 vs. all other groups.

or enteral route), parenteral GH (0.14 mg/kg/day), and a modified enteral diet in parenteral nutrition–dependent adult patients with gastrointestinal failure and short bowel syndrome (SBS) (180, 213, 214). After 3 weeks of combined diet-Gln-GH therapy, the treated patients gained minimal body fat, but significantly more lean body mass (4.3 ± 0.6 kg vs. 2.0 ± 0.2; $p < .03$) and more protein (1.4 ± 0.3 kg vs. 0.9 ± 0.1; $p < .03$) than individuals treated with standard therapy. In contrast, the patients receiving standard therapy deposited a greater proportion of body weight as extracellular water and body fat (180).

Markedly improved intestinal absorption of protein, carbohydrate, calories, sodium, and water occurred using this combined therapy in a subgroup of patients with SBS (Fig. 8.6), suggesting that this treatment enhanced bowel function, possibly through increased mucosal surface area and/or alterations in gut blood flow or transit time (213). A larger group of SBS patients was given the combined nutrient-growth factor therapy for 3 weeks, then were maintained on a Gln-supplemented modified diet (without

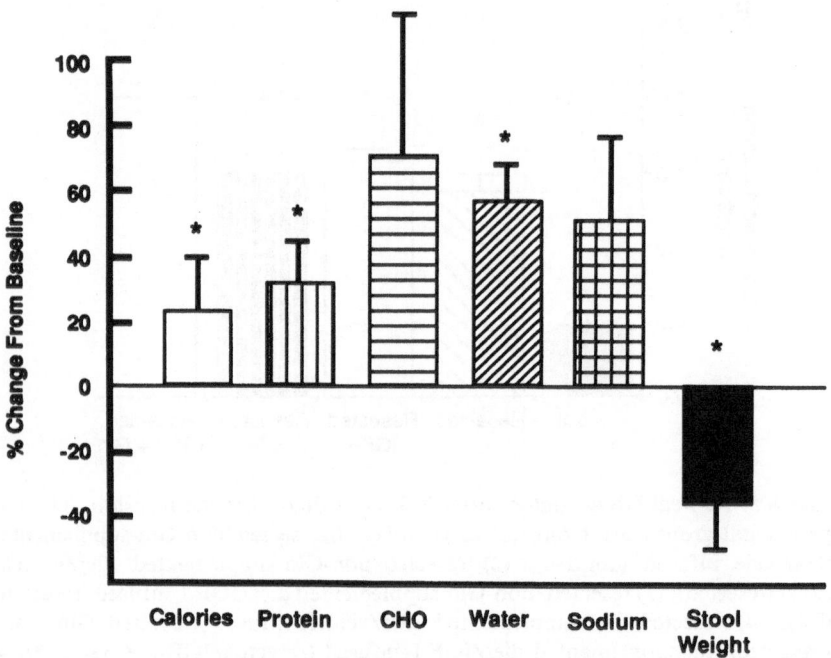

FIGURE 8.6. Enhanced intestinal nutrient absorption with combined Gln-enriched modified diet and recombinant GH administration in adults with long-standing short bowel syndrome. The percent change in nutrient absorption and stool weight from the initial baseline (pretreatment) period to the final week of study after 3 weeks of combined therapy is shown. Significantly improved intestinal absorption of calories, protein and water occurred and stool weight also fell significantly. *$p <$ .01 versus the baseline period.

GH) indefinitely. Therapy was associated with an 80% elimination or reduction in parenteral nutrition requirements after an average of 1 year of follow-up (214). Further work in progress to determine the molecular mechanisms and the nature of the apparent additive or synergistic effect of combined Gln and GH therapy. However, these studies illustrate the potential efficacy of combining gut-trophic and growth-promoting hormones and specific nutrients in a patient model of catabolic stress and intestinal adaptation.

Summary and Conclusions

Growth factors, general nutritional status, and specific nutrients are interactive in protein and tissue anabolism and wound healing. Exogenous administration of certain growth factors, such as GH, EGF, and IGF-I, appears to enhance the efficiency of nutrient utilization during cellular growth. Conversely, both general nutritional status and administration of specific nutrients are able to upregulate endogenous production of some peptide growth factors. Thus, specific growth factors appear to act synergistically with certain nutrients in tissue anabolism and repair. Growth factors and dietary components may also interact to facilitate wound healing by nonspecific mechanisms, such as via altering blood flow to tissues (Gln, GH, IGF-I) or by diminishing oxidative tissue damage (nutrient antioxidants).

Adequate nutritional status clearly seems to be important for optimal organ function and tissue anabolism. However, the role of dietary intake or underlying nutritional status is often not well controlled or characterized in most of the published studies on growth factor administration and wound healing. The available data suggest that the potential clinical efficacy of recombinant growth factor administration for wound healing may be increased with concomitant prevention of malnutrition during therapy, treatment of preexisting malnutrition, and/or provision of specific nutrients with growth-promoting effects.

References

1. Studley HO. Percentage of weight loss: a basic indicator of surgical risk in patients with chronic peptic ulcer. JAMA 1936;106:458–60.
2. Moore FD. Metabolic care of the surgical patient. Philadelphia: W.B. Saunders, 1959:58–9.
3. Cahill GF. Starvation in man. N Engl J Med 1970;282:668–75.
4. Daly JM, Vars HM, Dudrick SJ. Effects of protein depletion on strength of colonic anastomoses. Surg Gynecol Obstet 1972;134:15–21.
5. Wilmore DW. Catabolic illness: strategies for enhancing recovery. N Engl J Med 1991;325:695–702.

6. Albina JE. Nutrition and wound healing. In: Torosian MH, ed. Nutrition for the hospitalized patient: basic science and principles of practice. New York: Marcel-Dekker, 1995:57–83.

7. Beisel WR. Metabolic response to infection. Annu Rev Med 1975;26:9–20.

8. Winick M, Noble A. Cellular response in rats during malnutrition at various ages. J Nutr 1966;89:989–1003.

9. Irvin TT, Hunt TK. Effect of malnutrition on colonic healing. Ann Surg 1974;180:765–72.

10. Irvin TT. Effects of malnutrition and hyperalimentation on wound healing. Surg Gynecol Obstet 1978;146:33–7.

11. Spanheimer RG, Peterkofsky B. A specific decrease in collagen synthesis in acutely fasted, vitamin C-supplemented, guinea pigs. J Biol Chem 1985; 260:3955–62.

12. Steiner M, Bourges HR, Freedman LS, Gray SJ. Effect of starvation on the tissue composition of the small intestine in the rat. Am J Physiol 1968; 215:75–7.

13. Ziegler TR, Almahfouz A, Pedrini MT, Smith RJ. A comparison of rat small intestinal insulin and IGF-I receptors during fasting and refeeding. Endocrinology 1995;136:5148–54.

14. Dominioni L, Trocki O. Mochizuki H, Alexander JW. Prevention of severe postburn hypermetabolism and catabolism by immediate intragastric feeding. J Burn Care Rehabil 1984;5:106–12.

15. Zaloga GP, Bortenschlager L, Black KW, Prielipp R. Immediate postoperative enteral feeding decreases weight loss and improves wound healing after abdominal surgery in rats. Crit Care Med 1992;20:115–8.

16. Ziegler TR, Gatzen C, Wilmore DW. Strategies for attenuating protein-catabolic responses in the critically ill. Annu Rev Med 1994;45:459–80.

17. Scrimshaw NS, Taylor CE, Goodon JE. Interactions of nutrition and infection. Am J Med Sci 1973;237:367–403.

18. Windsor JA, Hill GL. Risk factors of postoperative pneumonia: the importance of protein depletion. Ann Surg 1988;207:290–6.

19. Haydock DA, Hill GA. Impaired wound healing in patients with varying degrees of malnutrition. JPEN J Parenter Enteral Nutr 1986;10:550–4.

20. Windsor JA. Underweight patients and the risk for major surgery. World J Surg 1993;17:165–72.

21. Lopes J, Russell DMcR, Whitwell J, Jeejeebhoy KN. Skeletal muscle function in malnutrition. Am J Clin Nutr 1982;36:602–10.

22. Jacobs Do, Kobayashi T, Imagire J, Grant C, Kesselly B, Wilmore DW. Sepsis alters skeletal muscle energetics and membrane function. Surgery 1991; 110:318–26.

23. Haydock DA, Hill GL. Improved wound healing responses in surgical patients receiving intravenous nutrition. Br J Surg 1987;74:320–3.

24. Schroeder D, Gillanders L, Mahr K, Hill GL. Effects of immediate postoperative enteral nutrition on body composition, muscle function and wound healing. JPEN J Parenter Enteral nutr 1991;15:376–83.

25. Windsor JA, Knight GS, Hill GL. Wound healing response in surgical patients: recent food intake is more important than nutritional status. Br J Surg 1988;75:135–7.

26. Alexander JW, McMillan BG, Stinnett JD, et al. Beneficial effects of

aggressive protein feeding in severely burned children. Ann Surg 1980; 192:505-17.

27. Müller JM, Brenner U, Dienst C, et al. Preoperative parenteral feeding in patients with gastrointestinal carcinoma. Lancet 1982;1:68-71.

28. The Veteran Affairs Total Parenteral Nutrition Cooperative Study Group. Perioperative total parenteral nutrition in surgical patients. N Engl J Med 1991;325:525-32.

29. American Society for Parenteral and Enteral Nutrition Board of Directors. Guidelines for the use of parenteral and enteral nutrition in adult and pediatric patients. JPEN J Parenter Enteral Nutr 1993;14(suppl 4):1SA-52SA.

30. Ziegler TR. New developments in specialized nutrition support. In: Bion JF, Burchardi H, Dellinger RP, Dobb GJ, eds. Current topics in intensive care. London: W.B. Saunders, 1995:144-74.

31. Lakshmi R, Lakshmi AV, Bamji MS. Skin wound healing in riboflavin deficiency. Bio Med Metab Biol 1989;42:185-91.

32. Dorup I. Magnesium and potassium deficiency: its diagnosis, occurrence and treatment in diuretic therapy and its consequences for growth, protein synthesis and growth factors. Acta Physiol Scand 1994;52:1-55.

33. Giugliano R, Millward DJ. The effects of severe zinc deficiency on protein turnover in muscle and thymus. Br J Nutr 1987;57:139-55.

34. Prasad AS. Zinc deficiency in human subjects. Prog Clin Biol Res 1983;129:1-33.

35. Ronaghy HA. The role of zinc in human nutrition. World Rev Nutr Diet 1987;54:237-54.

36. Meyer NA, Muller MJ, Herndon DN. Nutrient support of the healing wound. New Horizons 1994;2:202-14.

37. Pories WJ, Henzel JH, Rob CG, Strain WH. Acceleration of wound healing in man with zinc sulfate given by mouth. Lancet 1967;1:121-4.

38. Hallböök T, Lanier E. Serum zinc and healing of venous leg ulcers. Lancet 1972;1:780-2.

39. Chojkier M, Spanheimer R, Peterkovsky B. Specifically decreased collagen biosynthesis in scurvey dissociated from an effect on proline hydroxylation and correlated with body weight loss: in vitro studies in guinea pig calvarial bones. J Clin Invest 1983;72:826-35.

40. Hunt TK, Ehrlich P, Garcia JA, et al. Effect of vitamin A on reversing the inhibitory effect of cortisone on healing of open wounds in animals and man. Ann Surg 1969;170:633-40.

41. Levenson SM, Gruber CA, Rettura G, et al. Supplemental vitamin A prevents the acute radiation-induced defect in wound healing. Ann Surg 1984; 200:494-512.

42. Demetriou AA, Levenson SM, Rettura G, et al. Vitamin A and retinoic acid: induced fibroblast differentiation in vitro. Surgery 1985;98:931-34.

43. Levenson SM, Demetriou AA. Metabolic factors. In: Cohen IK, Diegelmann RF, Lindblad WJ, eds. Wound healing. Philadelphia: W.B. Saunders, 1992: 248-73.

44. Barbul A. Arginine: biochemistry, physiology and therapeutic implications. JPEN J Parenter Enteral Nutr 1986;10:227-38.

45. Ziegler TR, Smith RJ, Byrne TA, Wilmore DW. Potential role of glutamine supplementation in nutrition support. Clin Nutr 1993;12(suppl 1):S82-S90.

46. Barbul A, Rettura G, Wasserkrug HL, et al. Arginine stimulates lymphocyte immune responses in healthy humans. Surgery 1981;90:244–51.
47. Barbul A, Lazarou SA, Efron DT, et al. Arginine enhances wound healing and lymphocyte immune responses in humans. Surgery 1990;108:331–7.
48. Kirk SJ, Hurson M, Regan MC, et al. Arginine stimulates wound healing and immune function in elderly human subjects. Surgery 1993;114:155–60.
49. Daly JM, Reynolds J, Thom A, et al. Immune and metabolic effects of arginine in the surgical patient. Ann Surg 1988;208:512–23.
50. Besset A, Bonardet A, Rondouin G, Descomps B, Passouant P. Increase in sleep related growth hormone and prolactin secretion after chronic arginine aspartate administration in man. Acta Endocrinol 1982;99:18–23.
51. Smith RJ. Glutamine metabolism and its physiologic importance. JPEN J Parenter Enteral Nutr 1990;14:40S–4S.
52. Ziegler TR, Young LS. Therapeutic effects of specific nutrients. In: Rombeau JL, Rolandelli R, Caldwell MD, eds. Clinical nutrition: enteral and tube feeding, 3rd ed. Philadelphia: W.B. Saunders, 1996: in press.
53. Souba WW. Intestinal glutamine metabolism and nutrition. J Nutr Biochem 1993;4:2–9.
54. Stehle P, Mertes N, Puchstein Ch, et al. Effect of parenteral glutamine peptide supplements on muscle glutamine loss and nitrogen balance after major surgery. Lancet 1989;1:231–34.
55. Wernerman J, Hammarqvist F, Ali MR, Vinnars E. Glutamine and ornithine-alpha-ketoglutarate but not branched chain amino acids reduce the loss of muscle glutamine after surgical trauma. Metabolism 1989;38:63–6.
56. Ziegler TR, Young LS, Benfell K, et al. Clinical and metabolic efficacy of glutamine-supplemented parenteral nutrition following bone marrow transplantation: a randomized, double-blind, controlled study. Ann Intern Med 1992;116:821–8.
57. Van Der Hulst RRW, Van Kreel BK, von Meyenfeldt MF, et al. Glutamine and the preservation of gut integrity. Lancet 1993;341:1363–5.
58. Tremel H, Kienle B, Weilemann LS, Stehle P, Furst P. Glutamine dipeptide supplemented TPN maintains intestinal function in the critically ill. Gastroenterology 1994;107:1595–601.
59. Schloerb PR, Amare M. Total parenteral nutrition with glutamine in bone marrow transplantation and other clinical applications (a randomized, double-blind study). JPEN J Parenter Enteral Nutr 1993;17:407–13.
60. Scheltinga M, Young LS, Benfell K, et al. Glutamine-enriched intravenous feedings attenuate extracellular fluid expansion after a standard stress. Ann Surg 1991;214:385–95.
61. Ziegler TR, Bye RL, Persinger RL, Young LS, Wilmore DW. Glutamine-enriched parenteral nutrition increases circulating lymphocytes after bone marrow transplantation. JPEN J Parenter Enteral Nutr 1994;18:17S (abstr).
62. O'Riordain MG, Fearon KCH, Ross JA, et al. Glutamine-supplemented total parenteral nutrition enhances T-lymphocyte response in surgical patients undergoing colorectal resection. Ann Surg 1994;220:212–21.
63. Caldwell MD. Local glutamine metabolism in wounds and inflammation. Metabolism 1989;38(suppl 1):34–9.
64. Jain P, Khanna NK. Evaluation of anti-inflammatory and analgesic properties of L-glutamine. Agents Actions 1981;11:243–9.

65. Naik SR, Sheth UK. Effect of some amino acids on experimentally induced inflammation in rats. Indian J Pharmacol 1978;10:243-5.
66. Sies H, Stahl W, Sundquist AR. Antioxidant functions of vitamins: vitamins E and C, beta-carotene, and other carotenoids. Ann NY Acad Sci 1992; 669:7-20.
67. Hong RW, Rounds JD, Helton WS, Wilmore DW. Glutamine preserves liver glutathione after lethal hepatic injury. Ann Surg 1992;215:114-9.
68. Bray TM, Taylor CG. Enhancement of tissue glutathione for antioxidant and immune functions in malnutrition. Biochem Pharmacol 1994;47:2113-23.
69. Lash LH, Hagan TM, Jones DP. Exogenous glutathione protects intestinal epithelial cells from oxidative injury. Proc Natl Acad Sci USA 1986;83: 4461-5.
70. Jones DP, Kagan VE, Aust SD, Reed DJ, Omaye ST. Impact of nutrients on cellular lipid peroxidation and antioxidant defense system. Fund Appl Toxicol 1995;26:1-7.
71. Grimble RF. Nutritional antioxidants and modulation of inflammation: theory and practice. New Horizons 1994;2:175-85.
72. Wefers H, Sies H. The protection by ascorbate and glutathione against microsomal lipid peroxidation is dependent on vitamin E. Eur J Biochem 1988;174:353-7.
73. Coghlan JG, Flitter WD, Clutton SM, Ilsley CD, Rees A, Slater TF. Lipid peroxidation and changes in vitamin E levels during coronary artery bypass grafting. J Thorac Cardiovasc Surg 1993;106:268-74.
74. Goode HF, Cowley HC, Walker BE, Howdle PD, Webster NR. Decreased antioxidant status and increased lipid peroxidation in patients with septic shock and secondary organ dysfunction. Crit Care Med 1995;23:646-51.
75. Hammarqvist F, Luo J, Andersson K, Wernerman J. Glutathione and amino acid concentrations in ICU patients. JPEN J Parenter Enteral Nutr 1995; 19(suppl 1):19S (abstr).
76. Meister A. Glutathione deficiency produced by inhibition of its synthesis, and its reversal: applications in research and therapy. Pharmacol Ther 1991; 51:155-94.
77. Robinson MK, Rounds JD, Hong RW, Jacobs DO, Wilmore DW. Glutathione deficiency increases organ dysfunction after hemorrhagic shock. Surgery 1992;112:140-9.
78. Welbourne TC, King AB, Horton K. Enteral glutamine supports hepatic glutathione efflux during inflammation. J Nutr Biochem 1993;4:236-42.
79. Jensen JC, Schaefer R, Nwokedi E, et al. Prevention of chronic radiation enteropathy by dietary glutamine. Ann Surg Oncol 1994;1:157-63.
80. Uden S, Bilton D, Nathan L. Antioxidant therapy for recurrent pancreatitis: a placebo controlled trial. Aliment Pharmacol Ther 1990;4:357-71.
81. Madrerazo EG, Woronick CL, Hickingbotham N, et al. A randomized trial of replacement antioxidant vitamin therapy for neutrophil locomotory dysfunction in blunt trauma. J Trauma 1991;31:1142-50.
82. Youn Y-K, LaLonde C, Demling R. Trends in shock research: use of antioxidant therapy in shock and trauma. Circ Shock 1991;35:245-9.
83. Rabl H, Khoschsorur G, Colombo T, et al. A multivitamin infusion prevents lipid peroxidation and improves transplantation performance. Kidney Int 1993;43:912-7.
84. Matsuda T, Tanaka H, Williams S, et al. Reduced fluid volume requirement

for resuscitation of third-degree burns with high-dose vitamin C. J Burn Care Rehabil 1991;12:525–61.

85. Rabl H, Khoschsorur G, Petek W. Antioxidative vitamin treatment: effect on lipid and peroxidation and limb swelling after revascularization operations. World J Surg 1995;19:738–44.

86. Gottschlich MM, Jenkins M, Warden GD, et al. Differential effects of three dietary regimens on selected outcome variables in burn patients. JPEN J Parenter Enteral Nutr 1990;14:225–36.

87. Gottschlich MM, Warden GD. Vitamin supplementation in the patient with burns. J Burn Care Rehab 1990;11:275–9.

88. Berger MM, Cavadini C, Chiolero R, Guinchard S, Krupp S, Dirren H. Influence of large intakes of trace elements on recovery after major burns. Nutrition 1994;10:327–34.

89. Daly JM, Lieberman MD, Goldfine J, et al. Enteral nutrition with supplemental arginine, RNA, and omega-3 fatty acids in patients after operation: immunologic, metabolic, and clinical outcome. Surgery 1992;112:56–67.

90. Moore FA, Moore EE, Kudsk KA, et al. Clinical effects of an immune-enhancing diet for early postinjury enteral feeding. J Trauma 1994;37:607–15.

91. Bower RH, Cerra FB, Bershadsky B, et al. Early enteral administration of a formula (Impact) supplemented with arginine, nucleotides, and fish oil in intensive care unit patients: results of a multicenter, prospective, randomized, clinical trial. Crit Care Med 1995;23:436–49.

92. Bettger WJ, McKeehan WL. Mechanisms of cellular nutrition. Physiol Rev 1986;66:1–24.

93. Eagle H. Metabolic controls in cultured mammalian cells. Science 1965; 148:42–51.

94. Rubin AH, Chu B. Reversible regulation by magnesium in chick embryo fibroblast proliferation. J Cell Physiol 1978;94:13–9.

95. Rubin H. Inhibition of DNA synthesis in animal cells by ethylene diamine tetraacetate, and its reversal by zinc. Proc Natl Acad Sci USA 1972; 69:712–6.

96. Ley KD, Tobey RA. Regulation of initiation of DNA synthesis in Chinese hamster cells. II. Induction of DNA synthesis and cell division by isoleucine and glutamine in G_1-arrested cells in suspension culture. J Cell Biol 1970; 47:453–9.

97. Wylie AH, Kerr JFR, Currie AR. Cell death: the significance of apoptosis. Int Rev Cytol 1980;68:251–306.

98. Haussinger D, Roth E, Lang F, et al. Cellular hydration state: an important determinant of protein catabolism in health and disease. Lancet 1993; 341:1330–2.

99. Harp JB, Goldstein S, Phillips LS. Nutrition and somatomedin XXII. Molecular regulation of IGF-I by amino acid availability in cultured hepatocytes. Diabetes 1991;40:95–101.

100. D'Ercole AJ, Stiles AD, Underwood LE. Tissue concentrations of somatomedin C: further evidence for multiple sites of synthesis and paracrine or autocrine mechanisms of action. Proc Natl Acad Sci USA 1984;81:935–9.

101. Pierce GF, Mustoe TA. Pharmacologic enhancement of wound healing. Annu Rev Med 1995;46:467–81.

102. Hinton P, Allison SP, Littlejohn S, et al. Insulin and glucose to reduce catabolic response to injury in burned patients. Lancet 1971;1:767–9.

103. Woolfson AMJ, Heatley RV, Allison SP. Insulin to inhibit protein catabolism after injury. N Engl J Med 1979;30:14–7.

104. Shizgal HM, Posner B. Insulin and the efficacy of total parenteral nutrition. Am J Clin Nutr 1989;50:1355–63.

105. Deuel TF, Kawahara R, Mustoe TA, Pierce GF. Growth factors and wound healing: platelet-derived growth factor as a model cytokine. Annu Rev Med 1991;42:567–84.

106. Steed DL. The Diabetic Ulcer Study Group. Clinical evaluation of recombinant human platelet-derived growth factor (rhPDGF-BB) for the treatment of lower extremity diabetic ulcers. J Vasc Surg 1995;18:139–46.

107. Robson MC, Phillips LG, Thomason A, et al. Platelet-derived growth factor-BB in chronic pressure ulcers. Lancet 1992;339:23–5.

108. Mustoe TA, Pierce GF, Morishima C, Deuel TF. Growth factor induced acceleration of tissue repair through direct and inductive activities. J Clin Invest 1991;87:694–703.

109. Brown GL, Nanney LB, Griffen J, et al. Enhancement of wound healing by topical treatment with epidermal growth factor. N Engl J Med 1989;321:76–9.

110. Goodlad RA, Lee CY, Wright NA. Cell proliferation in the small intestine and colon of intravenously fed rats: effects of urogastrone-epidermal growth factor. Cell Prolif 1992;25:393–404.

111. Petschow BW, Carter DL, Hutton GD. Influence of orally administered epidermal growth factor on normal and damaged intestinal mucosa in rats. J Pediatr Gastroenterol Nutr 1993;17:49–58.

112. Chaet MS, Arya G, Ziegler MM, Warner BW. Epidermal growth factor enhances intestinal adaptation after massive small bowel resection. J Pediatr Surg 1994;29:1035–9.

113. Housley RM, Morris CF, Boyle W, et al. Keratinocyte growth factor induces proliferation of hepatocytes and epithelial cells throughout the rat gastrointestinal tract. J Clin Invest 1994;94:1764–77.

114. Pierce GF, Tarpley J, Yanagihara D, et al. PDGF-BB, TGF-β1, and basic FGF in dermal wound healing: neovessel and matrix formation and cessation of repair. Am J Pathol 1992;140:1375–88.

115. Ziegler TR, Jacobs DO. Anabolic hormones in nutritional support. In: Torosian MH, ed. Nutrition for the hospitalized patient: basic science and principles of practice. New York: Marcel-Dekker, 1995:207–32.

116. Steenfos HH, Jansson JO. Gene expression of insulin-like growth factor-I and IGF-I receptor during wound healing in rats. Eur J Surg 1992;158:327–31.

117. Gartner MH, Benson JD, Caldwell MD. Insulin-like growth factors I and II expression in the healing wound. J Surg Res 1992;52:389–94.

118. Clemmons DR, Underwood LE. Nutritional regulation of IGF-I and IGF binding proteins. Annu Rev Nutr 1991;11:393–412.

119. Tavakkol A, Elder JT, Griffiths CEM, et al. Expression of growth hormone receptor, insulin-like growth factor-I (IGF-I) and IGF-I receptor mRNA and proteins in human skin. J Invest Dermatol 1992;99:343–9.

120. Steenfos HH, Jansson JO. Growth hormone stimulates granulation tissue formation and insulin-like growth factor-I gene expression in wound chambers in the rat. J Endocrinol 1992;132:293–8.

121. Jorgensen PH, Bang C, Andreassen TT, Flyvbjerg A, Orskov H. Dose-response study of the effect of growth hormone on mechanical properties of skin graft wounds. J Surg Res 1995;58:295–301.

122. Christensen H, Oxlund H, Laurberg S. Postoperative biosynthetic human growth hormone increases the strength and collagen deposition of experimental colonic anastomoses. Int J Colorectal Dis 1991;6:133–8.
123. Christensen H, Flyvbjerg A, Orskov H, et al. Effect of growth hormone on the inflammatory activity of experimental colitis in rats. Scand J Gastroenterol 1993;28:503–11.
124. Suh DY, Hunt TK, Spencer EM. Insulin-like growth factor-I reverses the impairment of wound healing induced by corticosteroids in rats. Endocrinology 1992;131:2399–403.
125. Kratz G, Lke M, Gidlund M. Insulin-like growth factors -1 and -2 and their role in the re-epithelialization of wounds; interactions with insulin-like growth factor binding protein type 1. Scand J Plast Reconstr Surg Hand Surg 1994;28:107–12.
126. Jyung RW, Mustoe JA, Busby WH, Clemmons DR. Increased wound-breaking strength induced by insulin-like growth factor-I in combination with insulin-like growth factor binding protein-1. Surgery 1994;115:233–9.
127. Tsuboi R, Shi CM, Sata C, Cox GN, Ogawa H. Co-administration of insulin-like growth factor-I (IGF-I) and IGF binding protein-1 stimulates wound healing in animal models. J Invest Dermatol 1995;104:199–203.
128. Hamon GA, Hunt TK, Spencer EM. In vivo effects of systemic insulin-like growth factor-I alone and complexed with insulin-like growth factor binding protein-3 on corticosteroid suppressed wounds. Growth Regul 1993;3:53–6.
129. Greenhalgh DG, Hummel RP, Albertson S, Breeden MP. Synergistic actions of platelet-derived growth factors and insulin-like growth factors in vivo. Enhancement of tissue repair in genetically diabetic mice. Wound Rep Regen 1993;1:69–81.
130. McKeehan WL, McKeehan KA, Calkins D. Epidermal growth factor modifies CA^{+2}, MG^{+2}, and 2-oxocarboxylic acid, but not K^+ and phosphate ion requirement for multiplication of human fibroblasts. Exp Cell Res 1982; 140:25–30.
131. Lund PK. Nutritional control of genes encoding gastrointestinal peptides. In: Berdanier CD, Hargrove JL, eds. Nutrition and gene expression. Boca Raton, FL: CRC Press, 1993:91–116.
132. Donovan SM, Odle J. Growth factors in milk as mediators of infant development. Annu Rev Nutr 1994;14:147–67.
133. Baumrucker CR, Blum JW. Effects of dietary recombinant human insulin-like growth factor-I on concentrations of hormones and growth factors in the blood of newborn calves. J Endocrinol 1994;140:15–21.
134. Phillips LS, Unterman TG. Somatomedin activity in disorders of nutrition and metabolism. Clin Endocrinol Metab 1984;13:145–60.
135. Thissen J-P, Ketelslegers J-M, Underwood LE. Nutritional regulation of the insulin-like growth factors. Endocr Rev 1994;15:80–101.
136. Straus DS. Nutritional regulation of hormones and growth factors that control mammalian growth. FASEB J 1994;8:6–12.
137. Grant DB, Hambley J, Becker AD, Primstone BL. Reduced sulphation factor in undernourished children. Arch Dis Child 1973;48:596–600.
138. Hintz RL, Suskind R, Amatayakul K, Thanangkul O, Olson R. Plasma somatomedin and growth hormone values in children with protein-energy malnutrition. J Pediatr 1978;92:153–6.

139. Smith SR, Edgar PJ, Pozefsky T, Chetri MK, Prout TE. Growth hormone in adults with protein calorie malnutrition. Endocrinology 1974;39:53–62.
140. Ho KY, Veldhuis JD, Johnson ML, et al. Fasting enhances growth hormone secretion and amplifies the complex rhythms of growth hormone secretion in man. J Clin Invest 1988;81:968–75.
141. Vance ML, Hartman ML, Thorner MO. growth hormone and nutrition. Horm Res 1992;38:85–8.
142. Clemmons DR, Klibanski AM, Underwood LE, McArthur JW, Ridgway EC, Beitins IZ, Van Wyk JJ. Reduction of plasma immunoreactive somatomedin-C during fasting in humans. J Clin Endocrinol Metab 1981;53:1247–50.
143. Isley WL, Underwood LE, Clemmons DR. Dietary components that regulate serum somatomedin-C concentrations in humans. J Clin Invest 1983;71:175–82.
144. Isley WL, Underwood LE, Clemmons DR. Changes in plasma somatomedin-C in response to ingestion of diets with variable protein and energy content. JPEN J Parenter Enteral Nutr 1984;8:407–11.
145. Snyder DK, Clemmons DR, Underwood LE. Dietary carbohydrate content determines responsiveness to growth hormone in energy-restricted humans. J Clin Endocrinol Metab 1989;69:745–52.
146. Clemmons DR, Seek MM, Underwood LE. Supplemental essential aminoacids augment the somatomedin-C/insulin-like factor-I response to refeeding after fasting. Metabolism 1985;34:391–5.
147. Kimbrough T, Shernan S, Ziegler TR, Scheltinga M, Wilmore DW. Insulin-like growth factor I (IGF-I) response is comparable following intravenous and subcutaneous administration of growth hormone. J Surg Res 1991;51:472–76.
148. Bornfeldt KE, Arnqvist HJ, Enberg B, Mathews LS, Norstedt G. Regulation of insulin-like growth factor-I and growth hormone receptor gene expression by diabetes and nutritional state in rat tissues. J Endocrinol 1989;12:651–6.
149. Maiter D, Maes M, Underwood LE, Fliesen T, Gerard G, Ketalslegers JM. Early changes in serum concentrations of somatomedin-C induced by dietary protein deprivation in rats: contributions of growth hormone receptor and post-receptor defects. J Endocrinol 1988;118:113–20.
150. Ullrich AA, Gray AW, Tam T, et al. Insulin-like growth factor I receptor primary structure: comparison with insulin receptor suggests structural determinants that define functional specificity. EMBOJ 1986;5:2503–12.
151. Lowe WL, Adamo M, Werner H, Roberts CT, LeRoith D. Regulation by fasting of rat insulin-like growth factor I and its receptor: effects on gene expression and binding. J Clin Invest 1989;84:619–26.
152. Knopf R, Conn J, Fajans S, Floyd JC, Gutsche EM, Rull JA. Plasma growth hormone response to intravenous administration of amino acids. J Clin Endocrinol 1965;25:1140–3.
153. Merimee TJ, Lillicrop DA, Rabinowitz D. Effect of arginine on serum levels of human growth hormone. Lancet 1965;2:668–70.
154. Barbul A. Arginine: biochemistry, physiology, and therapeutic implications. JPEN J Parenter Enteral Nutr 1986;10:227–38.
155. Besset A, Bonardet A, Rondouin G, Descomps B, Passouant P. Increase in sleep related GH and Prl secretion after chronic arginine aspartate administration in man. Acta Endocrinol 1982;99:18–23.
156. Isidori A, Lo Monaco A, Cappa M. A study of growth hormone release in man after oral administration of amino acids. Curr Med Res Opin 1981;7:475–81.

157. Cossack ZT. Somatomedin-C and zinc status in rats as affected by zinc, protein and food intake. Br J Nutr 1986;56:163-9.
158. Droke EA, Spears JW, Armstrong JD, Kegley EB, Simpson RB. Dietary zinc affects serum concentrations of insulin and insulin-like growth factor-I in growing lambs. J Nutr 1993;123:13-9.
159. Roth HP, Kirchgebner M. Influence of alimentary zinc deficiency on the concentration of growth hormone (GH), insulin-like growth factor-I (IGF-I) and insulin in the serum of force-fed rats. Horm Metab Res 1994;26:404-8.
160. Tarnow P, Agren M, Steenfos H, Jansson J-O. Topical zinc oxide treatment increases endogenous gene expression of insulin-like growth factor-I in granulation tissue from porcine wounds. Scand J Plast Reconstr Surg 1994; 28:255-9.
161. Ninh NX, Thissen J-P, Maiter D, Adam E, Mulumba N, Ketelslegers J-M. Reduced liver insulin-like growth factor-I gene expression in young zinc-deprived rats is associated with a decrease in liver growth hormone (GH) receptors and serum GH-binding protein. J Endocrinol 1995;144:449-56.
162. Cossack ZT. Effect of zinc level in the refeeding diet in previously starved rats on plasma somatomedin-C levels. J Pediatr Gastroenterol Nutr 1988;7:441-5.
163. Tamada H, Nezu R, Matsuo M, Takagi Y, Okada A, Imamura I. Zinc-deficient diet impairs adaptive changes in the remaining intestine after massive small bowel resection in the rat. Br J Surg 1992;79:959-63.
164. Mantell MP, Ziegler TR, Roth BA, et al. Resection-induced colonic adaptation is augmented by IGF-I and associated with upregulation of colonic IGF-I mRNA. Am J Physiol 1995;269:G974-80.
165. Dorup I, Flyvbjerg A, Everts ME, Clausen T. Role of insulin-like growth factor-I and growth hormone in growth inhibition induced by magnesium and zinc deficiencies. Br J Nutr 1991;66:505-21.
166. Flyvbjerg A, Dorup I, Everts ME, Orskov H. Evidence that potassium deficiency induces growth retardation through reduced circulating levels of growth hormone and insulin-like growth factor-I. Metabolism 1991;40:769-75.
167. Rudman D, Millikan WJ, Richardson TJ, Bixler TJ, Stackhouse WJ, McGarrity WC. Elemental balances during intravenous hyperalimentation of underweight adult subjects. J Clin Invest 1975;55:94-104.
168. Molina PE, Fan J, Lang CH, Abumrad NN. Thiamine deficiency modulation of the IGF system response to growth hormone. Clin Nutr 1994;14(suppl 2):18.
169. Liljedahl S, Gemzell C, Plantin L, et al. Effect of human growth hormone in patients with severe burns. Acta Chir Scand 1961;122:1-14.
170. Wilmore DW, Moylan JA, Bristow BF, et al. Anabolic effects of human growth hormone and high caloric feedings following thermal injury. Surg Gynecol Obstet 1974;138:875-84.
171. Jiang ZM, He GZ, Zhang SY, et al. Low-dose growth hormone and hypocaloric nutrition attenuate the protein-catabolic response after major operation. Ann Surg 1989;210:513-24.
172. Vara-Thorbeck R, Guerrero JA, Rosell J, et al. Exogenous growth hormone: effects on the catabolic response to surgically produced acute stress and on postoperative immune function. World J Surg 1993;17:530-8.
173. Mjaaland M, Unneberg K, Larsson J, et al. Growth hormone after abdominal surgery attenuated forearm glutamine, alanine, 3-methylhistidine, and total amino acid efflux in patients receiving total parenteral nutrition. Ann Surg 1993;217:413-22.

174. Takaki K, Tashiro T, Yamamori H, et al. Recombinant human growth hormone and protein metabolism of burned rats and esophagectomized patients. Nutrition 1995;11:22–6.
175. Ziegler TR, Lazarus JM, Young LS, Hakim R, Wilmore DW. Effects of recombinant human growth hormone in adults receicing maintenance hemodialysis. J Am Soc Nephrol 1991;2:1130–5.
176. Schulman G, Wingard RL, Hutchison RL, et al. The effects of recombinant human growth hormone and intradialytic parenteral nutrition in malnourished hemodialysis patients. Am J Kidney Dis 1993;21:527–34.
177. Pape GS, Friedman M, Underwood LE, Clemmons DR. The effect of growth hormone on weight gain and pulmonary function in patients with chronic obstructive lung disease. Chest 1991;99:1495–500.
178. Mulligan K, Grunfeld C, Hellerstein MK, Schambelan M. Anabolic effects of recombinant human growth hormone in patients with wasting associated with human immunodeficiency virus infection. J Clin Endocrinol Metab 1993; 77:956–62.
179. Ziegler TR, Rombeau J, Young LS, et al. Administration of recombinant human growth hormone enhances the metabolic efficacy of parenteral nutrition: a double-blind, randomized, controlled study. J Clin Endocrinol Metab 1992;74:865–73.
180. Byrne TA, Morrissey TB, Gatzen C, et al. Anabolic therapy with growth hormone accelerates gain in lean tissue in surgical patients requiring nutritional rehabilitation. Ann Surg 1993;218:400–18.
181. Ziegler TR, Young LS, Manson J McK, Wilmore DW. Metabolic effects of recombinant human growth hormone in patients receiving parenteral nutrition. Ann Surg 1988;208:6–16.
182. Suchner U, Rothkopt MM, Stanislaus G, et al. Growth hormone and pulmonary disease. Metabolic effects in patients receiving parenteral nutrition. Arch Intern Med 1990;150:1225–30.
183. Pichard C, Kyle U, Chevrolet JC, et al. Recombinant growth hormone (rGH) effect on muscle function in ventilated chronic obstructive pulmonary disease (COPD). JPEN J Parenter Enteral Nutr 1994;18(suppl 1):35S.
184. Ziegler TR, Young LS, Ferrari-Baliviera E, Demling RH, Wilmore DW. Use of human growth hormone combined with nutritional support in a critical care unit. JPEN J Parenter Enteral Nutr 1990;14:574–81.
185. Douglas RG, Humberstone DA, Haystead A, Shaw JH. Metabolic effects of recombinant human growth hormone: isotopic studies in the postoperative state and during total parenteral nutrition. Br J Surg 1990;77:785–90.
186. Voerman HJ, Strack Van Schijndel RJM, Groeneveld ABJ, et al. Effect of recombinant human growth hormone in patients with severe sepsis. Ann Surg 1992;216:648–55.
187. Jeevanandam M, Ali MR, Holaday NJ, Peterson SR. Adjuvant recombinant human growth hormone normalizes plasma amino acids in parenterally fed trauma patients. JPEN J Parenter Enteral Nutr 1995;19:137–44.
188. Shernan SK, Demling RH, LaLonde C, Lowe D, Erlanson E, Wilmore DW. Growth hormone enhances re-epithelialization of human split-thickness skin graft donor sites. Surg Forum 1989;40:37–9.
189. Herndon DN, Barrow RE, Kunkle KR, et al. Effects of recombinant human growth hormone on donor site healing in severely burned children. Ann Surg 1990;212:424–9.

190. Gatzen C, Scheltinga MR, Kimbrough TD, Jacobs DO, Wilmore DW. Growth hormone attenuates the abnormal distribution of body water in critically ill surgical patients. Surgery 1992;112:181-7.
191. Kimbrough T, Shernan S, Ziegler TR, Scheltinga MS, Wilmore DW. Insulin-like growth factor I (IGF-I) response is comparable following intravenous and subcutaneous administration of growth hormone. J Surg Res 1991;51:472-6.
192. Dahn MA, Lange P, Jacobs LA. Insulin-like growth factor I production is inhibited in human sepsis. Arch Surg 1988;123:1409-14.
193. Belcher HJ, Mercer D, Judkins KC, et al. Biosynthetic human growth hormone in burned patients: a pilot study. Burns 1989;15:99-107.
194. Roth E, Valentini L, Semsroth M, et al. Resistance of nitrogen metabolism to growth hormone treatment in the early phase after injury in patients with multiple injuries. J Trauma 1995;38:136-41.
195. Boulware SD, Tamborlane W, Sherwin R. Diverse effects of insulin-like growth factor-I on glucose, lipid and amino acid metabolism. Am J Physiol 1992;262:130-33.
196. Clemmons DR, Smith-Banks A, Celniker AC, Underwood LE. Reversal of diet-induced catabolism by infusion of recombinant insulin-like growth factor-I (IGF-I) in humans. J Clin Endocrinnol Metab 1992;75:1192-7.
197. Kupfer SR, Underwood LE, Baxter RC, Clemmons DR. Enhancement of the anabolic effects of growth hormone and insulin-like growth factor I by use of both agents simultaneously. J Clin Invest 1993;91:391-6.
198. Thompson WA, Coyle SM, Lazarus D, Lowry SL. The metabolic effects of a continuous infusion of insulin-like growth factor (IGF-I) in parenterally fed men. Surg Forum 1991;42:23-5.
199. Chen SA, Bukar JG, Mohler MA, et al. Recombinant human IGF-I infusion results in transient improvement in nitrogen balance: evidence for IGF-I autoregulation. Presented at the 75th Annual Meeting of the Endocrine Society, Las Vegas, NV, 1993.
200. Cioffi WG, Gore DC, Rue LW, et al. Insulin-like growth factor-I lowers protein oxidation in patients with thermal injury. Ann Surg 1994;220:310-9.
201. Goeters C, Mertes N, Tacke J, et al. Repeated administration of recombinant human insulin-like growth factor-I in patients after gastric surgery: effects on metabolic and hormonal patterns. Ann Surg 1995;222:646-53.
202. Atkinson JB, Kosi M, Srikanth MS, Takano K, Costin G. Growth hormone reverses impaired wound healing in protein-malnourished rats treated with corticosteroids. J Pediatr Surg 1992;27:1026-8.
203. Majumdar APN. Postnatal undernutrition: effect of epidermal growth factor on growth and function of the gastrointestinal tract in rats. J Pediatr Gastroenterol Nutr 1984;3:618-25.
204. Jacobs DO, Evans DA, Mealy K, O'Dwyer S, Smith RJ, Wilmore DW. Combined effects of glutamine and epidermal growth factor (EGF) on the rat intestine. Surgery 1988;108:358-64.
205. Salloum RM, Stevens BR, Schultz GS, Souba WW. Regulation of small intestinal glutamine transport by epidermal growth factor. Surgery 1993;113:552-9.
206. Ko TC, Beauchamp RD, Townsend CM, Thompson JC. Glutamine is essential for epidermal growth factor-stimulated intestinal cell proliferation. Surgery 1993;114:147-54.
207. Ziegler TR, Benfell K, Smith RJ, et al. Safety and metabolic effects of

L-glutamine administration in humans. JPEN J Parenter Enteral Nutr 1990;14:137S–146S.
208. Welbourne TC. Increased plasma bicarbonate and growth hormone after an oral glutamine load. Am J Clin Nutr 1995;61:1058–61.
209. Hammarqvist F, Stromberg C, Decken von der A, et al. Biosynthetic human growth hormone preserves both muscle protein synthesis and the decrease in muscle free glutamine, and improves whole-body nitrogen economy after operation. Ann Surg 1992;216:184–91.
210. Nolan EM, Masters JN, Dunn A. Growth hormone regulation of hepatic glutamine synthetase mRNA levels in rats. Mol Cell Endocrinol 1990; 69:101–10.
211. Ziegler TR, Mantell MP, Rombeau JL, Smith RJ. Effects of glutamine and IGF-I administration on intestinal growth and the IGF pathway after partial small bowel resection. JPEN J Parenter Enteral Nutr 1994;18(suppl 1):20S.
212. Houdijk APJ, Van Leeuwen PAM, Boermeester MA, et al. Glutamine-enriched enteral diet increases splanchnic blood flow in the rat. Am J Physiol 1994;267:G1035–40.
213. Byrne TA, Morrissey TB, Nattakom TV, Ziegler TR, Wilmore DW. Growth hormone glutamine and a modified diet enhance nutrient absorption in patients with the severe short bowel syndrome. JPEN J Parenter Enteral Nutr 1995;19:296–302.
214. Byrne TA, Persinger RL, Young LS, Ziegler TR, Wilmore DW. A new treatment for patients with the short-bowel syndrome: growth hormone, glutamine and a modified diet. Ann Surg 1995;222:243–55.

Part III

Endogenous Growth Factors and Wound Healing

Part III

Endogenous Growth Factors and Wound Healing

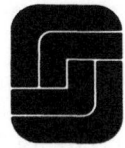

9

Fibroblast Growth Factor Receptors

David M. Ornitz and Gabriel Waksman

Fibroblast growth factor (FGF) was discovered in the 1970s as an activity that stimulates the proliferation of 3T3 cells (1). Currently, FGFs comprise a family of nine structurally related proteins (FGF-1 to -9) (reviewed in 2–6). FGFs are expressed in specific spatial and temporal patterns and are involved in developmental processes, angiogenesis, wound healing, and tumorigenesis (3, 4, 7). The purification of basic FGF (FGF-2) and other related growth factors has been facilitated by the discovery that FGFs have a high affinity for heparin (2). These growth factors can be assayed on a variety of cells or embryos, in vitro, resulting in growth, survival, or differentiation (8–11).

Recently, four distinct high-affinity FGF receptors have been cloned (corresponding to four distinct genes) (12–19). These receptors bind members of the FGF family of growth factors with varying affinity (19–22). Alternative messenger RNA (mRNA) splicing patterns lead to isoforms of these receptors that have unique ligand binding properties (21, 23). An additional mechanism regulating FGF activity involves heparin or heparan sulfate proteoglycans (HSPGs), molecules that are required for ligand-receptor interactions in vitro and possibly in vivo (18, 24). The proposed mechanism by which FGF activates its receptor involves the formation of a trimolecular complex between ligand, receptor, and a heparin-like molecule (24). The heparin–FGF-receptor complex facilitates receptor dimerization, which is required for the activation of downstream signaling pathways (25, 26).

This chapter discusses regulatory mechanisms that mediate FGF receptor activation and signaling, reviews mutations in FGFs and FGF receptors that have been engineered in mice, and reviews a series of mutations that have been discovered in three of the four FGF receptors that result in skeletal and craniofacial diseases in humans.

Primary Structure of the FGF Receptor

FGF receptors are members of the receptor tyrosine kinase superfamily (27). These proteins contain an extracellular ligand-binding domain, a single transmembrane domain, and an intracellular tyrosine kinase domain. Structural features of the FGF receptor must provide binding specificity for the nine FGF ligands, a mechanism to be activated by ligand, and a mechanism to activate downstream signaling pathways. The extracellular region is responsible for ligand-binding specificity and for ligand-mediated receptor dimerization. Upon receptor dimerization, the intracellular region becomes activated by one or more transphosphorylation events (28) and then becomes competent to interact with downstream signaling molecules.

The FGF receptor extracellular region contains three immunoglobulin (Ig)-like domains, a heparin-binding domain, and a stretch of seven conserved acidic amino acids (Fig. 9.1) (12). Alternative mRNA splicing in the extracellular domain creates several forms of the FGF receptor that have differential ligand-binding properties. One major splicing event results in the skipping of exons encoding the amino-terminal Ig-like domain (domain I) leading to a two Ig-like domain form of the receptor (Fig. 9.1) (29). The ligand-binding properties of the two and three Ig-like domain receptors are similar. However, the short form of the receptor may have higher affinity toward some FGFs than the long form (30). A change in splicing from the three Ig-like domain form of FGF receptor 1 to the two Ig-like domain receptor correlates with the progression of low-grade astrocytomas toward malignant astrocytomas (31) and with the progression of pancreatic tumors toward malignancy (32). Although this correlation in the expression of FGF

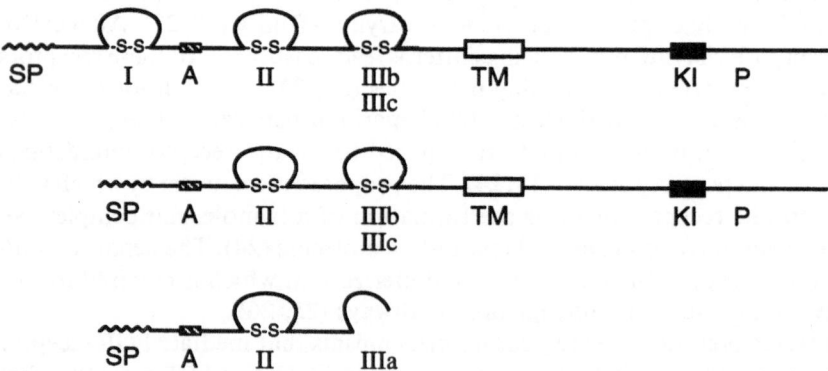

FIGURE 9.1. The primary structure of FGF receptors. Top: The full-length FGF receptor with three Ig-like domains. The major alternative splicing pathways will express either Ig-like domain IIIb or IIIc. The stippled region beginning in Ig-like domain III is the sequence subject to alternative splicing. Middle: Short form of the FGF receptor expressing Ig-like domains II and III. Bottom: Secreted form of the FGF-receptor expressing Ig-like domains II and IIIa. SP, signal peptide; A, acidic amino acid domain; I, II, III, Ig-like domains; TM, transmembrane domain; KI, kinase insert domain; P, site of putative receptor autophosphorylation; s-s, disulfide bond.

splice variants is not necessarily an etiologic event in the progression of these tumors, it may account for an increased responsiveness of these tumors to available ligand and give these cells a growth advantage.

Another RNA splicing event uses one of two unique exons and results in three alternative versions of Ig-like domain III (referred to as domains IIIa, IIIb, IIIc) (21, 29, 33). FGF receptors containing alternatively spliced Ig-like domains IIIb ("b") and IIIc ("c") are expressed on the cell surface and bind FGF ligands. The IIIa ("a") splice form of the FGF receptor terminates within Ig-like domain III to yield a secreted extracellular FGF binding protein (34) with no known signaling capability. Homologous isoforms of FGF receptors 1 to 4 (containing domains I, II, and IIIc) as well as alternatively spliced forms of FGF receptors 1 to 3 (containing domains I, II, and IIIb) have unique ligand-binding specificities (see below). Ligand-binding specificity is therefore determined both by sequence differences between homologous FGF receptors as well as by alternative splicing within a given FGF receptor. In addition to the splicing events discussed here, several other splicing events have been reported, both in the extra- and intracellular domains of FGF receptors 1 and 2 (35, 36). The biologic significance of these "minor" splicing events is not known.

The intracellular region of the FGF receptor can be divided into several regions (27). The region between the transmembrane domain and tyrosine kinase domain, referred to as the juxtatransmembrane region, is moderately conserved between the four FGF receptors (39–76%). The tyrosine kinase domain is split by a kinase insert sequence. The two tyrosine kinase domains are highly conserved (75–92%), while the kinase insert sequence is poorly conserved between the four FGF receptors (7–50%). The carboxy-terminal regions of the FGF receptors are only moderately conserved, sharing 42% to 62% amino acid identity (27). The capacity to signal a mitogenic response clearly differs among the FGF receptors. For example, in BaF3 cells, FGF receptors 1 and 2 signal well, FGF receptor 3 signals poorly, and FGF receptor 4 is inactive (33, 37–40). Presumably the less highly conserved regions of the intracellular domains confer specificity to the different FGF receptors toward downstream signaling molecules.

Alternative Splicing in Immunoglobulin-Like Domain III

DNA encompassing the carboxy-terminal half of Ig-like domain III in FGF receptors 1, 2, and 3 has a remarkable conservation in both the number and arrangement of the intron/exon boundaries (33, 41–43). Alternative splicing of these exons results in either "b" or "c" isoforms of the FGF receptor and dramatically effects ligand-receptor binding specificity (Fig. 9.2; Table 9.1) (23, 33). Expression of these various receptor isoforms

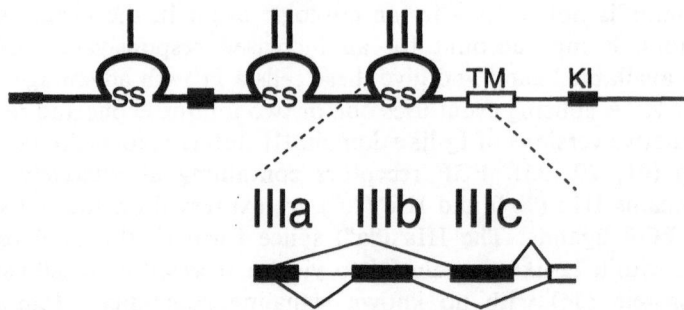

FIGURE 9.2. Alternative splicing of FGF receptors in the immunoglobulin-like domain III region. Alternatively spliced exons, IIIa, IIIb, and IIIc are shown. Abbreviations as in Fig. 9.1.

appears to be regulated in a tissue-specific manner (44–46). Although the expression patterns of FGF receptor 1, 2, and 3 are distinct, analysis of this splicing event demonstrates that utilization of either the "b" or "c" exon is dependent on the identity of the cell that synthesizes the mRNA. The "b" exon appears to be expressed in epithelial lineages, while the "c" exon is expressed in mesenchymal lineages (43, 44, 47). Thus, the exon that is utilized during mRNA splicing reflects the cells relationship to mesodermal and ectodermal lineages.

The tissue-specific expression of FGF receptor splice variants and of individual FGF ligands are critical elements that regulate the activation of the FGF receptor signaling pathways. Both misexpression of an FGF ligand or aberrant splicing of an FGF receptor can result in the activation of an autocrine signaling pathway and ensuing uncontrolled cell proliferation. For example, NIH3T3 fibroblasts normally express keratinocyte growth factor (KGF/FGF-7) and the "c" splice forms of FGF receptors 1 and 2. These cells do not exhibit a transformed phenotype because FGF-7 shows no binding activity for "c" splice forms of FGF receptors. In contrast, expression of the "b" splice variant of FGF receptor 2 in fibroblasts establishes an autocrine signaling pathway and is transforming for these cells (48). Switching in splice form expression from FGF receptor 2b to that of FGF receptor 2c has also been implicated in the progression of prostate cancer from a nonmalignant, stromal-dependent, epithelial tumor to an invasive, stromal-independent, undifferentiated tumor (44). This splice form change alters the ligand-binding profile of FGF receptor 2 for both FGF-2 and FGF-7, and is likely to contribute to the stromal-independence of the tumor. Concomitantly with this FGF receptor 2 isoform switch, upregulation of alternative ligands such as FGF-2 have been observed within these epithelial cells. This expression of alternate ligands by the tumor itself may induce a stimulatory autocrine loop that can also lead to tumor cell autonomy (44).

TABLE 9.1. Ligand-receptor specificity.

Receptor	Ig-like domain	Ligand[#]								
		aFGF FGF-1	bFGF FGF-2	int-2 FGF-3	k-FGF FGF-4	FGF-5	FGF-6	KGF FGF-7	AIGF FGF-8	GAF FGF-9
FGFR1 (flg)	I,II,IIIc	+++	+++		+++	++	++	-	-	+
	I,II,IIIb	+++	+++		+	-	-	-	-	-
	II,IIIc	+++	+++		+					-
	II,IIIb	+++	+	-						
	II,IIIa	+	++	++						
FGFR2 (bek)	I,II,IIIc	+++	++	-	+++	+	++	-	+	+++
	I,II,IIIb	+++	-	+	+	-	-	++	-	-
	II,IIIc	+						+++		
(KGFR)	II,IIIb	+++	+++					+++		
FGFR3	I,II,IIIc	+++	+++		+	+	-	-	++	+++
	I,II,IIIb	+++	-	-	-	-	-	-	-	++
	II,IIIc		+++	-						+++
	II,IIIb									
FGFR4	I,II,IIIc	+++	±,++	-	++	-	++	-	++	++
	II,IIIc	+++	+++		+++		++	-		

#Original FGF nomenclature is in the top row, the current FGF nomenclature is listed below, aFGF, acidic FGF; bFGF, basic FGF; int-2, mouse mammary tumor virus integration site; k-FGF, kaposi sarcoma FGF, also known as hst (FGF cloned from human stomach tumors); KGF, keratinocyte growth factor; AIGF, androgen induced growth factor; GAF, glia activating factor.
*Relative affinities for FGF ligands with different alternatively spliced forms of FGF receptors. Assays include receptor binding and mitogenic responsiveness. These data are compiled from several published and unpublished studies (see text). Blanks, unknown.

Ligand-Binding Specificities

Receptor-binding specificity is an essential mechanism for regulating FGF activity and is regulated by both alternative splicing of the FGF receptor and by sequence differences between the nine FGF ligands. Since the discovery of FGF receptors, investigators have been attempting to determine which ligand-receptor pairs are biochemically functional. More importantly, physiologically relevant ligand-receptor pairs must be identified. Knowledge of the paired interactions between the nine known FGFs and the major splice forms of the four known FGF receptors is essential to begin to discern the functions of FGFs during development.

Most if not all FGF receptors bind FGF-1 (aFGF) with high affinity (13, 20–22, 24, 33, 34, 36, 49–54). FGF-1 thus appears to be a universal FGF ligand and may functionally define a core binding domain of the FGF receptor molecule. In contrast to FGF-1, the best example of a highly specific FGF ligand is FGF-7 [keratinocyte growth factor (KGF)]. As discussed above, this ligand interacts exclusively with the "b" splice forms of FGF receptor 2 (FGF receptor 2b). However, FGF receptor 2b still can be activated by a number of other FGF ligands, including FGF-1, FGF-3, and FGF-4 (23, 38, 39). The ability to bind FGF-7 depends on the primary sequence of the "b" exon of FGF receptor 2. For example, FGF receptors 1b and 3b cannot be activated by FGF-7 and do not bind this ligand. FGF receptor 3 can, however, be engineered to bind FGF-7 simply by replacing the carboxyl terminal sequence of Ig-like domain III with the corresponding "b" exon of FGF receptor 2 (33). The "b" exons are poorly conserved between FGF receptor 2 and FGF receptor 3 and the net effect of FGF receptor 2 "b" exon sequence is to permit FGF-7 binding. One study using FGF receptors 1 and 2 indicates that additional sequences located in Ig-like domain II may also be required for FGF-7 binding (53). However, a second study demonstrates that FGF-7 binding only requires the "b" sequences from FGF receptor 2 (55). The requirement for Ig-like domain II sequence for FGF-7 binding will need further evaluation. The construction of chimeric molecules between FGF receptors 1 and 3 should help to resolve this issue.

The above-mentioned experiments suggest that the mechanism by which the FGF receptor 2 "b" exon confers FGF-7 binding is by allowing direct positive contacts between the FGF receptor and FGF-7. However, additional experiments utilizing tryptic digests of the FGF receptor 2 extracellular domain suggest that "b" sequences may function by masking a short conserved sequence (SD(P/A)QP), which may specifically block the binding of FGF-7 (55). The resolution of these two models will require specific mutations in the SD(P/A)QP sequence in an otherwise intact FGF receptor.

Receptor activation assays can be used to determine ligand specificity. Several cell types have been used to analyze the activity of expressed FGF receptors. These include *Xenopus* oocytes (42), CHO cells (56), L6 myoblast cells (21), MM14 myoblast cells (57, 58), Rat-2 cells (54), FDCP1 cells (54, 59), and BaF3 (24) cells. FDCP1 and BaF3 cells have the advantage of being dependent on interleukin-3 (IL-3) for growth. When expressing an FGF receptor, these cells can be made dependent on FGF for growth in the absence of IL-3. Table 9.1 shows a summary of the activity of the nine known FGF ligands and the alternatively spliced variances of the four known FGF receptors. These data demonstrate that all FGF receptors can be activated by FGF-1 (20, 33, 37–39, and unpublished data). In contrast, FGF-7 only activates the "b" splice forms of FGF receptor 2, while FGF-3 can activate the "b" splice forms of both FGF receptor 1 and FGF receptor 2 (39). The most specific receptor thus far identified is the "b" splice form of FGF receptor 3, which is activated only by FGF-1 and FGF-9 (38). The diversity in the binding specificity of FGF receptors and FGF clearly can lead to a large combinatorial set of possible interactions. In addition to the combinatorial interactions shown in Table 9.1, the possibility exists that heterodimers can form between FGF ligands and between FGF receptors. Heterodimers may further increase the repertoire of interactions between FGFs and FGF receptors. Furthermore, the interactions of FGF ligands with heparan sulfate proteoglycans may further affect or modulate specificity toward specific FGF receptors. These in vitro studies should lay the groundwork for determining specificity in FGF signaling. The important next step will be to determine physiologically and pathophysiologically relevant ligand-receptor pairs.

Glycosaminoglycan Interactions

For many years it has been known that FGFs bind the glycosaminoglycans heparin and heparan sulfate (3, 60). Heparin is a heterogeneously sulfated polysaccharide consisting of repeating disaccharide subunits of hexuronic acid and D-glucosamine. Heparin can stabilize FGF from both proteolytic and thermal degradation (61, 62). Additionally, bFGF is thought to undergo a conformational change upon binding to heparin (63). Heparan sulfate proteoglycans (HSPGs) are located on the cell surface and within the extracellular matrix. HSPGs serve as "low-affinity" ($K_d \approx 10^{-9}$ M), high-capacity, cell-surface FGF binding sites (60). The interaction of FGF with HSPGs has been established by demonstrating decreased binding of FGFs to cells deficient in cell-surface heparan sulfate (HS) (18). Additionally, treating cells with heparin-degrading enzymes or with inhibitors of sulfation decreases their ability to bind and respond to FGFs (64, 65). The affinity of FGFs for heparin-like molecules may severely limit the diffusion and release of growth factor into interstitial spaces (60, 66). FGFs may therefore exert their effects very close to their site of production, making the spatial and temporal patterns of expression of FGFs and FGF receptors an important biologic regulatory mechanism.

Recently, heparin and heparan sulfate proteoglycans have been directly implicated in the mechanism by which FGF activates the FGF receptor. In heparan sulfate proteoglycan-deficient cells that express FGF receptor 1, high-affinity FGF binding ($K_d \approx$ 2–20 $\times$ 10^{-11}M) requires heparin in the binding media (18, 64). Furthermore, heparin is required for FGF to bind to a soluble FGF receptor in a cell-free system and for FGF to activate its receptor when expressed in growth factor (IL-3) dependent lymphoid cell lines (20, 24, 33). The mechanism by which FGF interacts with its receptor may involve the formation of a low-affinity complex between FGF and the FGF receptor, which can then be stabilized by heparin. The increase in affinity between FGF and the FGF receptor in the presence of heparin is estimated to be approximately 4- to 10-fold (67, 68). Kinetic measurements demonstrate that heparin decreases the dissociation rate between FGF and the FGF receptor (by 22.7-fold) with little effect on initial binding (69). Consistent with these data, maximal DNA synthesis requires a minimum FGF exposure of 12 hours (70). This observation suggests that stable FGF-FGF receptor complexes are important for signaling a mitogenic response. However, in such mitogenic assays additional factors, such as FGF stability, must also be considered. Notably, transient activation of the FGF receptor (assayed by immediate early gene induction) may occur in the absence of heparin (67). Together, these studies suggest that to fully activate the FGF receptor a trimolecular complex forms between FGF, the FGF receptor, and heparin, but that in the absence of heparin less stable complexes between FGF and FGF receptor can still form resulting in partial receptor activation.

Heparin and heparan sulfate are very heterogeneous oligosaccharide polymers varying in molecular weight from 5000 to 100,000 kd (71). To understand the mechanism by which heparin activates FGF, binding and mitogenic assays have been used to examine both synthetic and size-fractionated heparin oligosaccharides for biologic activity. Size-fractionated heparin oligosaccharides, derived from chemically cleaved heparin, containing at least 8 to 10 sugar residues retain nearly full biologic activity, whereas heparin oligosaccharides containing six or fewer sugars are inactive (24, 72, 73). Tetra-, penta-, and hexa- saccharides derived from heparin nevertheless can bind to FGF and compete with its binding to native heparin and to heparan sulfate proteoglycans (73–76). Surprisingly, synthetic heparin oligosaccharides containing as few as two to three sugar residues also retain significant biologic activity (25). These synthetic heparan-derived di- and trisaccharides, heparin, and heparin-derived octasaccharides (and larger fragments) all bind to FGF, induce the formation of FGF dimers, and lead to FGF receptor dimerization (24–26; D. M. Ornitz and J. Xu, unpublished data).

Because dimerization of receptor tyrosine kinases is a necessary step for the activation of downstream signal transduction pathways (77), it is necessary to explain the activity of both large heparin fragments and small oligosaccharides in terms of ligand and receptor dimerization. Ligand dimerization assays demonstrate that heparin, a heparin-derived hexadeca-saccharide, and a heparan-derived trisaccharide can all induce FGF dimer-ization (24–26). A crystal structure of FGF with a synthetic heparan-derived trisaccharide shows that the trisaccharide binds at a previously identified heparin-binding site (site 1 in Fig. 9.3) and to two additional binding sites forming a dimer interface between two FGF molecules (at site 2 and 2' in Figs. 9.3 and 9.4). The role of trisaccharide binding may be to stabilize this dimer interface (25). In contrast, larger heparin molecules may have the same net effect on FGF; however, they may tether two FGF molecules together in a functional dimer using binding site 1 on respective FGF molecules (Fig. 9.4). Intermediate-sized heparin molecules (tetra- to hexa-saccharides) that are inactive may be too large to bind in the dimer interface (site 2, 2') yet too small to bridge two FGFs at site 1 (R. Sasisekhasam, personal communication) (Fig. 9.4).

In addition to the interactions between heparin and FGF it is also possible that heparin may bind directly to the FGF receptor, thus directly stabilizing FGF-FGF receptor interactions (78); however, the ability of heparin to bind directly to native FGF receptors is still controversial (25). Regardless of the precise mechanism, heparin and heparan sulfate proteoglycans appear to be essential modulators of FGF activity. Factors that affect proteoglycan biosynthesis and degradation may therefore also modulate FGF activity in vivo.

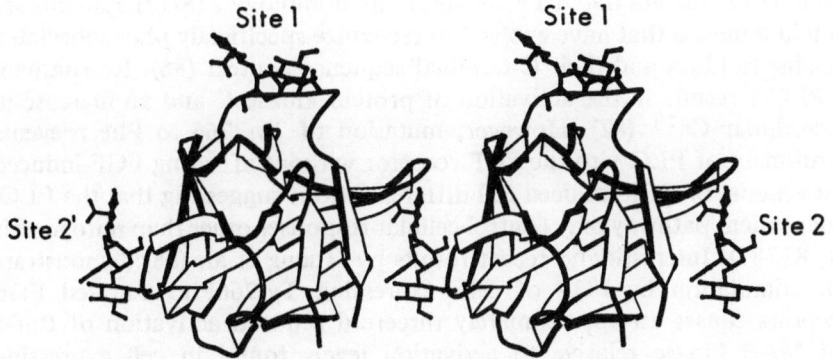

FIGURE 9.3. Crystal structure of FGF-2 complexed with a heparan-derived synthetic trisaccharide. Two FGF molecules are shown as ribbon diagrams. Each of these FGF molecules have three binding sites for trisaccharide (shown as a stick figure). Two of the binding sites (2 and 2') participate in the formation of a dimer interface between two FGF molecules.

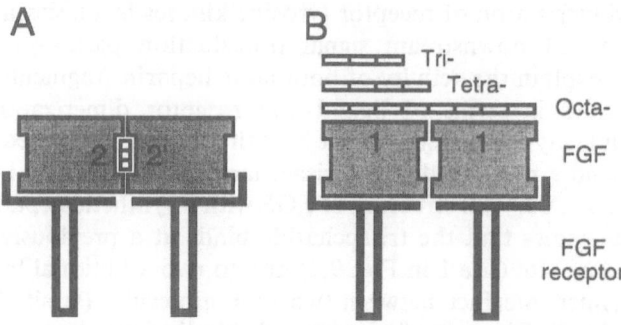

FIGURE 9.4. Model for the dimerization of FGF-2 in the presence of (A) synthetic trisaccharides or (B) heparin-derived oligosaccharides. Trisaccharides can fit within a pocket formed by two FGF molecules at binding sites 2 and 2'. Octasaccharides are large enough to tether two FGF molecules together at site 1. Tetra- to hexasaccharides can bind to site 1 but cannot link two FGF molecules. These intermediate-sized oligosaccharides may be too large to fit within the binding pocket formed by site 2 and 2'.

Signal Transduction

Following ligand binding and receptor dimerization, autophosphorylation activates the FGF receptor and allows it to bind to and transphosphorylate intracellular signal transduction proteins (79). The two primary pathways activated by FGF receptors are the Ras-Raf-MAP kinase pathway and the phospholipase C-γ (PLC-γ) pathway (80–84). PLC-γ is directly recruited to the intracellular domain of the FGF receptor through the binding of its SH2 domain to phosphorylated Tyr 766 (85). Src homology 2 (SH2) domains are protein domains that have evolved to recognize specifically phosphorylated tyrosine residues and their C-terminal sequence context (86). Recruitment of PLC-γ results in the activation of protein kinase C and an increase in intracellular Ca^{2+} (82). However, mutation of Tyr 766 to Phe prevents recruitment of PLC-γ to the FGF receptor without affecting FGF-induced mitogenesis, or FGF-induced cell differentiation, suggesting that the PLC-γ–dependent pathway may control cellular responses other than mitogenesis (81, 82, 87). Interestingly, recent results by Huang et al. (88) demonstrate that stimulation by FGF of cells expressing Tyr766Phe mutated FGF receptors causes an approximately threefold reduced activation of Raf-1 and MAP kinase relative to activation levels found in cell expressing wild-type FGF receptors, indicating a possible link between phosphatidylinositol hydrolysis and the MAP kinase pathway.

One mechanism by which the FGF signal may also be relayed to the MAP kinase cascade is via the activation of the guanosine triphosphate (GTP)-binding protein Ras (89). By analogy with other growth factor receptor tyrosine kinases, activation of FGF receptors may stimulate the formation of a complex consisting of the protein SHC (Src homologous and collagen), GRB-2, and the Ras activator protein mSOS (90). Ras-GTP then recruits the serine/threonine kinase Raf-1 to the plasma membrane, where Raf-1 becomes activated and promotes the sequential activation of the cascade of protein kinases (91). Although FGF-induced phosphorylation of SHC has been demonstrated, direct binding of SHC to the receptor has not (87). Moreover, recent reports suggest that activation of MAP kinases in the FGF system may involve yet uncharacterized pathways (83, 84, 92). For example, studies of the SH2-containing protein tyrosine phosphatase Syp and its involvement in *Xenopus* development showed that Syp signals upstream of the MAP kinase and downstream of the FGF receptors. However, no direct binding of Syp to the FGF receptor has been demonstrated, suggesting that interaction with yet unidentified proteins may be required.

Other proteins such as the protein tyrosine kinase Src (92) and phospholipase A_2 (83) have been shown to be involved in or associated with FGF signal transduction pathways. Association of Src with activated FGF receptors may be responsible for the tyrosine phosphorylation of cortactin during the middle to late G_1 phase of the cell cycle. Activation of cytosolic phospholipase A_2 by FGF may be a result of MAP kinase activation and is responsible for the release of arachidonate in endothelial cells.

The overall picture of signal transduction by FGF that emerges from these studies is that of a diversified range of pathways, reflecting the diversity of structures and biologic functions that characterize FGF and FGF receptors. The ability of FGFs to regulate mitogenic response, differentiation, and embryonic patterning may involve any or all of these signaling pathways or novel pathways. Importantly, sequence differences between the four FGF receptors, as well as alternative splicing, may significantly affect their ability to transmit a signal in diverse cell types and to interact with diverse signaling pathways (40; Ornitz, unpublished data).

Cell Growth and Development

The biologic response to FGFs vary depending on the cell type, tissue, and developmental stage. FGFs are required for survival and growth of 3T3 cells (93), endothelial cells (94), and receptor-expressing lymphoid cells (20, 24, 54). In primary culture FGF-2 is a necessary mitogen for growth plate chondrocytes and also functions to inhibit their terminal differentiation (95–97). In tissue culture, FGFs induce cells of neuroectodermal origin to express a more mature neuronal phenotype (98–102). FGF-2 is also effective in maintaining certain hematopoietic lineages in long-term primary bone marrow culture (103) and promotes the survival and possible differentiation of hematopoietic progenitor cells in vitro (104). FGF receptors 1 and 2 are expressed in some myeloid, erythroid, and megakaryocytic cell lines (95) and may therefore play a role in the growth and differentiation of these lineages. These diverse types of responses to FGFs (cell growth, survival, and differentiation) may result from the activity of alternative initial signaling pathways in different cell types, or from committed cells responding differentially to a common initial signaling pathway.

A large body of evidence shows that FGF pathways are essential for vertebrate embryogenesis. Early in development, FGF-2, FGF-3, and FGF-4 induce ventral mesoderm in *Xenopus* embryos (8, 11). Later in development, several studies demonstrate that FGF-2, -4, and possibly -8 are essential for limb development, a paradigm for patterning complex structures (105–108). Targeted disruptions of FGFs in mice also demonstrate that these growth factors are essential for cell growth and development. In mice homozygous for a disruption in the FGF-3 gene, inner ear defects as well as caudal vertebral defects are observed (109), suggesting that (a) FGF-3 may affect the rate of growth of cells that give rise to the tail bud; (b) FGF-3 may affect the relative rates of proliferation of cells within developing vertebrae; or (c) FGF-3 may affect the intercalation of mesodermal cells into the developing vertebral column (109). The inner ear phenotype may signify a role for FGF-3 in the induction of the endolymphatic duct from sites of FGF-3 synthesis in the hindbrain or in the otocyst. A null mutation in the FGF-5 gene results in viable mice with the surprising phenotype of long hair (110). This phenotype is identical to that seen in the angora mouse. Not surprisingly, careful analysis of the angora mutation revealed a deletion in the FGF-5 gene. Analysis of both the angora mouse and the FGF-5 null mouse suggests that FGF-5 is an essential regulator of hair cell growth, possibly by affecting the transition from an actively growing hair follicle to the stage of hair follicle regression (110, 111). Unlike with FGF-3 and FGF-5, a null mutation in the FGF-4 gene results in embryonic lethality (112). FGF-4 null embryos die shortly after uterine implantation. Examination of FGF-4 null blastocysts demonstrated poor proliferation of the inner cell mass. Because of this early embryonic lethality, roles for FGF-4 later in development remain unresolved and will need to be addressed by other means.

FGF receptor activity has been examined in mice by expressing dominant negative receptors using tissue-specific promoters and by modifying the endogenous genes by homologous recombination. A null mutation in the FGF receptor 1 gene results in early embryonic lethality (113, 114). These mice die around the time of gastrulation. Analysis of these animals demonstrate possible patterning defects in axial structures as well as general growth retardation. A null mutation in FGF receptor 2 (C. Deng, personal communication) also results in embryonic lethality. Embryonic death occurs in mid-gestation embryos; however, the precise etiology has not been determined. Null mutations in the FGF receptor 3 gene (J. Colvin, B. Bohne, and D. M. Ornitz, unpublished data) are viable; however, these mice develop severe defects in bone and cartilage growth and in the development of the organ of Corti of the inner ear. Unlike FGF receptors

1 to 3, null mutations in FGF receptor 4 (C. Deng, personal communication) demonstrate no apparent abnormalities.

Because null mutations in FGF receptors 1 and 2 result in embryonic lethality, other approaches are required to study the role of these receptors later in development and in adult physiology. The expression of dominant negative forms of the FGF receptors using tissue-specific promoters has been particularly informative. Targeting a dominant negative FGF receptor to the developing lung has revealed an essential role for FGF receptor 1 in branching morphogenesis (115). Targeting dominant negative forms of FGF receptors 1 and 2 to skin using keratin 10 and 14 promoters, respectively, has revealed a role for FGF signaling in epithelial development and wound healing (116, 117).

FGF Receptor Mutations in Human Disease

Recently, several human genetic diseases have been identified as having point mutations in the genes encoding FGF receptors 1, 2, and 3 (Fig. 9.5). These disorders result in the skeletal dysplasia syndromes: hypochondroplasia (Hch) (118), Achondroplasia (Ach) (119, 120) thanatophoric dysplasia (TD) (121), Crouzon syndrome (CS) (122, 123), Pfeffer syndrome (PS) (123–127), Jackson-Weiss syndrome (JWS) (128), and Apert syndrome (AS) (129). All these mutations are dominant and inheritable and can occur de novo.

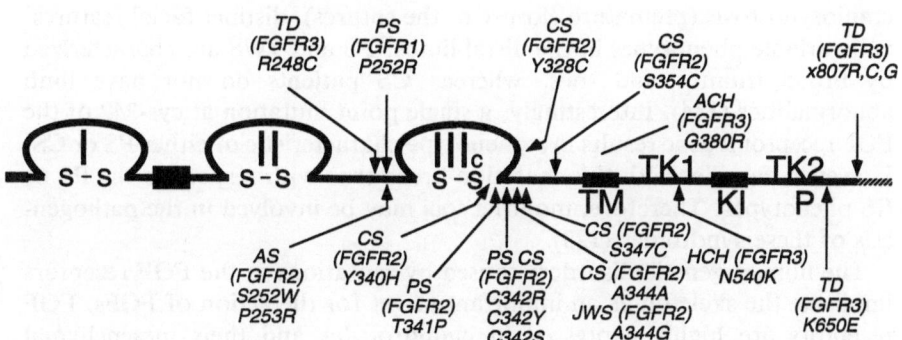

Figure 9.5. Mutations in the FGF receptor genes in human skeletal dysplasia. The FGF receptors involved are indicated (FGFR1, FGFR2, FGFR3). The specific syndrome (Ach, achondroplasia; AS, Apert syndrome; CS, Crouzon syndrome; Hch, hypochondroplasia; JWS, Jackson-Weiss syndrome; PS, Pfeiffer syndrome; TD, thanatophoric dysplasia) and the point mutation are indicated. The structural features of the FGF receptor gene are the same as in Fig. 9.1. The stippled line at the c-terminus represents an extension of FGF receptor 3 caused by a stop-codon mutation in some cases of TD.

Hch, Ach, and TD all result from dominant mutations in the FGF receptor 3 gene that maps to human chromosome 4p16.3 (118, 120, 121). Hch is a mild and relatively common skeletal disorder with clinical features similar to that of Ach. Ach, the most common form of genetic dwarfism, arises de novo in 20% of cases. Ach is characterized by rhizomelic shortening of the proximal, and to some extent, distal long bones. The cranium of Ach patients is characterized by frontal bossing, and the face is characterized by a depressed nasal bridge. Histologic examination reveals well-organized endochondral ossification (130). However, the rate of endochondral growth relative to periosteal ossification may be decreased. Rare homozygous cases of Ach usually result in neonatal lethality. These patients have similar features to that of Ach patients, except significantly more severe. Histologically, the endochondral growth zone is disorganized and narrow (131). However, other cartilaginous regions appear normal.

TD results from three dominant mutations in the FGF receptor 3 gene resulting in three closely related syndromes (121, 132). TD is the most common lethal-neonatal skeletal disorder and is clinically similar to homozygous Ach (133). Histologic analysis of TD growth plates indicates an abnormal ossification process. Islands of ossification form within the cartilaginous matrix of the growth plate (133). The common features of these syndromes and their increasing degree of severity suggests that these mutations in the FGF receptor 3 gene affects the activity of FGF receptor 3 in a graded and dose-dependent manner, with Hch < Ach < homozygous Ach ≤ TD.

PS, CS, JWS, and AS are clinically distinct syndromes characterized by craniosynostosis (premature closure of the sutures), distinct facial features, and variable phenotypes in the distal limbs. PS and JWS are characterized by broad thumbs and toes, whereas CS patients do not have limb abnormalities (134). Interestingly, a single point mutation at cys-342 of the FGF receptor 2 gene results in a phenotype characteristic of either PS or CS. However, families with this mutation breed true with respect to the PS or CS phenotypes. Therefore, modifier loci may be involved in the pathogenesis of these syndromes (123).

The human genetic disorders caused by mutations in the FGF receptors implicate the skeleton as an important target for the action of FGFs. FGF receptors are highly expressed in chondrocytes and their mesenchymal precursors. During limb morphogenesis, FGFs are found to have essential roles both in the progressive elongation of a developing limb and in the maintenance of spatial clues leading to the correct anatomic pattern of the limb. An abundance of evidence demonstrates that these effects of FGFs are transmitted and augmented through feedback signaling loops. Although incompletely defined, these circuits require BMP-2 (bone morphogenetic protein) for normal development (105, 106, 135–138). Similar feedback loops involving BMPs exist during the development of the vertebral column, perhaps suggesting a role of FGF receptors in the formation of the axial skeleton.

All of the identified mutations in FGF receptors 1 and 2 and one of the mutations identified in FGF receptor 3 are located in the extracellular region (Fig. 9.5). These mutations are clustered into two locations—the linker region between Ig-like domains II and III and the region surrounding the carboxy terminal part of Ig-like domain III. This clustering of point mutations in three different FGF receptors suggests that these sites are particularly important for regulating FGF receptor activity. It is likely that these mutations either change ligand-binding specificity, change ligand affinity, or modulate receptor dimerization and subsequent activation. Because all of these mutations are dominant the net effect of these mutations is likely to be a gain of function. However, if some of these mutations decrease ligand binding, they may function as dominant negative mutations. Biochemical analysis of these mutations should be able to distinguish between these mechanisms. In FGF receptor 3, but not in FGF receptors 1 and 2, point mutations have also been found in the transmembrane and intracellular region. The transmembrane mutation is likely to be activating because a similar mutation in the *neu* receptor tyrosine kinase is activating and results in cell transformation (139, 140). The intracellular mutations in FGF receptor 3 may also be activating or may alter substrate specificity. The discovery of several mutations in the intracellular region of FGF receptor 3 suggests that the signal transduction activity of this receptor may be particularly sensitive to specific downstream signaling molecules. This is consistent with the observed decreased signaling capacity of FGF receptor 3 (compared with FGF receptors 1 and 2) in BaF3 cells.

Conclusion

Mutations in both FGFs and FGF receptors demonstrate that FGF signaling pathways are essential for both embryonic development and for normal adult physiology. FGFs are important regulators of angiogenesis and wound healing. When inappropriately expressed, some FGFs cause cancer. The nine ligands and four receptors in this family form a complex signaling array. Not surprisingly, several mechanisms have evolved to regulate FGF signaling. These include cell type-specific alternative splicing of receptors, cell type-specific expression of receptors and ligands, selective binding of ligands to receptors, a glycosaminoglycan (GAG) cofactor requirement for ligand binding, and multiple signaling pathways that are differentially activated by the FGF receptors. Future studies will have to address the biochemical mechanisms regulating FGF receptor activity at all of these levels. Physiologically and pathophysiologically relevant ligand-receptor pairs will need to be identified and pharmacologic modulators of FGF activity will need to be developed.

References

1. Gospodarowicz D, Moran JS. Mitogenic effect of fibroblast growth factor on early passage cultures of human and murine fibroblasts. J Cell Biol 1975;66:451–7.
2. Basilico C, Moscatelli D. The FGF family of growth factors and oncogenes. Adv Cancer Res 1992;59:115–228.
3. Klagsbrun M. The fibroblast growth factor family: structural and biological properties. Prog Growth Fact Res 1989;1:207–35.
4. Thomas KA. Fibroblast growth factors. FASEB J 1987;1:434–40.
5. Tanaka A, Miyamoto K, Minamino N, et al. Cloning and characterization of an androgen-induced growth factor essential for the androgen-dependent growth of mouse mammary carcinoma cells. Proc Natl Acad Sci USA 1992;89:8928–32.
6. Miyamoto M, Naruo K, Seko C, Matsumoto S, Kondo T, Kurokawa T. Molecular cloning of a novel cytokine cDNA encoding the ninth member of the fibroblast growth factor family, which has a unique secretion property. Mol Cell Biol 1993;13:4251–9.
7. Folkman J, Klagsbrun M. Angiogenic factors. Science 1987;235:442–7.
8. Slack JMW, Darlington BG, Heath JK, Godsave SF. Mesoderm induction in early *Xenopus* embryos by heparin-binding growth factors. Nature 1987;326:197–200.
9. Schweigerer L, Neufeld G, Friedman J, Abraham JA, Fiddes JC, Gospoda-rowicz D. Capillary endothelial cells express basic fibroblast growth factor, a mitogen that promotes their own growth. Nature 1987;325:257–9.
10. Valles AM, Boyer B, Badet J, Tucker GC, Barritault D, Thiery JP. Acidic fibroblast growth factor is a modulator of epithelial plasticity in a rat bladder carcinoma cell line. Proc Natl Acad Sci USA 1990;87:1124–8.
11. Paterno GD, Gillespie LL, Dixon MS, Slack JMW, Heath JK. Mesoderm-inducing properties of INT-2 and kFGF: two oncogene-encoded growth factors related to FGF. Development 1989;106:79–83.
12. Lee PL, Johnson DE, Cousens LS, Fried VA, Williams LT. Purification and complementary DNA cloning of a receptor for basic fibroblast growth factor. Science 1989;245:57–60.
13. Dionne CA, Crumley G, Bellot F, et al. Cloning and expression of two distinct high-affinity receptors cross-reacting with acidic and basic fibroblast growth factors. EMBO J 1990;9:2685–92.
14. Ruta M, Burgess W, Givol D, et al. Receptor for acidic fibroblast growth factor is related to the tyrosine kinase encoded by the *fms*-like gene (FLG). Proc Natl Acad Sci USA 1989;86:8722–6.
15. Reid HH, Wilks AF, Bernard O. Two forms of the basic fibroblast growth factor receptor-like mRNA are expressed in the developing mouse brain. Proc Natl Acad Sci USA 1990;87:1596–600.

16. Hattori Y, Odagiri H, Nakatani H, et al. K-*sam*, an amplified gene in stomach cancer, is a member of the heparin-binding growth factor receptor genes. Proc Natl Acad Sci USA 1990;87:5983-7.
17. Safran A, Avivi A, Orr-Urtereger A, et al. The murine *flg* gene encodes a receptor for fibroblast growth factor. Oncogene 1990;5:635-43.
18. Yayon A, Klagsbrun M, Esko JD, Leder P, Ornitz DM. Cell surface, heparin-like molecules are required for binding of basic fibroblast growth factor to its high affinity receptor. Cell 1991;64:841-8.
19. Partanen J, Makela TP, Eerola E, et al. FGFR-4, a novel acidic fibroblast growth factor receptor with a distinct expression pattern. EMBO J 1991; 10:1347-54.
20. Ornitz DM, Leder P. Ligand specificity and heparin dependence of fibroblast growth factor receptors 1 and 3. J Biol Chem 1992;267:16305-11.
21. Werner S, Duan D-SR, de Vries C, Peters KG, Johnson DE, Williams LT. Differential splicing in the extracellular region of fibroblast growth factor receptor 1 generates receptor variants with different ligand-binding specificities. Mol Cell Biol 1992;12:82-8.
22. Mansukhani A, Dell'Era P, Moscatelli D, Kornbluth S, Hanafusa H, Basilico C. Characterization of the murine BEK fibroblast growth factor (FGF) receptor: activation by three members of the FGF family and requirement for heparin. Proc Natl Acad Sci USA 1992;89:3305-9.
23. Miki T, Bottaro DP, Fleming TP, et al. Determination of ligand-binding specificity by alternative splicing: two distinct growth factor receptors encoded by a single gene. Proc Natl Acad Sci USA 1992;89:246-50.
24. Ornitz DM, Yayon A, Flanagan JG, Svahn CM, Levi E, Leder P. Heparin is required for cell-free binding of basic fibroblast growth factor to a soluble receptor and for mitogenesis in whole cells. Mol Cell Biol 1992;12:240-7.
25. Ornitz DM, Herr AB, Nilsson M, Westman J, Svahn C-M, Waksman G. FGF binding and FGF receptor activation by synthetic heparin-derived di- and trisaccharides. Science 1995;268:432-6.
26. Spivak-Kroizman T, Lemmon MA, Dikic I, et al. Heparin-induced oligomerization of FGF molecules is responsible for FGF receptor dimerization, activation, and cell proliferation. Cell 1994;79:1015-24.
27. Johnson DE, Williams LT. Structural and functional diversity in the FGF receptor multigene family. Adv Cancer Res 1993;60:1-41.
28. Schlessinger J, Ullrich A. Growth factor signaling by receptor tyrosine kinases. Neuron 1992;9:383-91.
29. Johnson DE, Lu J, Chen H, Werner S, Williams LT. The human fibroblast growth factor receptor genes: a common structural arrangement underlies the mechanisms for generating receptor forms that differ in their third immunoglobulin domain. Mol Cell Biol 1991;11:4627-34.
30. Wang F, Kan M, Yan G, Xu J, McKeehan WL. Alternately spliced NH_2-terminal immunoglobulin-like loop I in the ectodomain of the fibroblast growth factor (FGF) receptor 1 lowers affinity for both heparin and FGF-1. J Biol Chem 1995;270:10231-5.
31. Yamaguchi F, Saya H, Bruner JM, Morrison RS. Differential expression of two fibroblast growth factor-receptor genes is associated with malignant progression in human astrocytomas. Proc Natl Acad Sci USA 1994;91:484-8.

32. Kobrin MS, Yamanaka Y, Friess H, Lopez ME, Korc M. Aberrant expression of type I fibroblast growth factor receptor in human pancreatic adenocarcinomas. Cancer Res 1993;53:4741-4.

33. Chellaiah AT, McEwen DG, Werner S, Xu J, Ornitz DM. Fibroblast growth factor receptor (FGFR) 3: alternative splicing in immunoglobulin-like domain III creates a receptor highly specific for acidic FGF/FGF-1. J Biol Chem 1994;269:11620-7.

34. Duan D-SR, Werner S, Williams LT. A naturally occurring secreted form of fibroblast growth factor (FGF) receptor 1 binds basic FGF in preference over acidic FGF. J Biol Chem 1992;267:16076-80.

35. Xu J, Nakahara N, Crabb JW, et al. Expression and immunochemical analysis of rat and human fibroblast growth factor receptor (flg) isoforms. J Biol Chem 1992;267:11792-803.

36. Dell K, Williams L. A novel form of fibroblast growth factor receptor 2. J Biol Chem 1992;267:21225-9.

37. MacArthur CA, Lawshé A, Xu J, et al. FGF-8 isoforms activate receptor splice forms that are expressed in mesenchymal regions of mouse development. Development 1995;121:3603-13.

38. Santos-Ocampo S, Colvin JS, Chellaiah AT, Ornitz DM. Expression and biological activity of mouse fibroblast growth factor-9 (FGF-9). J Biol Chem 1996;271:1726-31.

39. Mathieu M, Chatelain E, Ornitz D, et al. Receptor binding and mitogenic properties of mouse fibroblast growth factor 3 (FGF3); modulation of response by heparin. J Biol Chem 1995;270:24197-203.

40. Wang JK, Gao G, Goldfarb M. Fibroblast growth factor receptors have different signaling and mitogenic potentials. Mol Cell Biol 1994;14:181-8.

41. Champion-Arnaud P, Ronsin C, Gilbert E, Gesnel MC, Houssaint E, Breathnach R. Multiple mRNAs code for proteins related to the BEK fibroblast growth factor receptor. Oncogene 1991;6:979-87.

42. Johnson DE, Lee PL, Lu J, Williams LT. Diverse forms of a receptor for acidic and basic fibroblast growth factors. Mol Cell Biol 1990;10:4728-36.

43. Avivi A, Yayon A, Gibol D. A novel form of FGF receptor-3 using an alternative exon in the immunoglobulin domain III. FEBS Lett 1993; 330:249-52.

44. Yan G, Fukabori Y, McBride G, Nikolaropolous S, McKeehan WL. Exon switching and activation of stromal and embryonic fibroblast growth factor (FGF)-FGF receptor genes in prostate epithelial cells accompany stromal independence and malignancy. Mol Cell Biol 1993;13:4513-22.

45. Orr-Urtreger A, Bedford MT, Burakova T, et al. Developmental localization of the splicing alternatives of fibroblast growth factor receptor-2 (FGFR2). Dev Biol 1993;158:475-86.

46. Alarid ET, Rubin JS, Young P, et al. Keratinocyte growth factor functions in epithelial induction during seminal vesicle development. Proc Natl Acad Sci USA 1994;91:1074-8.

47. Gilbert E, Del Gatto F, Champion-Arnaud P, Gesnel M-C, Breathnach R. Control of BEK and K-SAM splice sites in alternative splicing of the fibroblast growth factor receptor 2 pre-mRNA. Mol Cell Biol 1993;13:5461-8.

48. Miki T, Fleming TP, Bottaro DP, Rubin JS, Ron D, Aaronson SA. Expression

of cDNA cloning of the KGF receptor by creation of a transforming autocrine loop. Science 1991;251:72–5.

49. Adenane J, Gaudray P, Dionne CA, et al. *BEK* and *FLG,* two receptors to members of the FGF family, are amplified in subsets of human breast cancers. Oncogene 1991;6:659–63.

50. Asai T, Wanaka A, Kato H, Masana Y, Seo M, Tohyama M. Differential expression of two members of FGF receptor gene family, FGFR-1 and FGFR-2 mRNA, in the adult rat central nervous system. Brain Res Mol Brain Res 1993;17:174–8.

51. Crumley G, Bellot F, Kaplow JM, Schlessinger J, Jaye M, Dionne CA. High-affinity binding and activation of a truncated FGF receptor by both aFGF and bFGF. Oncogene 1991;2255–62.

52. Cheon H-G, LaRochelle WJ, Bottaro DP, Burgess WH, Aaronson SA. High-affinity binding sites for related fibroblast growth factor ligands reside within different receptor immunoglobulin-like domains. Proc Natl Acad Sci USA 1994;91:989–93.

53. Zimmer Y, Givol D, Yayon A. Multiple structural elements determine ligand binding of fibroblast growth factor receptors. J Biol Chem 1993;268: 7899–903.

54. Bernard O, Li M, Reid HH. Expression of two different forms of fibroblast growth factor receptor 1 in different mouse tissues and cell lines. Proc Natl Acad Sci USA 1991;88:7625–9.

55. Wang F, Kan M, Xu J, Yan G, McKeehan WL. Ligand-specific structural domains in the fibroblast growth factor receptor. J Biol Chem 1995; 270:10222–30.

56. Mansukhani A, Moscatelli D, Talarico D, Levytska V, Basilico C. A murine fibroblast growth factor (FGF) receptor expressed in CHO cells is activated by basic FGF and Kaposi FGF. Proc Natl Acad Sci USA 1990;87:4378–82.

57. Kudla AJ, John ML, Bowen-Pope DF, Rainish B, Olwin BB. A requirement for fibroblast growth factor in regulation of skeletal muscle growth and differentiation cannot be replaced by activation of platelet-derived growth factor signaling pathways. Mol Cell Biol 1995;15:3238–46.

58. Templeton TJ, Hauschka SD. FGF-mediated aspects of skeletal muscle growth and differetiation are controlled by a high affinity receptor, FGFR1. Dev Biol 1992;154:169–81.

59. Li M, Bernard O. FDC-P1 myeloid cells engineered to express fibroblast growth factor receptor 1 proliferater and differentiate in the presence of fibroblast growth factor and heparin. Proc Natl Acad Sci USA 1992; 89:3315–9.

60. Moscatelli D. High and low affinity binding sites for basic fibroblast growth factor on cultured cells: absence of a role for low affinity binding in the stimulation of plasminogen activator production by bovine capillary endothelial cells. J Cell Physiol 1987;131:123–30.

61. Gospodarowicz D, Chen J. Heparin protects acidic and basic FGF from inactivation. J Cell Physiol 1986;128:475–484.

62. Volkin DB, Tsai PK, Dabora Jm, Gress JO, Burke CJ, Linhardt RJ, et al. Physical stabilization of acidic fibroblast growth factor by polyanions. Arch Biochem Biophys 1993;300:30–41.

63. Prestrelski SJ, Fox GM, Arakawa T. Binding of heparin to basic fibroblast growth factor induces a conformational change. Arch Biochem Biophys 1992;293:314-9.
64. Rapraeger AC, Krufka A, Olwin BB. Requirement of heparan sulfate for bFGF-mediated fibroblast growth and myoblast differentiation. Science 1991;252:1705-8.
65. Olwin B, Rapraeger A. Repression of myogenic differentiation by aFGF, bFGF, and K-FGF is dependent on cellular heparan sulfate. J Cell Biol 1992;118:631-9.
66. Flaumenhaft R, Moscatelli D, Rifkin DB. Heparin and haparan sulfate increase the radius of diffusion and action of basic fibroblast growth factor. J Cell Biol 1990;111:1651-9.
67. Roghani M, Mansukhani A, Dell'Era P, et al. Heparin increases the affinity of basic fibroblast growth factor for its receptor but is not required for binding. J Biol Chem 1994;269:3976-84.
68. Pantoliano MW, Horlick RA, Springer BA, et al. Multivalent ligand-receptor binding interactions in the fibroblast growth factor system produce a cooperative growth factor and heparin mechanism for receptor dimerization. Biochemistry 1994;33:10229-48.
69. Nugent MA, Edelman ER. Kinetics of basic fibroblast growth factor binding to its receptor and heparan sulfate proteoglycan: a mechanism for cooperativity. Biochemistry 1992;31:8876-83.
70. Zhan W, Hu W, Friesel R, Maciag T. Long term growth factor exposure and differential tyrosine phosphorylation are required for DNA synthesis in BALB/c 3T3 cells. J Biol Chem 1993;268:9611-20.
71. Casu B. Structure and biological activity of heparin. Adv Carbohydr Chem Biochem 1985;43:51-134.
72. Ishihara M, Tyrrell D, Stauber G, Brown S, Cousens L, Stack R. Preparation of affinity-fractionated, heparin-derived oligosaccharides and their effects on selected biological activities mediated by basic fibroblast growth factor. J Biol Chem 1993;268:4675-83.
73. Aviezer D, Levy E, Safran M, et al. Differential structural requirements of heparin and heparan sulfate proteoglycands that promote binding of basic fibroblast growth factor to its receptor. J Biol Chem 1994;269:114-21.
74. Vlodavsky I, Ishai-Michaeli R, Mohsen M, et al. Modulation of neovascularization and metastasis by species of heparin. In: Lane DA, et al., ed. Heparin and related polysaccharides. New York: Plenum Press, 1992:317-27.
75. Maccarana M, Casu B, Lindahl U. Minimal sequence in heparin/heparan sulfate required for binding of basic fibroblast growth factor. J Biol Chem 1993;268:23898-905.
76. Bârzu T, Lormeau J-C, Petitou M, Michelson S, Choay J. Heparin-derived oligosaccharides: affinity for acidic fibroblast growth factor and effect on its growth-promoting activity for human endothelial cells. J Cell Physiol 1989;140:538-48.
77. Ullrich A, Schlessinger J. Signal transduction by receptors with tyrosine kinase activity. Cell 1990;61:203-12.
78. Kan M, Wang F, Xu J, Crabb JW, Hou J, McKeehan WL. An essential heparin-binding domain in the fibroblast growth factor receptor kinase. Science 1993;259:1918-21.

79. Lemmon MA, Schlessinger J. Regulation of signal transduction and signal diversity by receptor oligomerization. TIBS 1994;19:459–63.
80. Campbell JS, Wenderoth MP, Hauschka SD, Krebs EG. Differential activation of mitogen-activated protein kinase in response to basic fibroblast growth factor in skeletal muscle cells. Proc Natl Acad Sci USA 1995;92:870–4.
81. Mohammadi M, Dionne CA, Li W, et al. Point mutation in FGF receptor eliminates phosphatidylinositol hydrolysis without affecting mitogenesis. Nature 1992;358:681–4.
82. Peters KG, Marie J, Wilson E, et al. Point mutation of an FGF receptor abolishes phosphatidylinositol turnover and Ca^{2+} flux but not mitogenesis. Nature 1992;358:678–81.
83. Sa G, Murugesan G, Jaye M, Ivashchenko Y, Fox PL. Activation of cytosolic phospholipase A2 by basic fibroblast growth factor via p42 mitogen-activated protein kinase-dependent phosphorylation pathway in endothelial cells. J Biol Chem 1995;270:23600–6.
84. Tang TL, Freeman RMJ, O'Reilly AM, Neel BG, Sokol SY. The SH2-containing protein-tyrosine phosphatase SH-PTP2 is required upstream of MAP kinase for early Xenopus development. Cell 1995;80:473–83.
85. Mohammadi M, Honneger AM, Rotin D, et al. A tyrosine-phosphorylated carboxy-terminal peptide of the fibroblast growth factor receptor (Flg) is a binding site for the SH2 domain of phospholipase C-γ1. Mol Cell Biol 1991;11:5068–78.
86. Pawson T, Schlessinger J. SH2 and SH3 domains. Curr Biol 1993;3:434–42.
87. Spivak-Kroizman T, Mohammadi M, Hu P, Jaye M, Schlessinger J, Lax I. Point mutation in the fibroblast growth factor receptor eliminates phosphatidylinositol hydrolysis without affecting neuronal differentiation of PC12 cells. J Biol Chem 1994;269:14419–23.
88. Huang J, Mohammadi M, Rodriges GA, Schlessinger J. Reduced activationof RAF-1 and MAP kinase by fibroblast growth factor receptor mutant deficient in stimulation of phosphatidylinositol hydrolysis. J Biol Chem 1995; 270:5065–72.
89. Blumer KJ, Johnson GL. Diversity in function and regulation of MAP kinase pathways. TIBS 1994;19:236–40.
90. Marengere LE, Songyang Z, Gish CD, et al. SH2 domain specificity and activity modified by a single residue. Nature 1994;369:502–5.
91. Avruch J, Zhang X-F, Kyriakis JM. Raf meets Ras: completing the framework of a single transduction pathway. TIBS 1994;19:279–83.
92. Zhan X, Plourde C, Hu X, Friesel R, Maciag T. Association of fibroblast growth factor receptor-1 with c-src correlates with association between c-src and cortactin. J Biol Chem 1994;12:20221–4.
93. Tamm I, Kikuchi T, Zychlinsky A. Acidic and basic fibroblast growth factors are survival factors with distinctive activity in quiescent BALB/c 3T3 murine fibroblasts. Proc Natl Acad Sci USA 1991;88:3372–6.
94. Jaye M, Howk R, Burgess W, et al. Human endothelial cell growth factor: cloning, nucleotide sequnce, and chromosome localization. Science 1986; 233:541–5.
95. Katoh O, Hattori Y, Sato T, et al. Expression of the heparin-binding growth factor receptor genes in human megakaryocytic leukemia cells. Biochem Biophys Res Commun 1992;183:83–92.

96. Wroblewski J, Edwall-Arvidsson C. Inhibitory effects of basic fibroblast growth factor on chondrocyte differentiation. J Bone Miner Res 1995; 10:735–42.

97. Iwamoto M, Shimazu A, Nakashima K, Suzuki F, Kato Y. Reduction of basic fibroblasts growth factor receptor is coupled with terminal differentiation of chondrocytes. J Biol Chem 1991;266:461–7.

98. Birren S, Anderson D. A v-myc-immortalized sympathoadrenal progenitor cell line in which neuronal differentiation is initiated by FGF but not NGF. Neuron 1990;4:189–201.

99. Claude P, Parada I, Gordon K, D'Amore P, Wagner J. Acidic fibroblast growth factor stimulates adrenal chromoffin cells to proliferate and to extend neurites, but is not a long-term survival factor. Neuron 1988;1:783–90.

100. Murphy M, Drago J, Bartlett P. Fibroblast growth factor stimulates the proliferation and differentiation of neural precursor cells in vitro. J Neurosci Res 1990;25:463–75.

101. Pruss R, Bartlett P, Gavrilovic J, Lisak R, Rattray S. Mitogens for glial cells: a comparison of the response of cultured astrocytes, oligodendrocytes, and Schwann cells. Dev Brain Res 1982;2:19–35.

102. Stemple D, Mahanthappa N, Anderson D. Basic FGF induces neuronal differentiation, cell division, and NGF dependence in chromaffin cells: a sequence of events in sympathetic development. Neuron 1988;1:517–25.

103. Wilson LE, Rifkin DB, Kelly F, Hannocks M-J, Gabrilove JL. Basic fibroblast growth factor stimulates myelopoiesis in long-term human bone marrow cultures. Bloo 1991;77:954–60.

104. Gabbianelli M, Sargiacomo M, Pelosi E, Testa U, Isacchi G, Peschle C. "Pure" human hematopoietic progenitors: premissive action of basic fibroblast growth factor. Science 1990;249:1561–4.

105. Laufer E, Nelson CE, Johnson RL, Morgan BA, Tabin C. Sonic hedgehog and Fgf-4 act through a signaling cascade and feedback loop to integrate growth and patterning of the developing limb bud. Cell 1994;79:993–1003.

106. Niswander L, Tickle C, Vogel A, Booth I, Martin GR. FGF-4 replaces the apical ectodermal ridge and directs outgrowth and patterning of the limb. Cell 1993;75:579–587.

107. Cohn MJ, Izpisúa-Belmonte JC, Abud H, Heath JK, Tickle C. Fibroblast growth factors induce additional limb development from the flank of chick embryos. Cell 1995;80:739–46.

108. Heikinheimo M, Lawshé A, Shackleford GM, Wilson DB, MacArthur CA. FgF-8 expression in the post-gastrulation mouse suggests roles in the development of the face, limbs and central nervous system. Mech Dev 1994;48:129–38.

109. Mansour S, Goddard J, Capecchi M. Mice homozygous for a targeted disruption of the proto-oncogene int-2 developmental defects in the tail and inner ear. Development 1993;117:13–28.

110. Hébert JM, Rosenquist T, Götz J, Martin GR. FGF5 as a regulator of the hair growth cycle: evidence from targeted and spontaneous mutations. Cell 1994;78:1017–25.

111. Pennycuik PR, Raphael KA. The angora locus (go) in the mouse: hair morphology, duration of growth cycle and site of action. Genet Res (Camb) 1984;44:283–91.

112. Feldman B, Poueymirou W, Papaioannou VE, DeChiara TM, Goldfarb M. Requirement of FGF-4 for postimplantation mouse development. Science 1995;267:246–9.
113. Yamaguchi TP, Harpal K, Henkemeyer M, Roussant J. FGFR-1 is required for embryonic growth and mesodermal patterning during mouse gastrulation. Genes Dev 1994;8:3032–44.
114. Deng C-X, Wynshaw-Boris A, Shen MM, Daugherty C, Ornitz DM, Leder P. Murine FGFR-1 is required for early postimplantation growth and axial organization. Genes Dev 1994;8:3045–57.
115. Peters K, Werner S, Liao X, Wert S, Whitsett J, Williams L. Targeted expression of a dominant negative FGF receptor blocks branching morphogenesis and epithelial differentiation of the mouse lung. EMBO J 1995; 13:3296–301.
116. Werner S, Smola H, Liao X, et al. The function of KGF in morphogenesis of epithelium and reepithelialization of wounds. Science 1994;266:819–22.
117. Werner S, Weinberg W, Liao X, et al. Targeted expression of a dominant-negative FGF receptor mutant in the epidermis of transgenic mice reveals a role of FGF in keratinocyte organization and differentiation. EMBO J 1993; 12:2635–43.
118. Bellus GA, McIntosh I, Smith EA, et al. A recurrent mutation in the tyrosine kinase domain of fibroblast growth factor receptor 3 causes hypochondroplasia. Nat Genet 1995;10:357–9.
119. Rousseau F, Bonaventure J, Legeal-Mallet L, et al. Mutations in the gene encoding fibroblast growth factor receptor-3 in achondroplasia. Nature 1994;371:252–4.
120. Shiang R, Thompson LM, Zhu Y-Z, et al. Mutations in the transmembrane domain of FGFR3 cause the most common genetic form of dwarfism, achondroplasia. Cell 1994;78:335–42.
121. Tavorimina PL, Shiang R, Thompson LM, et al. Thanatophoric dysplasia (types I and II) caused by distinct mutations in fibroblast growth factor receptor 3. Nat Genet 1995;9:321–8.
122. Reardon W, Winter RM, Rutland P, Pulleyn LJ, Jones BM, Malcolm S. Mutations in the fibroblast growth factor receptor 2 gene cause Crouzon syndrome. Nat Genet 1994;8:98–103.
123. Rutland P, Pulleyn LJ, Reardon W, et al. Identical mutations in the FGFR2 gene cause both Pfeiffer and Crouzon syndrome phenotypes. Nat Genet 1995;9:173–6.
124. Schell U, Hehr A, Feldman GJ, et al. Mutations in FGFR1 and FGFR2 cause familial and sporadic Pfeiffer syndrome. Human Mol Genet 1995; 4:323–8.
125. Robin NH, Feldman GJ, Mitchell HF, et al. Linkage of Pfeiffer syndrome to chromosome 8 centromere and evidence for genetic heterogeneity. Hum Mol Genet 1994;3:2153–8.
126. Muenke M, Schell U, Hehr A, et al. A common mutation in the fibroblast growth factor receptor 1 gene in Pfeiffer syndrome. Nat Genet 1994;8:269–74.
127. Lajeunie E, Ma HW, Bonaventure J, Munnich A, LeMerrer M. FGFR2 mutations in Pfeiffer syndrome. Nat Genet 1995;9:108.
128. Jabs EQ, Li X, Scott AF, et al. Jackson-Weiss and Crouzon syndromes are

allelic with mutations in fibroblast growth factor receptor 2. Nat Genet 1994;8:275–279.

129. Wilkie AOM, Slaney SF, Oldridge M, et al. Apert syndrome results from localized mutations of FGFR2 and is allelic with Crouzon syndrome. Nat Genet 1995;9:165–72.

130. Rimoin DL, Hughes GN, Kaufman RL, Rosenthal RE, McAlister WH, Silberberg R. Endochondral ossification in achondroplastic dwarfism. N Engl J Med 1970;283:28–35.

131. Stanescu R, Stanescu V, Maroteaux P. Homozygous achondroplasia: morphologic and biochemical study of cartilage. Am J Med Genet 1990;37:412–21.

132. Narcy F, Sanak M. Stop codon FGFR3 mutations in thanatophoric dwarfism type I. Nat Genet 1995;10:11–12.

133. Horton WA, Hood OJ, Machado MA, Ahmed S, Griffey ES. Abnormal ossification in thanatophoric dysplasia. Bone 1988;9:53–61.

134. McKusick VA. Mendelian inheritance in man: catalogs of autosomal dominant, autosomal recessive, and X-linked phenotypes, 8th ed. Baltimore: Johns Hopkins University Press, 1988.

135. Erlebacher A, Filvaroff EH, Gitelman SE, Derynck R. Toward a molecular understanding of skeletal development. Cell 1995;80:371–8.

136. Johnson RL, Riddle RD, Tabin CJ. Mechanisms of limb patterning. Curr Opin Genet Dev 1994;4:535–42.

137. Niswander L, Martin GR. FGF-4 and BMP-2 have opposite effects on limb growth. Nature 1993;361:68–71.

138. Niswander L, Jeffrey S, Martin GR, Tickle C. A positive feedback loop coordinates growth and patterning in the vertebrate limb. Nature 1994; 371:609–12.

139. Weiner DB, Liu J, Cohen JA, Williams WV, Greene MI. A point mutation in the *neu* oncogene mimics ligand induction of receptor aggregation. Nature 1989;339:230–1.

140. Bargmann CI, Hung M-C, Weinberg RA. Multiple independent activations of the *neu* oncogene by a point mutation altering the transmembrane domain of p185. Cell 1986;45:649–57.

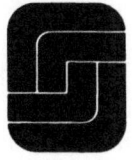

10

Arginine and Nitric Oxide (NO) Interactions in the Healing Wound

JORGE E. ALBINA

The appearance, accumulation, degradation, and biologic activity of different cytokines at sites of injury and inflammation have attracted considerable attention. These signal peptides synthesized by inflammatory cells are justifiably thought to convey fundamental intercellular messages that regulate the process of repair.

The presence of cytokines is not, by any means, the only distinctive feature of the extracellular space of wounds. It has been shown in this regard that wound fluid is a veritable "third space" that, among other distinctive features, contains less glucose and oxygen, more lactate, and a different amino acid composition than plasma (1). These compositional differences between plasma and wound fluid reflect specifics of substrate flux between both compartments and the local metabolism of plasma-borne substrates by the inflammatory cells of the wound. Most importantly, it appears that some of the substrates and metabolites accumulating in the wound space share with the cytokines the ability to elicit specific cellular responses and are, thus, coregulatory of repair.

The amino acid composition of wound fluid differs from that of plasma. Most prominent among the specific alterations in amino acid composition that distinguish wound fluid are those resulting from the expression of two different enzymes of arginine metabolism — arginase and nitric oxide synthase — in the wound space (2, 3). Evidence recently obtained indicates that molecules with potential regulatory roles to the process of repair are derived from the local metabolism of arginine within the wound through these two enzymes.

The nitric oxide synthases (NOS) catalyze the catabolism of arginine to citrulline and NO, this last a short-lived moiety associated with a variety of biologic effects (reviewed in 4). Arginase, while also utilizing arginine as a substrate, results in the formation of different products: ornithine and urea. This chapter presents current knowledge on the expression of both pathways in wounds and discusses their potential relevance to the process of tissue repair.

Most of the data reported here were obtained from experimental wounds in rats. The presence of these distinct enzymes of arginine metabolism and the particulars of their temporal segregation have not been investigated in humans to any significant extent. Results, then, that form the basis of this chapter were obtained mainly from the dead-space wound created in rats through the subcutaneous implantation of sterile polyvinyl alcohol sponges (2). This model allows for the harvesting of the sponges and subsequent isolation of viable wound cells or of wound fluid over time. Data to be shown are not unique to this model. Almost identical findings were obtained in muscle wound models or using the Schilling-Hunt stainless steel mesh cylinder (2).

Examination of extracellular fluid obtained from these experimental wounds provided evidence for the temporally restricted expression of NOS and arginase that was mentioned earlier. Evidence in this regard was given by changes in the concentrations of arginine and its enzyme-specific metabolites in wound fluid over time that are shown in Figure 10.1. Data in this figure, derived from wound fluid and plasma obtained from animals with implanted polyvinyl alcohol sponges, show that wound fluid and plasma arginine concentrations are lower than the normal fasting plasma arginine level in the rat (approximately 200 μM) for the initial 12 hours after wounding. While the arginine plasma concentration returns to normal by 24 hours, that in wound fluid remains below the corresponding plasma concentration for 72 hours. Following a brief period of identity between plasma and wound fluid arginine levels, the concentration of this amino acid in wound fluid decreases progressively and profoundly. In many experiments arginine is undetectable in wound fluid harvested 10 to 15 days after injury (3).

An explanation for the early (6 to 72 hours after wounding) decline in wound fluid arginine concentration is given by the accumulation of citrulline and NO_2^-, two metabolites of the NOS reaction, in wound fluid. The late and persistent reduction in arginine content appears to be explained by its local metabolism through arginase. This is so because ornithine, the product of arginine metabolism through arginase, accumulates in wound fluid to concentrations almost sixfold those found in normal rat plasma. Moreover, analysis of wound fluid also revealed the presence and accumulation of arginase activity, most prominently in wounds harvested from day 5 after injury (3).

That the composition of wound fluid accurately reflects the local metabolism of arginine in the wound at the different time points was established using whole sponge cultures. In these experiments, the previously implanted sponges were harvested over time and cultured in media containing surfeit arginine (4 mM). Results obtained, shown in Figure 10.2, closely resemble those from wound fluid analysis in that citrulline accumulates only in cultures of sponges harvested during the initial 24 to 48 hours after injury and ornithine in cultures of sponges obtained at later times.

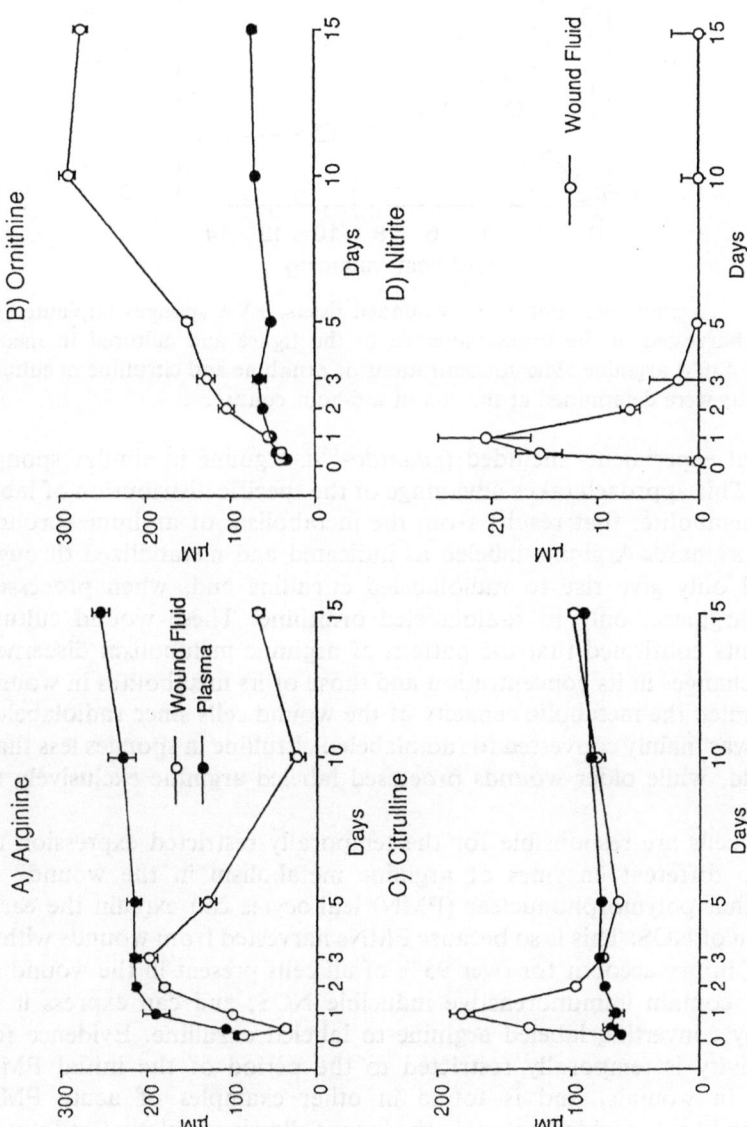

FIGURE 10.1. Evidence for the temporally segregated metabolism of arginine through nitric oxide synthase and arginase in experimental wounds in rats. Animals received polyvinyl alcohol (PVA) sponge implants that were harvested at the times indicated in the figure. Data represents the concentrations of the indicated substrates in wound fluid and plasma of wounded animals.

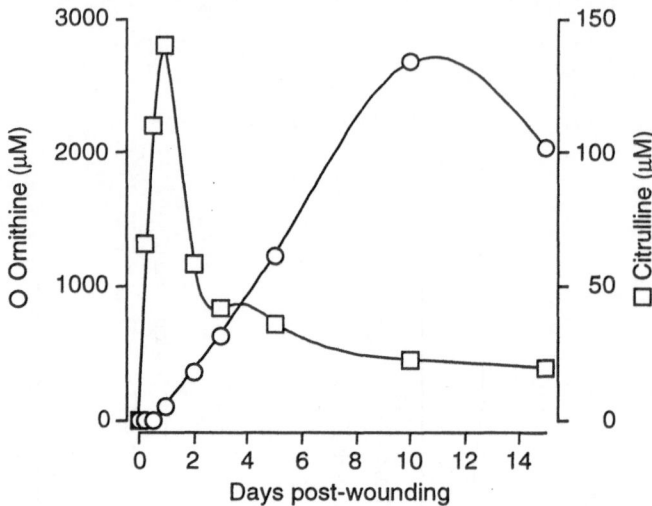

FIGURE 10.2. Arginine metabolism by wounded tissue. PVA sponges implanted in rats were harvested at the times indicated in the figure and cultured in media containing 4 mM arginine. The concentrations of ornithine and citrulline in culture supernatants were determined at the end of a 6-hour culture.

Additional experiments included [*guanido*-[14]-L-arginine in similar sponge cultures. This approach takes advantage of the specific distribution of label among metabolites that results from the metabolism of arginine through NOS or arginase. Arginine labeled as indicated and metabolized through NOS will only give rise to radiolabeled citrulline and, when processed through arginase, only to radiolabeled ornithine. These wound culture experiments confirmed that the pattern of arginine metabolism discerned through changes in its concentration and those of its metabolites in wound fluid revealed the metabolic capacity of the wound cells since radiolabeled arginine was mainly converted to radiolabeled citrulline in sponges less than 2 days old, while older wounds processed labeled arginine exclusively to ornithine.

Which cells are responsible for the temporally restricted expression of these two different enzymes of arginine metabolism in the wound? It appears that polymorphonuclear (PMN) leukocytes can explain the early expression of NOS. This is so because PMNs harvested from wounds within 2 days of injury account for over 95% of all cells present in the wound at the time, contain immunoreactive inducible NOS, and can express it in culture by converting labeled arginine to labeled citrulline. Evidence for NOS activity is temporally restricted to the period of the initial PMN infiltrate in wounds, and is found in other examples of acute PMN infiltration like that which occurs in the lungs following sublethal endotoxin administration, where the activity of NOS in the tissues is increased for less than 24 hours (5).

The production of NO by the PMNs that constitute the very early inflammatory infiltrate of the wound could explain some of the events known to follow tissue injury. It is reasonable, for example, to propose that NO-mediated vasodilatation could mediate the hyperemia associated with the acute inflammation. Additionally, it has been reported that inhibitors of NOS suppress the appearance of edema following the injection of substance P (6), carrageenan, or dextra (7), thus supporting a role of NO in the development of Celsus's tetrad at the site of injury. Contrasting with this proinflammatory role of NO in early repair, NO also reduces platelet aggregation and adhesiveness (8), leukocyte adherence to vascular endothelia (9, 10), and microvascular permeability (11). Inhibition of NOS in PMNs in vitro was also shown to result in an increase in the expression of the adhesion molecules CD11/CD18 (9). These effects of NO could be interpreted as potentially downregulatory of inflammatory responses. Further work is needed in this area to fully understand the specific role of PMN-derived NO in the early stages of inflammation and repair.

There is controversy regarding the end result of the reaction of NO with other reactive species, most particularly with O_2^-. In combining, NO and O_2^- result in the production of peroxynitrite (ONOO) (12–16). This reaction occurs with extraordinary velocity, with a rate constant approaching the diffusion-controlled limit. In fact, the affinity of NO for O_2^- is larger than that of the former for heme compounds and the latter for superoxide dismutase. As a result of their reaction, then, NO and O_2^- can be mutually eliminated. Indeed, evidence in the literature demonstrates that O_2^- scavengers, for example, can enhance the biologic activity of NO by prolonging its half-life. In a similar fashion, NO can quench O_2^- and thus act as an antioxidant. The reaction, then, of NO and O_2^- could serve to decrease the biologic activity of both compounds. However, the product of their reaction, ONOO, either by itself or through its putative by-products $OH^{\bullet}$ or $HOONO^{\bullet}$, is a potent oxidant that can attack a variety of biologic targets. It appears, then, from the preceding discussion that local circumstances should determine the outcome of the concurrent production of NO and O_2^-. It is quite easily conceivable that the PMNs accumulating in a restricted area of injury or inflammation could produce sufficient NO, O_2^-, or ONOO to result in significant collateral damage to surrounding tissues.

Returning to the biphasic pattern of arginine metabolism in the wounds, arginase is the predominant, and almost exclusive, enzyme capable of catabolizing this amino acid during the period of predominant macrophage infiltration. Macrophages, in turn, are the most likely source of arginase at that time. That macrophages contain this enzyme and that arginase activity characterizes areas of chronic inflammation has long been known.

Edlbacher and Merz (17) first described in 1927 the presence of arginase in granulation tissue. Dry and others (reviewed in 18) proposed an important role for macrophage arginase in the regulation of immune responses. In this context, arginase actively secreted from macrophages would consume extracellular arginine at different sites and different circumstances of immune activation, like those resulting from tumor development or parasitic or viral infection. By catabolizing arginine to levels incompatible with the metabolic requirements of the tumor cells or the infectious agents, arginase-dependent arginine deprivation would limit tumor growth or assist in infection control. Alternatively, macrophage-derived arginase could be immunosuppressive by preventing lymphocyte proliferation, also through an identical mechanism of substrate deprivation. Can a similar role be conceived for extracellular arginase in wounds? First, work from this and other laboratories failed to find evidence for the active secretion of arginase (18). While arginase has been often listed as a secretory protein of macrophages, data obtained from wounds correlates best with the hypothesis that the release of arginase from macrophages is a by-product of cell lysis within the wound. This conclusion emerges from the strict correlation of arginase activity in wound fluid with the lactic dehydrogenase activity in the fluid, which is a clear marker for cell lysis (3). It does not appear, then, that macrophage arginase release is a specific response triggered by stimuli found in wounds. Second, while it is conceivable that the low arginine content of the wound fluid could become limiting for the proliferation of cells involved in the healing response, this is contrary to the simple fact that fibroblasts are known to proliferate in wounds. It can, however, be proposed that arginase activity and arginine concentrations are not uniformly distributed throughout the wound. In this connection, it has been clearly shown that oxygen tensions in a healing wound change as a function of distance from neo-vessels (19). While the central, macrophage-rich area of the wound is virtually anoxic, peripheral areas of fibroblast proliferation and neovascularization contain higher tensions of oxygen. It could, in a similar fashion, be that arginase activity mainly resides in the macrophage core of the wound where it truly restricts fibroblast proliferation and premature repair. Vessel-rich areas of active granulation of the wound could possess, in contrast, less if any arginase and maintain arginine concentrations sufficient to support reparative cell division.

A teleologic explanation for the high arginase activity in wounds can alternatively be built on the role of one of its products, ornithine, in the synthesis of collagen. In this connection, ornithine is a synthetic precursor for proline. Due to the high proline and hydroxyproline content of collagen, its accelerated synthesis during repair can be predicted to increase the local demand for proline. It has been demonstrated that the size of the locally available proline pool determines the rate of collagen synthesis in conditions of rapid collagen deposition and that the local synthesis of proline from its precursors, namely ornithine, glutamate, and glutamine, is accelerated under these circumstances to accommodate the relative deficiency of preformed proline (20, 21). It is conceivable, then, that a similar relative proline deficiency exists in healing wounds, and that the massive production of ornithine from arginine through arginase serves to alleviate this deficiency by the subsequent conversion of ornithine to proline. Indeed, results reported from this laboratory confirmed that wound-derived fibroblasts can take up and convert ornithine to proline and incorporate ornithine-derived proline into secretory proteins (22). Therefore, arginase may facilitate the process of repair by increasing the availability of ornithine for its conversion and incorporation as proline into collagen.

While the examination of the amino acid composition of wound fluid presents a tidy picture of early NOS activity and late arginase activity, macrophages harvested from the wound produce abundant citrulline in culture. Data in Table 10.1 show results of experiments where rat wound-derived macrophages were harvested 10 days following injury; resident peritoneal or *C. parvum*–activated peritoneal macrophages were cultured in the presence of radiolabeled arginine for 24 hours. As can be seen in the table, wound macrophages in culture were capable of producing more citrulline than resident peritoneal macrophages and virtually as much as their activated counterparts. Interestingly, while all three macrophage types contain intracellular arginase activity, only wound-derived cells manifested this enzyme activity in culture by producing radiolabeled urea from radioactive arginine.

The preceding data indicate that wound macrophages, while fully capable of expressing NOS in culture, do not appear to express this enzyme in wounds in vivo. Several hypotheses were tested in investigating the lack of NOS activity in macrophage-infiltrated wounds. The most obvious and immediate was that the dramatic arginine depletion caused by its catabolism by arginase deprived NOS of substrate. Indeed, culture of any macrophage in arginine-deficient medium markedly reduces the amount of citrulline and NO_2^- produced. Wound cores are hypoxic-anoxic environments. Because the synthesis of NO consumes molecular oxygen, it seemed reasonable to predict that reductions in oxygen tension would decrease arginine flux through NOS. Experiments performed, then, to explore the relationship between oxygen availability and NO production demonstrated that culture of macrophages obtained from wound or from the peritoneal cavity at oxygen tensions below 37 torr (5% O_2) reduced the production of NO and

TABLE 10.1. Arginine metabolism by wound-derived, resident peritoneal or *C. parvum*–activated rat peritoneal macrophages.

Macrophage type	Urea	Citrulline
Wound-derived	4.5 ± 0.1	5.8 ± 0.3
Resident peritoneal	0.1 ± 0.1	1.4 ± 0.1
C. parvum–activated peritoneal	0.1 ± 0.1	5.4 ± 0.5

Rat wound-derived macrophages harvested 10 days after injury and resident peritoneal or *C. parvum*–activated peritoneal macrophages were cultured in media containing [*guanido*-^{14}C]-L-arginine. The distribution of radiolabel into urea and citrulline was determined at the end overnight culture. Data are nmol/h/10^6 cells and were calculated from the radioactivity in the products and the specific radioactivity of arginine at the beginning of culture.

that arginine flux through NOS was completely suppressed in anoxic cultures (23).

These experiments provided additional fascinating information. Wound-derived macrophages, but not resident or *C. parvum*-elicited peritoneal macrophages, remarkably enhanced their arginase activity when cultured in an anoxic environment (23). In regard to wound macrophages, therefore, anoxia suppressed NOS activity both directly through lack of oxygen and indirectly by accelerating arginine consumption through arginase. All macrophage types studied enhanced their tumor necrosis factor-α (TNF-α) and interleukin-6 (IL-6) release in anoxic cultures. Anoxia appeared thus to provide some activating signal to the macrophages. Interestingly, and connecting these findings with those in the literature, it has been shown that anoxia promotes the release of angiogenic factors from macrophages and that TNF-α may mediate angiogenesis (24, 25). Lastly, immunoblotting for NOS in wound macrophages demonstrated that they contain little immunoreactive NOS when freshly harvested, that they increase their NOS content during overnight culture, and that this increase is markedly enhanced in anoxic cultures (23).

These findings warrant further discussion. First, they indicate that culture in serum-free medium for less than 12 hours results in a manyfold increase in the immunoreactive NOS content of the wound-derived macrophages. This increase does not appear to result from the adherence of the cells to plastic since it also occurs in cells cultured in suspension. Studies under way will explore whether it is the retrieval of the cells from the wound environment that removes a suppressive signal curtailing the appearance of NOS protein in the cells in vivo. The most likely candidates for such a suppressive role are transforming growth factor-β (TGF-β) and corticosterone, both potent inhibitors of the induction of NOS. Their potential suppressive role in vivo on the expression of NOS by wound macrophages is currently being investigated. A second observation, derived from studies using anoxic cultures, is that conditions inimical to the expression of NOS, including anoxia, arginine deprivation, or the inclusion in culture media of an inhibitor of NOS, lead to marked increases in the NOS content of the cells. While evidence for a feedback inhibitory effect of NO on the activity of NOS has been reported (26, 27), current data indicate that the production of NO could actually lead to a decrease in the NOS protein of the cells. The molecular level at which this control could be effected is presently being explored.

Wound macrophages do not appear to express NOS in vivo, and multiple elements, including extracellular arginase activity, a depleted arginine pool, and hypoxia, virtually guarantee that little if any NO will be produced during the macrophage phase of wound healing.

Work in progress indicates, in addition, that NOS can easily be induced by interferon-γ (IFN-γ), TNF-α, and other cytokines in wound-derived fibroblast. These cells, however, do not express NOS when freshly obtained from experimental wounds. Why is this so? NO has gained recognition as a mediator of macrophage antitumor and anti-infectious actions. In this connection, abundant data correlate the production of reactive nitrogen intermediates by macrophages and their capacity to lyse or arrest the growth of some tumor cell lines and to kill certain intracellular parasites. It is, however, also true that NO is profoundly toxic for the cell that produces it. Work from this laboratory has shown that the production of NO by macrophages correlates with decreases in the production of O_2^-, phagocytic capacity, electron transport chain activity, and total protein synthesis (28, 29). Moreover, continued production of NO by macrophages or fibroblasts results in the death of the producing cells (30, 31). Beyond these deleterious effects of NO on its producer cell, NO is immunosuppressive. Evidence from this and other laboratories (32–35) indicates that macrophage-derived NO suppresses T-cell proliferation and may even result in apoptosis in the targeted lymphocytes. It may well be, then, that it is because of its antiproliferative and cytotoxic activities that NO production in healing wounds is significantly curtailed.

Conclusion

Arginine is the only amino acid whose utilization in wounds exceeds its availability. It serves as a substrate to two distinct enzymes, NOS and arginase, in a temporally segregated fashion. The early phase, characterized by the presence of NOS, coincides with the appearance of PMNs in the wounds. In this context, NO may serve to regulate acute inflammation. Later, when macrophages populate the wound, arginase becomes the predominant enzyme of arginine metabolism in wounds and by-products of this reaction may support collagen synthesis in the wound. The expression of NOS by wound macrophages is, as described above, severely curtailed through a variety of mechanisms. These mechanisms may ensure that the toxic effects of NO do not derail the process of repair.

References

1. Albina JE, Shearer J, Mastrofrancesco B, Caldwell MD. Amino acid metabolism after λ-carrageenan injury to rat skeletal muscle. Am J Physiol 1986;250:E24–30.
2. Albina JE, Mills CD, Barbul A, et al. Arginine metabolism in wounds. Am J Physiol 1988;254:E459–67.
3. Albina JE, Mills CD, Henry WL Jr, Caldwell MD. Temporal expression of different pathways of L-arginine metabolism in healing wounds. J Immunol 1990;144:3877–80.
4. Moncada S, Palmer RMJ, Higgs EA. Nitric oxide: physiology, pathophysiology, and pharmacology. Pharmacol Rev 1991;43:109–42.
5. Abate JA, Albina JE. Temporal expression of nitric oxide synthase in post-

endotoxin rat lung. In: Moncada S, Marletta MA, Hibbs JB Jr, Higgs EA, eds. The biology of nitric oxide. 2. Enzymology, biochemistry and immunology. Proceedings of the 2nd International Meeting on the Biology of Nitric Oxide; 1991 Sept. 30–Oct. 2; London. Colchester: Portland Press, 1992;197-9.

6. Hughes SR, Williams TJ, Brain SD. Evidence that endogenous nitric oxide modulates oedema formation induced by substance P. Eur J Pharmacol 1990;191:481-4.

7. Ialenti A, Ianaro A, Moncada S, Di Rosa M. Modulation of acute inflammation by endogenous nitric oxide. Eur J Pharmacol 1992;211:177-82.

8. Radomski MW, Palmer RMJ, Moncada S. An L-arginine/nitric oxide pathway present in human platelets regulates aggregation. Proc Natl Acad Sci USA 1990;87:5193-7.

9. Kubes P, Suzuki M, Granger DN. Nitric oxide: an endogenous modulator of leukocyte adhesion. Proc Natl Acad Sci USA 1991;88:4651-5.

10. Kubes P, Kanwar S, Niu X-F, Gaboury JP. Nitric oxide synthesis inhibition induces leukocyte adhesion via superoxide and mast cells. FASEB J 1993; 7:1293-9.

11. Kurose I, Kubes P, Wolf R, et al. Inhibition of nitric oxide production: mechanisms of vascular albumin leakage. Circ Res 1993;73:164-71.

12. Beckman JS, Beckman TW, Chen J, Marshall PA, Freeman BA. Apparent hydroxyl radical production by peroxynitrite: implications for endothelial injury from nitric oxide and superoxide. Proc Natl Acad Sci USA 1990;87:1620-4.

13. Radi R, Beckman JS, Bush KM, Freeman BA. Peroxynitrite oxidation of sulfhydryls: the cytotoxic potential of superoxide and nitric oxide. J Biol Chem 1991;266:4244-50.

14. Hogg N, Darley-Usmar VM, Wilson MT, Moncada S. Production of hydroxyl radicals from the simultaneous generation of superoxide and nitric oxide. Biochem J 1992;281:419-24.

15. Beckman JS, Chen J, Ischiropoulos H, Crow JP. Oxidative chemistry of peroxynitrite. Methods Enzymol 1994;233:229-40.

16. Pryor WA, Squadrito GL. The chemistry of peroxynitrite: a product from the reaction of nitric oxide with superoxide. Am J Physiol 1995;268:L699-722.

17. Edlbacher S, Merz KW. Über den stoffwechsel der tumoren. Z Physiol Chem 1927;171:252-63.

18. Schneider E, Dy M. The role of arginase in the immune response. Immunol Today 1985;6:136-40.

19. Hunt TK. Prospective: a retrospective perspective on the nature of wounds. In: Barbul A, Pines E, Caldwell M, Hunt TK, eds. Growth factors and other aspects of wound healing. Biological and clinical implications. Proceedings of the Second International Symposium on Tissue Repair; 1987 May 13-17; Tarpon Springs (FL). New York: Alan R. Liss, 1987:xiii-xx.

20. Kershenobich D, Fierro FJ, Rojkind M. The relationship between the free pool of proline and collagen content in human liver cirrhosis. J Clin Invest 1970;49:2246-9.

21. Rojkind M, Diaz de León L. Collagen biosynthesis in cirrhotic rat liver slices: a regulatory mechanism. Biochim Biophys Acta 1970;217:512-22.

22. Albina JE, Abate JA, Mastrofrancesco B. Role of ornithine as a proline precursor in healing wounds. J Surg Res 1993;55:97-102.

23. Albina JE, Henry WL Jr, Mastrofrancesco B, Martin BA, Reichner JS.

Macrophage activation by culture in an anoxic environment. J Immunol 1995; in press.

24. Knighton DR, Hunt TK, Scheuenstuhl H, Halliday BJ. Oxygen tension regulates the expression of angiogenesis factor by macrophages. Science 1983; 211:1283-5.

25. Leibovich SJ, Polverini PJ, Shepard HM, Wiseman DM, Shively V, Nuseir N. Macrophage-induced angiogenesis is mediated by tumour necrosis factor-α. Nature 1987;329:630-2.

26. Rogers NE, Ignarro LJ. Constitutive nitric oxide synthase from cerebellum is reversibly inhibited by nitric oxide formed from L-arginine. Biochem Biophys Res Commun 1992;189:242-9.

27. Griscavage JM, Fukuto JM, Komori Y, Ignarro LJ. Nitric oxide inhibits neuronal nitric oxide synthase by interacting with the heme prosthetic group. J Biol Chem 1994;269:21644-9.

28. Albina JE, Caldwell MD, Henry WL Jr, Mills CD. Regulation of macrophage functions by L-arginine. J Exp Med 1989;169:1021-9.

29. Albina JE, Mills CD, Henry WL Jr, Caldwell MD. Regulation of macrophage physiology by L-arginine: role of the oxidative L-arginine deiminase pathway. J Immunol 1989;143:3641-6.

30. Albina JE, Cui S, Mateo RB, Reichner JS. Nitric oxide-mediated apoptosis in murine peritoneal macrophages. J Immunol 1993;150:5080-5.

31. Werner-Felmayer G, Werner ER, Fuchs D, Hausen A, Reibnegger G, Wachter H. Tetrahydrobiopterin-dependent formation of nitrite and nitrate in murine fibroblasts. J Exp Med 1990;172:1599-607.

32. Hoffman RA, Langrehr JM, Billiar TR, Curran RD, Simmons RL. Alloantigen-induced activation of rat splenocytes is regulated by the oxidative metabolism of L-arginine. J Immunol 1990;145:2220-6.

33. Albina JE, Henry WL Jr. Suppression of lymphocyte proliferation through the nitric oxide synthesizing pathway. J Surg Res 1991;50:403-9.

34. Albina JE, Abate JA, Henry WL Jr. Nitric oxide production is required for murine resident peritoneal macrophages to suppress mitogen-stimulated T cell proliferation. J Immunol 1991;147:144-8.

35. Albina JE, Henry WL Jr. Cytokine network regulating macrophage-mediated suppression through nitric oxide synthase products. In: Moncada S, Marletta MA, Hibbs JB Jr, Higgs EA, eds. The biology of nitric oxide. 2. Enzymology, biochemistry and immunology. Proceedings of the 2nd International Meeting on the Biology of Nitric Oxide; 1991 Sept. 30-Oct. 2; London. Colchester: Portland Press, 1992:210-3.

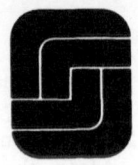

11

Endogenous Growth Factors and Nutrients in the Healing Wound

Wes J. Arlein and Michael D. Caldwell

This chapter focuses on the temporal sequence of endogenous growth factors and nutrients in the healing wound. We propose that the function and proliferation of wound cells are dependent on the concentration of substrates, hormones, growth factors, cytokines, matrix, etc. in the local wound environment and less dependent on serum factors. The consistent proliferative effect of early wound fluid and inhibitory effect of late wound fluid is supportive of this hypothesis (1).

This stimulation of proliferation by wound fluid is consistent with current concepts that extracellular factors determined whether quiescent cells begin to proliferate and whether proliferating cells in the G_1 phase will continue to cycle or become quiescent (2). The G_1 state of the cell cycle has been divided into competence, entry, and progression subphases (3). Competence has been produced in untransformed fibroblasts by platelet-derived growth factor (PDGF) (4, 5). In the absence of amino acids the cell cycle stops at the competence subphase (2). Competent cells progress toward the S phase in the presence of epidermal growth factor (EGF), insulin, insulin-like growth factors, or plasma (4–7). Only insulin-like growth factor-I (IGF-I) has been shown to be required for the progression subphase of 3T3 fibroblasts (6, 7).

Although Carrell (8) first described the stimulation of fibroblast proliferation by wound cells in 1922, only recently have the factors responsible for this proliferation begun to be elucidated. Many of the cell cycle regulatory growth factors and nutrients discussed above have been identified in wounds. Classical metabolism and immunology has delineated altered fuel sources, macromolecule synthesis, and amino acid metabolism in the wound. Analysis of temporal and spatial variations in messenger RNA (mRNA) and protein using the newest developments in molecular biology and immunology have sparked major advances in our understanding of growth factors in the wound. To follow is both a review of what is currently known about the endogenous growth factors and nutrients in the healing wound as well as an analysis of the temporal relationships among these factors.

Growth Factors

Epidermal Growth Factor

Epidermal growth factor (EGF) is a 53 amino acid polypeptide shown to affect keratinocyte migration and stimulate DNA, RNA, and protein synthesis in a variety of cell types (9). It was first identified in salivary glands by Cohen (10) in 1962. As EGF is present in saliva and animals lick their wounds, it has been postulated that EGF has a role in wound healing (11). EGF is released by platelets, suggesting a role in early wound healing. Exogenously applied EGF has been shown to speed epithelialization in burn and surgical wounds (12–14).

We measured the time course of EGF messenger RNA in healing wounds (15). Using the polymerase chain reaction (PCR), we detected message for EGF in unwounded skin, polymorphonuclear leukocytes (PMN), and wounded skin. The amount of message in scar varied over time with a bimodal peak at a half day and 15 days post-wounding and a nadir at 3 days post-wounding. Peaks of EGF message were considerably higher than message in unwounded skin. Although PMNs expressed EGF message, levels were much lower than in scar samples, making it unlikely that PMNs contribute significantly to EGF expression in the wound.

Rappollee and colleagues (16) also examined EGF message in a wound model. Glass adherent cells were isolated from Hunt-Schilling chambers 6 days after they were implanted subcutaneously. These adherent cells were 50% to 80% macrophages. Using PCR, this cell population was found to express EGF message. However, no EGF transcript was found in either a highly purified macrophage culture or in macrophage cell lines. These data suggest non–macrophage adherent cells as the source of the EGF message.

Whereas EGF message has been found consistently in wounds, EGF protein data is more equivocal. Ono and associates (17) in Japan measured cytokines in wound fluid from human skin graft donor sites. EGF was examined by human EGF (hEGF)-specific radioimmunoassay using anti-hEGF serum developed by the investigators. Human EGF antibodies were purified, ^{125}I labeled, and used in a standard radioimmunoassay. No EGF was identified in the donor fluid using this method. A major limitation of these data is the absence of a positive control for EGF. Other cytokines were measured in this study by standard commercially available immunoassays.

Grayson and colleagues (18) found appreciable levels of EGF in skin graft donor fluid. Similarly to the study of Ono et al. (17), split-thickness skin graft donor sites in humans were covered with an occlusive dressing. Wound fluid was harvested on the first postoperative day and every day thereafter until no more fluid could be obtained. EGF was measured by standard enzyme immunoassay (mouse primary monoclonal, rabbit anti-mouse peroxidase labeled secondary). EGF levels in donor fluid were elevated as compared with serum with a nadir at days 2 to 3 and peaks at days 1 and 4 (Fig. 11.1).

Wenczak and colleagues (19) investigated EGF receptor (EGF-R) protein in human burn wounds. Protein was detected by immunohistochemistry in excised wound, both partial and full thickness. EGF-R was detected in the migrating epithelial sheet and hair follicles in the early burn wounds. Late burn wound showed less superficial staining but continued moderately positive staining in sweat glands and hair follicles. EGF-R functional status was confirmed by radiolabeled EGF binding.

From the above studies, we conclude that EGF is translated in the wound with an initial early peak and a late peak. This EGF message is not synthesized by wound macrophages or PMNs. As Ono et al.'s (17) study may be flawed by lack of a positive control, we believe EGF protein is present in wound fluid as demonstrated by Grayson et al. (18). EGF product has a similar bimodal distribution to message with an early peak at 1 day and a nadir at days 2 to 3. EGF-R is prominent in the early burn wound in the migrating epithelial sheet. The temporal correlation of message and product for EGF suggests translation within the wound.

Fibroblast Growth Factor

Fibroblast growth factor (FGF) has both acidic and basic forms. Basic FGF is the more potent and in general more studied of the two forms. Basic FGF

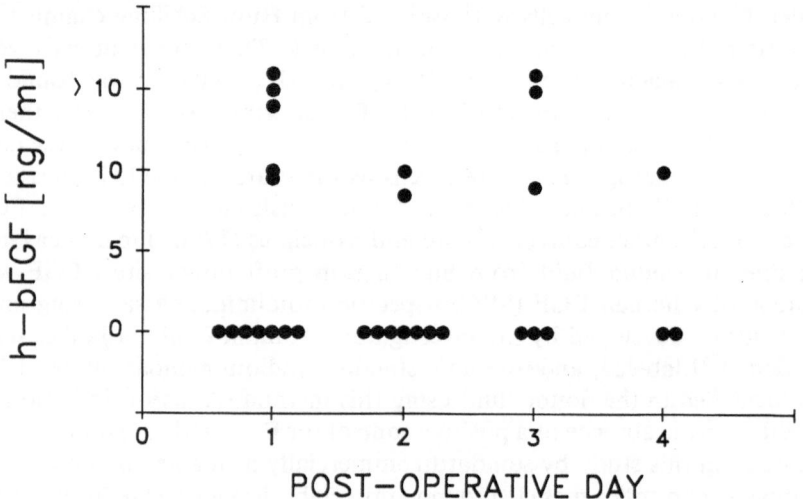

FIGURE 11.1. Each point represents the concentration of EGF measured from a patient's wound fluid on that particular postoperative day (POD). Horizontal lines represent the mean values for all patients on that particular POD. Control serum had no detectable levels of EGF. $p < .007$ for POD 4 compared with POD 2 and 3; $p = .05$ for POD 1 compared with POD 2. (From Grayson LS, Hansbrough JF, et al. Quantitation of cytokine levels in skin graft donor site wound fluid. Burns 1993;19(5):401–405, with permission.)

(bFGF) is a potent mitogen, angiogenic agent, and chemoattractant. It affects all cells involved in wound healing (20). Basic FGF is stored in inactive form in extracellular matrix and cell cytoplasm and in cell injury is activated (Gibran). It does not have a signal sequence and thus is likely released secondary to cell damage and subsequent cytolysis and proteolysis (21). Normal skin contains bFGF and it immunolocalizes to the dermal-epidermal junction, capillaries, and dermal appendages (22, 23). Because it is found in normal skin and is released with injury, bFGF has been postulated to play a prominent role in wound and burn healing. Exogenous bFGF has been shown to accelerate dermal and epidermal healing (24).

Werner and colleagues (25) measured mRNA in the healing wound for the whole family of FGFs including acidic FGF, bFGF, keratinocyte growth factor (KGF), and FGF3-6. They also investigated message for FGF receptors (FGFR1-3). Message was examined by either RNase protection or, for KGF and FGFR-2, in situ hybridization. RNA was obtained from biopsies of full-thickness excisional wounds from a half day to 7 days after wounding. Message for a-FGF, bFGF, FGF-5, and KGF were all increased post-wounding as compared with unwounded skin. No message for either FGF3, 4, or 6 was found in either normal or wounded skin. bFGF message peaked at fourfold induction 5 days post-wounding. a-FGF, bFGF, and FGF-5 message all returned to baseline 7 days post-wounding. Message for KGF was induced 160-fold within 24 hours after wounding and was still 100-fold elevated 7 days post-wounding. FGFR message levels did not change appreciably post-wounding. In situ hybridization for KGF and its receptor (a splice variant of FGFR-2) showed KGF to be produced primarily in the dermis and hypodermis and its receptor confined predominantly in the epidermis.

Using Hunt-Schilling chambers, Steenfos and associates (26) investigated endogenous growth factors (protein) in chamber granulation tissue. Basic FGF was detected by immunohistochemistry in all types of inflammatory cells. Staining was variable and predominantly cytoplasmic. Faint immunoreactivity in the extracellular matrix was present. Addition of exogenous PDGF or EGF did not change the immunostaining intensity or location. Kurita et al. also used immunohistochemistry to identify bFGF in the wound. Their wound model was punch biopsies in mice. Contrary to Steenfos, they found immunoreactive FGF in epithelial cells but not in the inflammatory infiltrate. Given the pronounced staining of these inflammatory cells in vitro, the authors suggest that the in vivo staining may somehow be masked and likely varies depending on which bFGF antibody is used.

Gibran and colleagues (27) studied bFGF antigen using immunolocalization as well. They investigated human excised burn wounds, both partial and full thickness. Strong bFGF staining was found extracellularly in the area of tissue destruction; no bFGF was in the extracellular matrix containing viable cells or in normal skin. Intense staining was found days 4 to 11 post-burn (4 days was the earliest time examined) and was absent extracellularly 30 days post-burn. bFGF specificity was confirmed by competition assays and Western immunoblot with three different anti-bFGF antibodies.

Grayson and associates (18) also looked for bFGF in their covered skin graft donor site model (see above for details). Donor site fluid contained bFGF protein detected by enzyme immunoassay in 5 of 13 donor sites. No variation with time in bFGF levels could be detected. Control serum had no detectable bFGF.

Chen and colleagues (28) investigated the interrelationship between fibroblast proliferation factors and urokinase production factors in the wound. Their experimental model involved Yorkshire White pigs in which full-thickness wounds were made, covered by an occlusive dressing, and wound fluid underneath the dressing harvested. They found that whereas the mitogen for fibroblasts in wound fluid was not effected by a neutralizing antibody to FGF, anti-FGF antibody neutralized urokinase production. The wound urokinase production was heat labile, as is FGF.

From the above studies we conclude that both acidic and basic FGF are transcribed within a few days post-wounding. This augmentation in transcription, however, is relatively small compared with the massive 160-fold KGF induction at 24 hours, implying that KGF has a large role in early wounding and is likely translated in the wound. Basic FGF protein is found in high concentration in areas of tissue destruction in burns and less consistently in donor fluid. It likely is present in the inflammatory infiltrate, although this finding is equivocal. As basic FGF is not secreted, its release in early wound healing may be from cytolysis and it may therefore have a larger role in wounds with extensive tissue destruction. FGF is responsible for wound urokinase production.

Insulin-Like Growth Factor

The insulin-like growth factors (IGFs) consist of IGF-1 and IGF-2 and are also known as somatomedins. They are polypeptide proteins of approximately 7500 daltons and are potent mitogens for many cells. Somatomedins increase DNA synthesis and RNA synthesis and stimulate the transport of amino acids and glucose into the cell (29). They are primarily under the control of growth hormone in vivo, but do have other stimuli (30, 31). IGF-2 has been found in high concentrations in fetal tissue and thus has been proposed to be a fetal growth factor (32–35). Given their role as mitogens, anabolic agents and collagen stimulators, they have been postulated to play a role in wound healing.

Spencer and colleagues (36) investigated the role of somatomedins in wound healing. They removed fibroblasts from Hunt-Schilling chambers 21 days post–subcutaneous implantation in the rat. Using solution hybridization they found 15 IGF-I mRNA copies per cell in active fibroblasts inside the chambers as compared with seven in less active fibroblasts outside the chamber. By comparison, the liver, the largest producer of somatomedins, has 30 copies or IGF-I per cell. They also measured IGF-I protein using radioimmunoassay as a function of time post–chamber implantation in the rabbit. They found less IGF-I in wound fluid than in serum and no variation in wound fluid levels over time.

Our group has also investigated IGF message in the healing wound. We used two models—one sponge model (subcutaneously implanted sponges) and one incisional (4 cm dorsal incision)—and measured IGF mRNA in the cellular infiltrate and scar, respectively (37). Message was semi-quantitated with PCR using [³H] deoxyguanosine triphosphate (dGTP). Both in the scar and in the cellular infiltrate IGF-I message increased markedly over time, with levels by day 3 post-wounding markedly higher than that in serum (Figs. 11.2 and 11.3). PMN had a lower mRNA copy number than wound fibroblasts derived from day 5 sponges. Two mRNA were found for IGF-2, one expected at 383 base pairs (bp) and one unexpected at 650 bp. The 283-bp transcript increased markedly over time in both cellular infiltrate, and scar and was significantly greater than in unwounded skin by day 5 post-wounding. The 650-bp fragment has fewer copies in the wound than in normal skin.

Stefanos and colleagues (26) used immunohistochemistry to measure

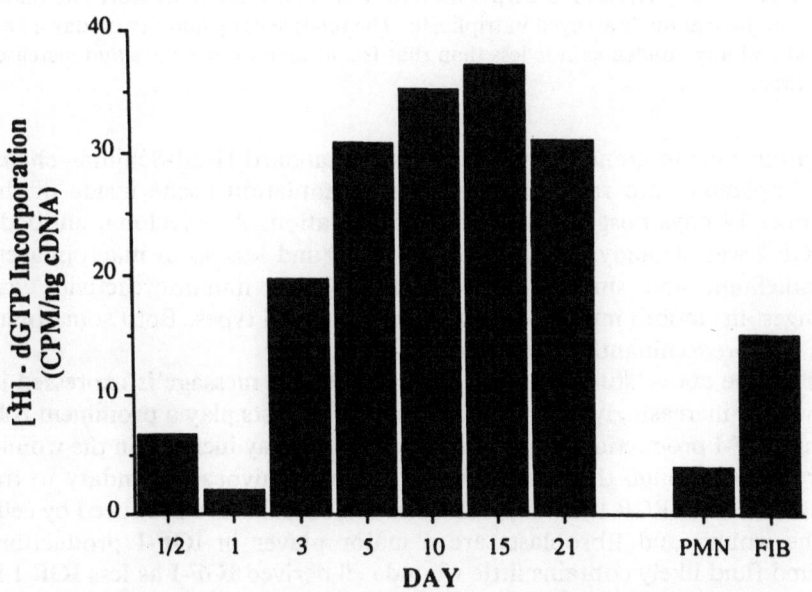

FIGURE 11.2. The [³H] deoxyguanosine triphosphate (dGTP) incorporation for IGF-1 message, expressed as cpm/ng cDNA in the total cellular infiltrate. The results show temporal variation with low levels at the early time points and higher levels at later times points after wounding. Low copy number is also seen in PMN and a higher level in fibroblasts (FIB). (From Grayson LS, Hansbrough JF, et al. Quantitation of cytokine levels in skin graft donor site wound fluid. Burns 1993; 19(5):401–405, with permission.)

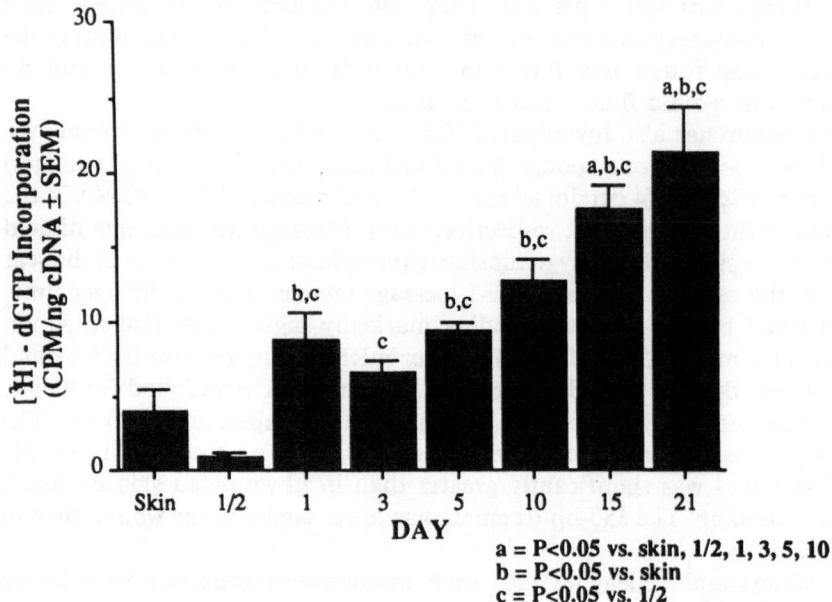

FIGURE 11.3. The [^{3}H]dGTP incorporation for IGF-1 message in the scar. The values are from three animals assayed in triplicate. The relative copy number on day a half wound and unwounded skin is less than that found on all other days and increases over time.

somatomedins in granulation tissue. Using standard Hunt-Schilling chambers implanted into rats, they harvested granulation tissue inside of the chamber 14 days post–subcutaneous implantation. A polyclonal antibody to IGF-I was strongly positive in fibroblasts and less so in macrophages, endothelium, and smooth muscle cells. IGF-II immunoreactivity was strongest in smooth muscle, less so in the other cell types. Both somatomedins had predominantly cytoplasmic staining.

From the above studies we conclude that IGF-I message is expressed in the wound increasingly over time. Wound fibroblasts play a prominent role in this IGF-I production. IGF-II transcripts also may increase in the wound over time, although this finding is a bit more equivocal secondary to the presence of two PCR transcripts. Both somatomedins are produced by cells in the wound and fibroblasts are a major player in IGF-I production. Wound fluid likely contains little wound cell derived IGF-I as less IGF-1 is found in wound fluid than in serum.

Macrophage Colony Stimulating Factor

Macrophage colony stimulating factor (M-CSF) is a homodimer of two identical polypeptide chains linked by a disulfide bridge. Varying degrees of glycosylation result in molecular weights between 45 and 90 kd. The main source of M-CSF is the monocyte or macrophage, although fibroblasts can constitutively produce it. Although M-CSF stimulates macrophage colony formation, its major role may be in stimulating the production of tumor necrosis factor (TNF) and interferon and increasing macrophage cytotoxic activity (38).

Ford and associates (39) have measured the stimulation of colony formation by wound fluid. Using the colony-forming assay, they found stimulation of colony production over that of serum on all days post-wounding studied (days 3, 5, 8, and 13). Colonies were predominantly macrophage colonies. Specific bioassays for multi-CSF [interleukin-3 (IL-3)], granulocyte-macrophage colony stimulating factor (GM-CSF), and granulocyte CSF failed to detect these factors. M-CSF levels as measured by radioimmunoassay were high throughout the time period studied and could account for all of the CSF bioactivity measured. Ford et al. concluded that M-CSF likely has a prominent role in the healing wound.

Platelet-Derived Growth Factor

Platelet derived growth factor (PDGF) is one of several growth factors contained in the α-granule of the platelet. It is a 30-kd basic protein consisting of two peptide chains A and B, which form two homodimers (AA or BB) or a heterodimer (AB) (40). PDGF is a mitogen and chemoattractant for fibroblasts and smooth muscle cells. At low concentrations (0.5 to 1.0 ng/ml) it causes fibroblast migration, and at slightly higher concentrations it causes fibroblast replication (41). A similar peptide is produced by macrophages and endothelial cells (42–44).

Rappolee and associates (16) studied the production of PDGF message by wound macrophages. As detailed above, they harvested cells from wound cylinders in mice 6 days postimplantation. Glass adherent cells (mostly macrophages) were analyzed by PCR for growth factor message. Wound macrophages expressed PDGF-α mRNA. In addition they tested the P388D1 macrophages cell line and thiogycollate-elicited mouse peritoneal macrophages stimulated with lipopolysaccharide (LPS) and found they also expressed PDGF mRNA.

Antoniades and colleagues (45) studied PDGF and PDGF receptor (PDGF-R) messages by in situ hybridization using a Yorkshire pig partial-thickness wound model. Fibroblasts and epithelial cells did not constitutively express PDGF mRNA; fibroblasts normally express PDGF-R receptor. They found marked increase in message in epithelial cells and fibroblasts for both hormone and receptor within 1 day of injury. Levels were either low or nondetectable 9 days post-wounding. Using immuno-histochemistry, they also identified PDGF and PDGF-R like proteins 1 day postinjury. These proteins were identified in both the epithelial layer and connective tissue layer, paralleling the message data.

Although no PDGF protein has been detected in wound fluid, PDGF-like peptides with PDGF activity has been found. Grayson and associates (18) measured PDGF protein in fluid from covered skin graft donor sites in humans. PDGF, detected by commercially available radioimmunoassay, was not found in wound fluid in any of 13 patients tested.

Native PDGF was not detected by Matsuoka and Grotendorst (46) in wound fluid. Their wound model was human postmastectomy wound drainage. Antibodies against PDGF and PDGF A- and B-chain components were prepared using standard techniques. Specificity and sensitivity were tested and were excellent. No PDGF chain or protein was detected in any of the six wound fluid samples tested. Western blots revealed two peptides with PDGF activity, one 16 to 17 kd and one 34 to 36 kd in all six patients (native human PDGF is 30 kd). The smaller peptide peaked early (day 1 post-wounding) the larger late (day 7 post-wounding). Data suggested that the 16- to 17-kd protein acted through the PDGF receptor.

From the above studies we conclude that PDGF (or a PDGF-related factor) and the PDGF receptor are transcribed in the wound by multiple cells including fibroblasts and epithelial cells. Although authentic native PDGF has not been identified in wound fluid, numerous studies show a PDGF-related factor with PDGF chemoattractant and mitogenic properties. PDGF activity increases markedly by day 1 post-wounding and returns to baseline 7 days postinjury. This PDGF-related protein is likely 16 to 17 kd and acts through the PDGF receptor.

Tumor Necrosis Factor-α

Tumor necrosis factor-α (TNF-α), also known as cachectin, is a 17-kd protein initially synthesized as a prohormone prior to secretion. TNF is produced by macrophages, monocytes, lymphocytes, and keratinocytes. Cachectin lowers transmembrane potential in muscle and may be responsible for the third spacing seen in sepsis. In addition, it has a marked catabolic affect on many cell types. T-cell–mediated responses are enhanced with TNF-α and T cells treated with TNF show an enhanced proliferation to IL-1. Cachectin is a mitogen for fibroblasts and increases fibroblast collagenase (47). Given TNF's production by macrophages and its role in inflammation and catabolism, it has been postulated to play a role in early wound healing.

TNF-α protein has been found in wound fluid; TNF-α message has not been investigated (18, 39). Grayson et al. (18) used commercially available enzyme-linked immunosorbent assay (ELISA) kit to measure TNF-α levels over time in donor fluid. They found increasing concentrations of TNF-α over time (days 1 to 4 measured) with elevated levels in all 13 patients studied. TNF-α was measured by Ford et al. (39) in wound fluid obtained from sponges implanted subcutaneously in mice. TNF was measured by cytotoxicity assays with standard curves generated with recombinant TNF-α.

TNF-α levels in this study peaked 3 days after wounding and decreased thereafter. From these studies, we conclude that TNF-α likely has a role in the early (days 1 to 4 postinjury) wound. Whether or not it is transcribed, its cell of origin and its specific effects have yet to be elucidated.

Transforming Growth Factor-α

Transforming growth factor-α (TGF-α) is a member of the epidermal growth factor family. It has homology to EGF and binds to the EGF receptor. In a wide variety of cell lines, TGF-α acts as a mitogenic for EGF responsive cells. TGF-α is secreted by macrophages, keratinocytes, and fibroblasts and may have important functions in the regulation of inflammation. Most studies have not found a significant difference in potency or activity between TGF-α and EGF. However, TGF-α may be more potent in promoting angiogenesis and in keratinocyte colony formation (48). Given its prominent role as a director of inflammation, TGF-α has been postulated to play a role in the healing wound.

Rappollee et al. (16), as detailed above, investigated mRNA of growth factors in wound macrophages. Using quantitative PCR, they found transcripts for TGF-α in glass-adherent cells from all wound chambers. They also found transcripts in the macrophage cell line P388D1 and the copy number increased with LPS treatment. TGF-α protein concentration as measured by ELISA in wound fluid was 51 ng/L. Both highly purified macrophages and a macrophage cell line did not constitutively express TGF-α antigen. Both expressed the protein after LPS stimulation.

Our group also investigated TGF-α message and protein in the wound. Using a subcutaneously implanted sponge model, we found a peak of message at days 3 and 5 as detected by competitive PCR (49). TGF-α protein peaked at day 10 as measured by radioimmunoassay. As protein temporally followed message, we concluded that TGF-α is likely transcribed in the wound.

Ono et al. (17) found TGF-α in 5-day-old covered human skin graft donor sites by ELISA. Mean TGF-α concentration was 2.04 ng/ml. They found a negative correlation of TGF-α levels with the age of the patient from whom the graft was taken.

From the above studies, we conclude that TGF-α is transcribed and translated within the wound. The wound macrophage likely plays a large role in this TGF-α production. TGF-α is present in skin graft donor site wounds, wound chambers, and wound sponges, suggesting a prominent role in wound healing.

TGF-β

The original transforming growth factor-β (TGF-β) was a 25-kd homodimeric peptide purified from human platelets. There are now known to be many other isoforms of the peptide, the most studied of which are TGF-β2 and TGF-β3 (the original is TGF-β1). These three isoforms have extensive homology and similar potency. The TGF-βs have profound effects on cell growth and differentiation. They are potent chemoattractants for inflammatory cells, fibroblasts, smooth muscle cells, and T cells. TGF-β is found in the α-granule of the platelet and is secreted after injury (50). Exogenously applied TGF-β has been shown to enhance wound healing in animals (51). Numerous studies have investigated the role of endogenous TGF-β in the wound.

Schmid and colleagues (52) investigated message for TGF-β1, 2, and 3 and the TGF-β type II receptor in a human nonhealing wound model. In situ hybridization as well as immunocytochemistry was performed on biopsies from chronic nonhealing decubitus ulcer in elderly patients with normal skin and an acute burn wound used as controls. Strong constitutive expression of TGF-β3 was seen in keratinocytes in intact epidermis. No TGF-β1 or β2 mRNA was seen in intact skin. TGF-β3 message continued to be strongly expressed in both chronic and acute wounds in the epidermis and migrating epithelial sheet (acute wound). Importantly, TGF-β1 was found in the keratinocytes of the re-epithelialization front of the acute wound but not found at all in the chronic decubitus ulcers. TGF-β2 was not detected in any wound biopsies. TGF-β type II receptors were detected in both normal, acute, and chronic wounds in the epidermis. They suggested from this study that "constitutive expression of TGF-β3 is important for maintenance of epidermal differentiation and that an induction of TGF-β1 expression is essential for re-epithelialization in human skin wounds."

Cromack et al. (53) measured TGF-β protein levels over time in rat wound fluid harvested from Hunt-Schilling chambers. This study from 1986 predated the discovery of the TGF-β isoforms. Cromack et al. used both a biologic colony forming assay and a radioreceptor binding assay to measure TGF-β. Biologically active TGF-β first appeared in wound chambers 3 days post-wounding, peaked at 7 days post-wounding, and then gradually declined. One possible limitation of the study cited by the authors was the persistent PMN predominance in the cellular infiltrate, suggesting chronic inflammation and likely a result of daily aspiration of the wound cylinders.

Kane and colleagues (54) investigated TGF-β1 protein using immunocytochemistry in both a human blister model and partial-thickness porcine wound model. They used two previously described antibodies to TGF-β1, anti-CC and anti-LC. Anti-LC was constitutively expressed in the numerous layers of the epidermis in both models (human more intense than porcine). There was no significant change in anti-LC staining post-wounding in either model. Anti-CC was not expressed in normal skin. In the human blister wound within 24 hours anti-CC had increased and was concentrated in the keratinocytes adjacent to the wound. By day 3 the staining had changed, with fewer peri-wound keratinocytes staining and in both models marked staining in the migrating epithelial sheet. By day 7, when re-epithelialization has been completed, both models show a marked decrease in anti-CC staining. Kane et al. then investigated a human incisional wound model following myeloplasty and found that this anti-CC expression appeared as early as 5 minutes following injury and was concentrated in the incisional margin.

Numerous other studies have shown a prominent role for TGF-β in wounding. McMullen et al. (55) investigated TGF-β1–3 isoforms in ovine excisional and incisional models. They found characteristic changes in immunohistochemical localization of these isoforms in the wounded skin, the extracellular matrix, and the inflammatory infiltrate. Even by day 21 immunostaining had not returned to normal with immunoreactive fibroblasts (for all isoforms) in a dense, immunostained extracellular matrix. This finding was more prominent in the excisional wound model. Shah and colleagues (56), using an incisional model in rats, investigated the effect of neutralizing antibodies to the TGF-β isoforms. They found a synergistic effect on anti-TGF-β1 and TGF-β2 with reduced scarring and reduced macrophage infiltration, neovascularization, and collagen deposition. Considerable less effect was seen with either isoform alone.

From the above studies we conclude that TGF-β has a prominent role in wound healing. TGF-β1 and -3 message is transcribed in the wound. Message for TGF-β3 is constitutively expressed; TGF-β1 message is not found in normal skin and is induced in the migrating epithelial sheet. TGF-β1 protein likely undergoes a conformational change post-wounding as evidenced by a change in staining with two TGF-β1 isoforms. The isoform identified by anti-CC antibody initially is found in the keratinocytes around the wound and then shifts to less replicating epidermis and the migrating epithelial sheet. This induction of anti-CC occurs as early as 5 minutes post-wounding. Finally, the combination of neutralizing antibodies to TGF-β1 and TGF-β2 is synergistic when exogenously added and reduces scarring.

Table 11.1 summarizes the temporal variation of growth factor message and product in the wound. As some of the data are equivocal, this table is only a rough guide.

Nutrients

Amino Acids in Wound Fluid

Rationale for the Changes in Amino Acid Concentration

We have investigated the temporal changes in amino acids in wound fluid and attempted to provide a rationale for this change (57). Our model is

TABLE 11.1. Temporal variation in growth factor message and product.

Growth factor	Message peak (post-wounding)	Cell or origin	Protein peak (post-wounding)	Cell of origin
EGF	Days 1/2 and 5	Not macrophages or PMNs	Days 1 and 5	In wound fluid
KGF	24 hours	Dermal	?	?
bFGF	Day 5	?	Day 4	Areas of tissue destruction
IGF-1	Day 3	Fibroblasts?	?	Fibroblasts
IGF-2	Day 5	?	?	Smooth muscle
M-CSF	?	?	No peak	In wound fluid
PDGF	Day 1	Macrophage?	Day 1	Multiple cells, but not in wound fluid
TNF-α	?	?	Days 3–4	?
TGF-α	Days 3–5	Macrophage?	Day 10	In wound fluid
TGF-β1	?	Keratinocytes	Days 1–7	Keratinocytes and other cells

wound fluid derived from subcutaneously implanted sponges in Fisher rats. Amino acids are quantitated by a Durrum D-500 amino acid analyzer.

In general amino acids accumulate over time in the wound. Notable exceptions are cysteine, tryptophan, arginine, and citrulline. The increase in serine and leucine may be explained by an increase in these amino acids in the serum. The remainder of the amino acids are concentrated in wound fluid. Phenylalanine, threonine, glutamine, proline, alanine, valine, methionine, leucine, isoleucine, histidine, and asparagine plus aspartic acid accumulation in the wound are possibly due to proteolysis. The temporal increase in taurine, glutamic acid, and aspartic acid may be due to cytolysis. Decreasing arginine and accumulation of ornithine is related to an increase in extracellular arginase accompanying macrophage lysis (58). Proline and hydroxyproline may accumulate as a result of collagen synthesis and turnover. Glycine, alanine, valine, and lysine accumulate out of proportion to what would be expected from proteolysis, suggesting either increased synthesis, decreased degradation, or release from other pools.

Ornithine as a Proline Precursor

Albine and colleagues (59) investigated the local synthesis of collagen in wounds by focusing on proline production from ornithine. They found increased concentration of proline and its metabolic precursors ornithine, glutamate, and glutamine in wound fluid using a subcutaneously implanted polyvinyl alcohol sponge model in rats. They then investigated the incorporation of radiolabeled proline precursors into protein-bound proline and found, predictably, that proline was the preferential precursor. Other precursors in order of contribution to protein-bound proline were ornithine, arginine, and glutamine. No glutamate was converted into protein-bound proline. In a wound fibroblast culture system, ornithine was not found to be an efficient competitive inhibitor to proline in proline incorporation into protein, for even at the greatest excess of ornithine tested, ornithine incorporation was <30% that of preformed proline. More ornithine was converted to free proline than protein-bound proline and this conversion was increased by increasing concentrations of free proline. From this study they concluded that direct incorporation of ornithine into protein-bound proline is a relatively minor pathway.

Glutamine Metabolism

Glutamine is considered to be a major fuel for many cells including enterocytes, reticulocytes, stimulated lymphocytes, fibroblasts in culture, and malignant cells (60–67). These cells all share the common characteristics of rapid growth rates, poor glucose oxidative capacity, and high glutaminase activity. Given the cell types that use glutamine as well as their characteristics, we postulated a significant role for glutamine in the wound (68).

Our wound model was λ-carrageenan–injected rodent hindlimbs. By 12 hours there was a decrease in intracellular glutamine in the wound that progressed to a 50% reduction by 24 hours. Glutamine levels had returned to preinjury values by 10 days postinjection. Glutamine synthetase activity increased with a peak corresponding to the nadir of glutamine concentration and suggesting induction of glutamine synthetase by low ambient glutamine concentrations. Wounded muscle was found to produce more $[^{14}C]O_2$ and more glutamate from U-$[^{14}C]$ glutamine than nonwounded muscle. When peritoneal macrophages were co-incubated with skeletal muscle in numbers equal to those found in wounded tissue, the co-incubated complex reproduced the glutamine oxidation found in injured muscle. Inflammatory cells isolated from subcutaneously implanted polyvinyl alcohol sponges also consumed glutamine. From the above studies we proposed that the local depression in tissue glutamine concentration followed injury was the result of glutamine utilization by the inflammatory cells.

Arginine Metabolism

Wounded muscle contains less free arginine and more ornithine than nonwounded muscle in the λ-carrageenan wound model (69). Our further investigations characterized the mechanism of altered arginine metabolism in Hunt-Schilling chambers, 1-carrageenan–injected muscle, and subcutaneously implanted polyvinyl alcohol sponges (58). All three models showed decreased arginine, increased ornithine, and increased arginase. Peritoneal macrophages were assayed for arginase. Resident peritoneal macrophages contained little arginase and this was not increased by LPS; 1-carrageenan–stimulated peritoneal macrophages had a tenfold induction in arginase with further augmentation by LPS. Arginase was not detectable in the supernatants of these cultures, and when labeled arginine was added to these cultures labeled citrulline was the principal product produced (likely from arginine deaminase). Lysed macrophage cultures, however, contained large amounts of arginase with corresponding large increases in radiolabeled urea. From the above studies we concluded that the arginase increase in the wound was independent of injured muscle and may be the result of macrophage lysis.

Collagen and Glycosaminoglycan Precursors

Dolychuk and Bowness (70) investigated the time course of collagen and noncollagenous glycoprotein synthesis from their precursors in the wound. They created full-thickness wounds in rats and harvested wounds at various times post-wounding. They incubated these wounds with radiolabeled sulfate (incorporated into glycosaminoglycan) and either radiolabeled fucose (incorporated into insoluble glycoproteins) or radiolabeled proline (incorporated into collagen). Wounds were solubilized and the above molecules measured. Structural glycoprotein synthesis was found to peak at days 2 to 3 post-wounding; glycosaminoglycan peaked at day 5. Collagen peaked at day 5 post-wounding, consistent with previous published reports of maximal collagen synthesis at this time period. These data support the hypothesis that significant metabolic activity including matrix synthesis precedes the period of maximal collagen synthesis.

Fukasawa and colleagues (71) investigated the effect of macrophage factors on uptake of collagen and glycosaminoglycan precursors in a wound model. They abraded the peritoneum of rabbits to produce an injury and harvested the cells from the abraded area. They took these cells (morphologically similar to fibroblasts) that they called tissue repair cells (TRCs) and cultured them with macrophage-conditioned media derived from peritoneal exudate cells. Macrophage-conditioned media caused proliferation of the TRCs as well as increased incorporation of glucosamine and proline, precursors of glycosaminoglycans and collagen, respectively. However, glucosamine and proline incorporation per cell was unchanged, showing no metabolic effect of the macrophage conditioned media.

Glucose Metabolism

Tischler and Fagan (72) used a rat hindleg blunt wound model to investigate carbohydrate and amino acid metabolism. Uptake of glucose, glycolysis, and glucose oxidation were increased in injured muscle as compared with contralateral uninjured muscle, which served as a control. Insulin increased glucose uptake and glycolysis but had no effect on glucose oxidation. Alanine synthesis from leucine was found to be increased in injured muscle; no difference was found in glutamine or glutamate synthesis.

Shangraw and Turinsky (73) investigated local glycolysis and amino acid release in burns. Their model was isolated soleus muscle underlying a nonlethal scald burn in rats. Burned muscle was found to have a higher lactate pyruvate ratio, higher glucose uptake, and greater alanine, glutamic acid, and tyrosine release. Hypoxia only partly explained these augmentations. Alanine release in burned muscle likely was secondary to increased glycolysis; the release of other amino acids studied may be secondary to proteolysis.

Although lactate is consistently elevated in wounds, we postulated wound aerobic glycolysis based on improved glycolysis with increasing oxygen concentrations, improved blood flow to injured extremities, and normal oxygen consumption in wounded tissue (33). We used an isolated λ-carrageenan-injected rat hindlimb wound model to test this hypothesis. Oxygen consumption was equal to that in unwounded controls, as was pyruvate and glucose oxidation. Glucose uptake as a function of glucose concentration reached a early plateau between 5 and 10 mM perfusate glucose concentration; in nonwounded limbs glucose uptake continued to increase with increasing glucose concentrations. Lactate production in wounded muscle was consistently higher at all glucose concentrations. Further study of a simulated wound combining macrophages and normal muscle showed that 70% of the glucose uptake, 87% of the lactate produced from exogenous glucose, and 52% of the total lactate production from wounded tissue could be accounted for by macrophages present in the healing wound.

We have shown from the above review that endogenous growth factors and nutrients play a prominent role in the healing wound. Although we have focused on individual growth factors and nutrients in the wound in isolation, clearly many of these factors in this complicated system interact. Future and current research are focusing on these interactions (see Chapter 8).

References

1. Mills CD, Pricolo VE, Albina JE, Caldwell MD. Concomitant macrophage and fibroblast/lymphocyte inhibition by wound fluid: the "Arginine-deficiency of inflammation" is a partial explanation. Presented at 3rd International Symposium on Tissue Repair: clinical and experimental approaches to dermal and epidermal repair: normal and chronic wounds, 1990.
2. Pardee AB. G1 events and regulation of cell proliferation. Science 1989; 246:603–8.
3. Temin HM. Stimulation by serum of multiplication of stationary chicken cells. J Cell Physiol 1971;78(2):161–70.
4. Denhardt DT, Edward DR, Parfett CLJ. Gene expression during the mammalian cell cycle. Biochim Biophys Acta 1986;865:83–125.
5. Cross F, Weintraub H, Roberts J. Simple and complex cell cycles. Annu Rev Cell Biol 1989;5:341–96.
6. Leof EB, Van Wyk JJ, O'Keefe EJ, Pledger WJ. Epidermal growth factor (EGF) is required only during the traverse of early G1 in PDGF density-arrested BALB/c-3T3 cells. Exp Cell Res 1983;147:202–8.

7. Yang HC, Pardee AB. Insulin-like growth factor I regulation of transcription and replicating enzyme induction necessary for DNA synthesis. J Cell Physiol 127:410-6.

8. Carrell A. Growth-promoting function of leukocytes. J Exp Med 1992;36:385.

9. Carpenter G, Wahl MI. The epidermal growth factor family. In: Sporn MB, Roberts AB, eds. Peptide growth factors and their receptors. New York: 1990:69-171.

10. Cohen S. Isolation of a mouse submaximally gland protein accelerating incisor eruption and eyelid opening in the newborn animal. J Biol Chem 1962;237: 1555.

11. Nail M, Graeme RB, O'Brien BM. The effect of epidermal growth factor on wound healing in mice. J Surg Res 1982;33:164-9.

12. Franklin JD, Lynch JB. Effects of topical applications of growth factor on wound healing. Plast Reconstr Surg 1979;64(6):766-70.

13. Nanney LB. Epidermal growth factor-induced effects on wound healing. Clin Res 1987;35:706A.

14. Brown GL, Nanney LB, Griffin J, et al. Enhancement of wound healing by topical treatment with epidermal growth factor. N Engl J Med 1989;321:76-9.

15. Gartner MH, Benson JD, Caldwell MD. Time course of epidermal growth factor mRNA expression in healing wounds using polymerase chain reaction. Surg Forum 1994;42:643-5.

16. Rappolee DA, Mark D, Banda MJ, Werb Z. Wound macrophages express TGF-a and other growth factors in vivo: analysis by mRNA phenotyping. Science 241:708-11.

17. Ono I, Gunji H, Suda K, Iwatsuki K, Kaneko F. Evaluation of cytokines in donor site wound fluids. Scand J Plast Reconstr Hand Surg 1994;28:269-73.

18. Grayson LS, Hansbrough JF, Zapata-Sirvent RL, Dore CA, Morgan JL, Nicolson MA. Quantitation of cytokine levels in skin graft donor site wound fluid. Burns 1993;19:401-5.

19. Wenczak BA, Lynch JB, Nanney LB. Epidermal growth factor receptor distribution in burn wounds. J Clin Invest 1992;90:2392-401.

20. Gospodarowicz D, Neufeld G, Schweigerer L. Fibroblast growth factor: structure and biological properties. J Cell Physiol 1987;5(suppl):15-26.

21. Muthukrishnan L, Warder E, McNeil PL. Basic fibroblast growth factor is efficiently released from a cytosolic storage site through plasma membrane disruptions of endothelial cells. J Cell Physiol 1991;148:1-16.

22. Cordon-Cardo C, Vlodavsky I, Haimovitz-Friedman A, Hicklin D, Fuks Z. Expression of basic fibroblast growth factor in normal human tissues. Lab Invest 1990;63(6):832-40.

23. Schulze-Osthoff K, Risau W, Vollmer E, Sorg C. In situ detection of basic fibroblast growth factor by highly specific antibodies. Am J Pathol 1990; 137:85-92.

24. Greenhalgh DG, Sprugel KH, Murray MJ, Ross R. PDGF and FGF stimulate wound healing in the genetically diabetic mouse. Am J Pathol 1990; 136(6):1235-46.

25. Werner S, Peters KG, Longaker MT, Fuller-Pace F, Banda MJ, Williams LT. Large induction of keratinocyte growth factor expression in the dermis during wound healing. Proc Natl Acad Sci USA 1992;89:6896-900.

26. Stefanos H, Lossing C, Hansson HA. Immunohistochemical demonstration of endogenous growth factors in wound healing. Wounds 1990;2(6):218-26.

27. Gibran NS, Isik FF, Heimbach DM, Gordon D. Basic fibroblast growth factor in the early human burn wound. J Surg Res 1994;56:226–34.
28. Chen WYJ, Rogers AA, Lydon MJ. Characterization of biologic properties of wound fluid collected during early stages of wound healing. J Invest Dermatol 1992;99:559–64.
29. Spencer EM. The somatomedins. In: Greenspand FS, Forsham PH, eds. Basic and clinical endocrinology. Los Altos, CA: 1986:89–99.
30. Schlechter NL, Russell SM, Spencer EM, Nicoll CS. Evidence suggesting that the direct growth-promoting effects of growth hormone in cartilage in vivo is mediated by local production of somatomedins. Proc Natl Acad Sci USA 1986;83:7932–4.
31. Copeland KC, Johnson DM, Kuehl TJ, Castracane VD. Estrogen stimulated growth hormone and somatomedin-C in castrate and intact female baboons. J Clin Invest 1984;58:698–703.
32. Bowsher R, Lee W, Apathy J, O'Brien PJ, Ferguson AL, Henry DP. Measurement of insulin-like growth factor in physiological fluids and tissues. I. An improved extraction procedure and radioimmunoassay for human and rat fluids. Endocrinology 1991;128:805–14.
33. Caldwell MD. Carbohydrate and energy metabolism in healing wounds. In: Barbul A, Pines E, Caldwell M, Hunt TK, eds. Growth factors and other aspects of wound healing. Biological and clinical implications. Proceedings of the Second International Symposium on Tissue Repair, 1987, May 13–17. New York: Liss, 1988:183–213.
34. Lee W, Bowsher R, Apathy J, Smith MC, Henry DP. Measurement of insulin-like growth factor-II in physiological fluids and tissues. II. Extraction and quantification in rat tissues. Endocrinology 1991;128:815–22.
35. Stempien M, Fong N, Rail L, Bell G. Sequence of a placental cDNA encoding the mouse insulin-like growth factor II precursor. DNA 1986:357–61.
36. Spencer EM, Skover G, Hunt TK. Somatomedins: Do they play a pivotal role in wound healing? In: Burbul A, Pines E, Caldwell M, Hunt TK, eds. Growth factors and other aspects of wound healing. Biological and clinical implications. Proceedings of the Second International Symposium on Tissue Repair, 1987, May 13–17. New York: Liss, 1988:103–16.
37. Gartner MH, Benson JD, Caldwell MD. Insulin-like growth factors I and II expression in the healing wound. J Surg Res 1992;52:389–94.
38. Olofsson TB. Growth regulation of hematopoetic cells. Acta Oncol 1991; 30:889–902.
39. Ford HR, Hoffman RA, Wing EJ, Magee M, McIntyre L, Simmons RL. Characterization of wound cytokines in the sponge matrix model. Arch Surg 1989;124:1422–8.
40. Raines EW, Bowen-Pope DF, Ross R. Platelet-derived growth factor. In: Sporn MB, Roberts AB, eds. Peptide growth factors and their receptors, I. New York: Springer-Verlag, 1990:173–5.
41. Ross R. Platelet-derived growth factor. Annu Rev Med 1987;38:71–9.
42. Smimokado K, Raines EW, Madtes DK, Barret TB, Benditt EP, Ross R. A significant part of macrophage derived growth factor consists of at least 2 forms of PDGF. Cell 1985;43:277–86.
43. Martinet Y, Bitterman PB, Mornex J-F, Grotendorst GR, Martin GR, Crystal RG. Activated human monocytes express the c-cis proto-oncogene and release a mediator showing PDGF-like activity. Nature (Lond) 1986;319:158–60.

44. Barret TB, Gajdusek CM, Schwartz SM, McDougall JK, Benditt EP. Expression of the cis gene by endothelial cells in culture and in-vivo. Proc Natl Acad Sci USA 1984;81:6772–4.
45. Antoniades HM, Galanopoulos T, Neville-Golden J, Kiritsy CP, Lynch SE. Injury induces in vivo expression of platelet-derived growth factor (PDGF) and PDGF receptor mRNA in skin epithelial cells and PDGF mRNA in connective tissue fibroblasts. Proc Natl Acad Sci USA 1991;88:565–9.
46. Matsuoka J, Grotendorst GR. Two peptides related to platelet-derived growth factor are present in human wound fluid. Proc Natl Acad Sci USA 1989; 86:4416–20.
47. Beutler B. Cachectin/tumor necrosis factor and lymphotoxin. In: Sporn MB, Roberts AB, eds. Peptide growth factors and their receptors, II. New York: Springer-Verlag, 1990:39–70.
48. Carpenter G, Wahl MI. The epidermal growth factor family. In: Sporn MB, Roberts AB, eds. Peptide growth factors and their receptors, II. New York: Springer-Verlag, 1990:69–172.
49. Gartner MH, Aberle LA, Richards JR, Caldwell MD. Interrelationships between growth factor messenger RNA and protein product in the healing wound. Surg Forum 1992;43:683–5.
50. Roberts AB, Sporn MB. The transforming growth factor-β's. In: Sporn MB, Roberts AB, eds. Peptide growth factors and their receptors, I. New York: Springer-Verlag, 1990:419–72.
51. Cox D, Kunz S, Cerletti N, McMaster G, Buerk R. Wound healing in aged animals — effects of locally applied transforming growth factor-$\beta2$ in different model systems. In: Steiner R, Weisz PB, Langer R, eds. Angiogenesis. Basel: Birkhaeuser-Verlag, 1992:287–95.
52. Schmid et al. TGF-βs and TGFβ type II receptor in human epidermis: differential expression in acute and chronic skin wounds. J Pathol 1993; 171:191–7.
53. Cromack DT, Sporn MB, Roberts AB, Merino MJ, Dart LL, Norton JA. Transforming growth factor β levels in rat wound chambers. J Surg Res 1987;42:622–8.
54. Kane CJM, Hebda PA, Mansbridge JN, Hanwalt PC. Direct evidence for spatial and temporal regulation of transforming growth factor b1 expression during cutaneous wound healing. J Cell Physiol 1991;148:157–73.
55. McMullen H, Longaker MT, Cabrera R, et al. Spatial and temporal expression of transforming growth factor-β isoforms during ovine excisional and incisional wound repair. Wound Rep Reg 1994;3:141–56.
56. Shah M, Foreman DM, Ferguson MWJ. Neutralization of TGF-b1 and TGF-b2 or exogenous addition of TGF-b3 to cutaneous rat wounds reduces scarring. J Cell Sci 1995;108:985–1002.
57. Caldwell MD, Mastrofrancesco B, Shearer J, Bereiter D. The temporal change in amino acid concentration within wound fluid — a putative rationale. In: Clinical and experimental approaches to dermal and epidermal repair: normal and chronic wounds. New York: Wiley-Liss, 1991:205–22.
58. Albine JE, Mills CD, Barbul A, et al. Arginine metabolism in wounds. Am J Physiol 1988;254:E459–67.
59. Albine JE, Abate JA, Mastrofrancesco B. Role of ornithine as a proline precursor in healing wounds. J Surg Res 1993;55:97–102.

60. Windmueller HG, Spaeth AE. Uptake and metabolism of plasma glutamine by the small intestine. J Biol Chem 1974;249:5070-9.
61. Watford M, Lund P, Krebs HA. Isolation and metabolic characteristics of rat and chicken enterocytes. Biochem J 1979;178:589-96.
62. Rapoport S, Rost J, Schultze M. Glutamine and glutamate as respiratory substrate of rabbit reticulocytes. Eur J Biochem 1971;23:166-70.
63. Ardawi MSM, Newsholme EA. Maximum activities of some enzymes of glycolysis, the tricarboxylic acid cycle and ketone-body and glutamine utilization pathways in lymphocytes of the rat. Biochem J 1982;201:743-8.
64. Donnelly M, Scheffer IE. Energy metabolism in respiration deficient and wild type Chinese hamster fibroblasts in culture. J Cell Physiol 1976;89:39(abstr).
65. Zielke HR, Aielke CL, Ozand PT. Glutamine: a major energy source for cultured mammalian cells. Fed Proc Fed Am Soc Exp Biol 1984;43:121-5.
66. Kovacevic Z, Morris HP. The role of glutamine in the oxidative metabolism of malignant cells. Cancer Res 1973;32:326(abstr).
67. Reitzer LJ, Wice BM, Kennell DJ. Evidence that glutamine, not sugar is the major energy source for cultured HeLa cells. J Biol Chem 1979;254:2669-76.
68. Caldwell MD. Local glutamine metabolism in wounds and inflammation. Metabolism 1989;38(8)(suppl 1):34-9.
69. Albine JE, Shearer J, Mastrofrancesco B, Caldwell MD. Amino acid metabolism after 1-carrageenan injury to rat skeletal muscle. Am J Physiol 1986;250(endocrinol metab 13):E24-30.
70. Dolychuk KN, Bowness JM. The early metabolism of noncollagenous glycoproteins during wound healing. J Surg Res 1981;31:218-24.
71. Fukasawa M, Bryant SM, Orita H, Campeau JD, Dizerega GS. Modulation of proline and glucosamine incorporation into tissue repair cells by peritoneal macrophages. J Surg Res 1989;46:166-71.
72. Tischler ME, Fagan JM. Response to trauma of protein, amino acid, and carbohydrate metabolism in injured and uninjured rat skeletal muscles. Metabolism 1983;32(9):853-68.
73. Shangraw RE, Turinsky JT. Local response of muscle to burns: relationship of glycolysis and amino acid release. J Parenter Enteral Nutr 1981;5(3):193-9.

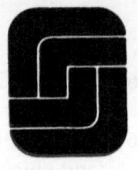

12

Epidermal Growth Factor in Wound Healing: A Model for the Molecular Pathogenesis of Chronic Wounds

ROY W. TARNUZZER, SHAWN P. MACAULEY, BRUCE A. MAST, JANE S. GIBSON, MICHAEL C. STACEY, NAOMI TRENGROVE, LYLE L. MOLDAWER, FRANK BURSLEM, AND GREGORY S. SCHULTZ

General Background of Skin Wound Healing

Wound healing in the skin is a complex biological process that has been extensively characterized at the light microscope level. However, regulation of skin wound healing is only partially understood at the molecular level. Skin wound healing can be divided into three general phases: (a) the inflammatory phase, (b) the repair phase, and (c) the remodeling phase. There is considerable temporal overlap of these stages of healing and the entire process lasts for several months (1, 2).

The process of wound healing begins when the skin is injured intentionally (e.g., a surgical incision) or unintentionally (accidental trauma). Injury to blood vessels initiates blood clotting and platelet degranulation (Fig. 12.1). Contained within the alpha granules of platelets are several growth factors including platelet-derived growth factor (PDGF) (3), insulin-like growth factor-I (IGF-I) (4), epidermal growth factor (EGF) (5), and transforming growth factor-β (TGF-β) (6). The burst of growth factors released from platelets quickly diffuses from the wound into the surrounding tissue and blood system. TGF-β released from platelets chemotactically recruits inflammatory cells into the injured area, which initiates the inflammatory phase that peaks during the first 2 to 3 days. Neutrophils are the first major inflammatory cell to enter the wound. Neutrophils in the wound secrete more proinflammatory cytokines, engulf and destroy bacteria, and release proteases including the matrix metalloproteinases (MMPs), elastase and collagenase (7, 8, 9), which remove damaged extracellular matrix components. This early burst of protease activity in the wound is important in debriding the wound and is distinct from the later release of MMPs from fibroblasts during the remodeling phase of healing. Monocytes

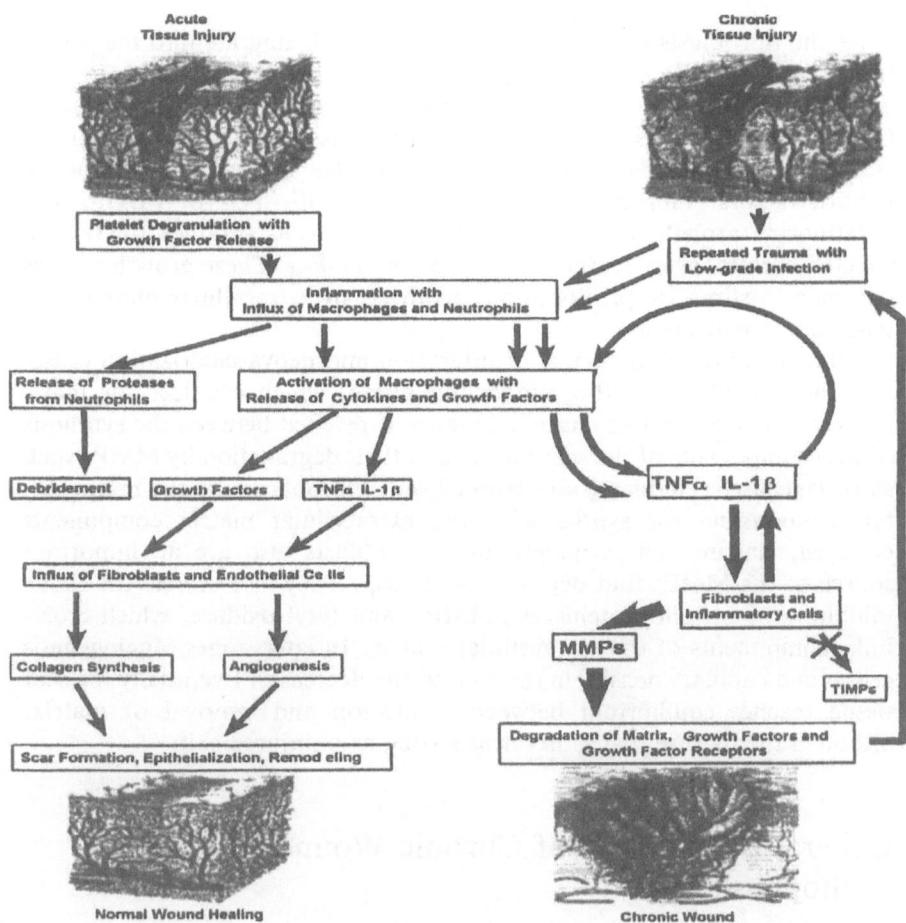

FIGURE 12.1. Molecular pathophysiology of chronic wounds.

are chemotactically drawn into the wound by TGF-β or fragments of fibronectin about a day later than neutrophils and become activated macrophages (10). Macrophages also secrete proinflammatory cytokines including tumor necrosis factor-α (TNF-α) and interleukin-1 (IL-1) and engulf and destroy bacteria. Macrophages also synthesize and secrete additional growth factors including TGF-β, transforming growth factor-α (TGF-α), leukocyte-derived growth factor (LDGF, a PDGF-like protein), basic fibroblast growth factor (bFGF), and heparin-binding epidermal growth factor (HB-EGF). If the wound does not become infected and is not subjected to repeated trauma or ischemia, the neutrophils disappear, probably by undergoing apoptosis, and the inflammatory phase begins to decline. The growth factors secreted by macrophages continue to stimulate migration of fibroblasts, epithelial cells, and vascular endothelial cells into the wound, setting up the repair phase of wound healing.

As the fibroblasts and vascular endothelial cells migrate into the site of injury, they begin to proliferate, and the cellularity of the wound increases. The repair phase often lasts several weeks. As the number of macrophages in the wound begins to decrease, other cells in the wound such as fibroblasts, endothelial cells, and keratinocytes continue to synthesize growth factors. Fibroblasts secrete IGF-1, bFGF, TGF-β, PDGF, and keratinocyte growth factor (KGF). Endothelial cells produce bFGF and PDGF. Keratinocytes synthesize TGF-β and TGF-α. These growth factors continue to stimulate proliferation, synthesis of extracellular matrix proteins, and angiogenesis.

After the initial scar forms, proliferation and neovascularization cease, and the wound enters the remodeling phase, which can last for many months. During this last phase, a balance is reached between the synthesis of new components of the scar matrix and their degradation by MMPs such as collagenase, gelatinase, and stromelysin. Fibroblasts are the major cell type responsible for synthesis of the extracellular matrix components collagen, elastin, and proteoglycans. Fibroblasts also are an important source of the MMPs that degrade the matrix. They also secrete the tissue inhibitors of metalloproteinases (TIMPs) and lysyl oxidase, which cross-links components of the extracellular matrix. In later stages, angiogenesis ceases and capillary density in the wound site decreases. Eventually the scar tissue reaches equilibrium between deposition and removal of matrix, although the mature scar is never as strong as uninjured skin.

General Background of Chronic Wound Pathophysiology

Most skin wounds heal without difficulty, but in some people with predisposing factors an acute wound fails to heal, resulting in a chronic wound. There are several types of chronic wounds that are recognized clinically, including diabetic foot ulcers, decubitus ulcers, venous stasis ulcers, and arterial insufficiency ulcers. However, based on our biochemical analyses of the molecular environment of acute and chronic human wounds, we propose there is a common molecular pathophysiology of chronic human wounds that prevents the wounds from healing. Although chronic wounds appear to be rather heterogeneous superficially, they are similar in that each is characterized by repeated tissue injury due to one or more of the following: recurring trauma, ischemia, or low-grade bacterial contamination (Fig. 12.1). For example, diabetic foot ulcers typically occur when there is repeated trauma to an area of the foot due to lack of sensation caused by neuropathy. This leads to local tissue ischemia and tissue injury with breakdown of the skin, which leads to secondary bacterial contamination from the open wound and inflammation. Pressure ulcers (decubitus) have a similar pattern of events. Repeated tissue injury from ongoing pressure and shear forces occurs in insensate areas when the pressure in the tissue exceeds capillary perfusion pressure. This leads to local ischemia and the sequence of tissue breakdown, bacterial contamination of the open wound, and inflammation. Venous stasis ulcers are characterized by venous hypertension and edema in the lower extremity. This stems from faulty venous valves, which produce elevated venous pressure within the leg. When the venous pressure exceeds the capillary perfusion pressure of skin, local tissue injury due to ischemia occurs. When this is combined with a minor local trauma, the sequence of tissue breakdown, bacterial contamination of the open wound, and inflammation occurs. Ischemic ulcers of the lower extremity secondary to arterial insufficiency follow a similar pattern. Minor trauma leads to an open wound that fails to heal because of poor oxygen perfusion. Bacterial contamination of the open wound occurs and inflammation follows. Once these different types of wounds have reached the point where the skin barrier is broken, bacterial colonization occurs. We propose that a common cascade pathway is initiated that prevents healing.

Inflammatory molecules from bacteria such as endotoxin, platelet products such as TGF-β or fragments of extracellular matrix molecules such as fibronectin stimulate inflammatory cells (neutrophils and macrophages) to enter the wound. The next step is the prolonged secretion of TNF-α and IL-1β by macrophages and neutrophils and other wound cells such as keratinocytes, fibroblasts, and vascular endothelial cells. The prolonged secretion of TNF-α is amplified because TNF-α stimulates its own synthesis (11) and stimulates the synthesis of IL-1β (12). Elevated levels of TNF-α and IL-1β then synergistically stimulate synthesis of MMPs by inflammatory cells and wound tissue cells while suppressing synthesis of TIMPs (13, 14). Elevated levels of activated MMPs degrade important components of the extracellular matrix (ECM) such as fibronectin and collagen, and perhaps more importantly, degrade growth factors and their receptors on cells in the wound. The proteolytic destruction of essential ECM components and growth factor/receptor systems prevents healing from progressing by interrupting the integrated sequence of processes that are necessary for healing including migration and mitosis of tissue cells and regeneration of the ECM. Furthermore, proteolytic degradation fragments of ECM molecules such as fibronectin are chemotactic for inflammatory cells and help to amplify the cytokine cycle.

It is important to note that both acute and chronic wounds begin with a similar proinflammatory cytokine response to the tissue injury that includes release of TNF-α and IL-1β. In healing wounds, however, tissue injury is a single occurrence, and the stimulus for the inflammatory stage is limited and transient. The normal sequence of inflammatory events then follows, with neutrophils and macrophages removing bacteria and denatured ECM components from the wound. The macrophages, fibroblasts, vascular endothelial cells, and keratinocytes secrete growth factors that promote epithelialization, ECM production, angiogenesis, and scar formation. In chronic wounds that fail to heal, however, tissue injury is recurrent and the proinflammatory cytokine cascade becomes prolonged and amplified, leading to elevated levels of proteases. The increase in proteases leads to destruction of ECM, growth factors, and receptors, which prevents the wounds from entering the repair phase and ultimately healing.

Current treatments for chronic wounds are only partially successful. Treatment protocols are generally limited to nonspecific and generalized attempts to reduce the conditions that initially lead to the injury rather than to treatments to correct the molecular pathophysiology responsible for the failure of the wound to heal. For example, frequently used treatments include physical devices such as special shoes designed to reduce tissue trauma, antibiotics to reduce bacterial contamination, and dressings designed to remove necrotic or ischemic tissue. However, even with appropriate use of these agents, chronic wounds frequently fail to heal or heal very slowly. This may be because dressings and treatments only indirectly and suboptimally alter the molecular environment of chronic wounds by decreasing tissue injury or bacterial colonization but are ineffective in altering the pathophysiology of most chronic wounds by blocking the activity of cytokines or proteases.

The Role of Endogenous EGF Family Proteins in Wound Healing

Epidermal growth factor (EGF) was the first true growth factor to be biochemically characterized and was named for its ability to stimulate mitosis and hypertrophy of the epidermis when injected subcutaneously into neonatal mice (5). EGF is synthesized as a single chain, 1207 amino acid, transmembrane precursor protein and is proteolytically cleaved to generate a soluble 53 amino acid protein. EGF contains three intrachain, disulfide loops that are essential for maintaining the biologically active conformation. This three-loop structure is characteristic for the members of the EGF family of proteins. Since the identification of EGF, several additional proteins with structural similarities to EGF have been identified in humans. These include TGF-α (15), amphiregulin (AR) (16), and HB-EGF (17). Each of these growth factors binds to the same receptor protein on target cells, the EGF receptor.

The first major process that occurs after a skin injury is the formation of a blood clot in the injured area and degranulation of platelets (1, 2). Platelets contain prepackaged growth factors including EGF, PDGF, TGF-β, and IGF-I that are released at the site of skin injury in active forms even as the blood clot is forming. Thus, EGF is present in skin wounds from the earliest point after injury, suggesting that it is important in helping to initiate the cascade of processes that occur in normal wound healing.

Several biological actions of EGF and other members of this growth factor family suggest they play important roles in local wound repair. EGF and TGF-α are potent mitogens for epidermal cells, fibroblasts, and vascular endothelial cells in vitro, which are the three major cell types involved in healing skin wounds. EGF and TGF-α promote migration of cultured human keratinocytes (18, 19), and EGF is chemotactic for corneal cells (20) and for vascular endothelial cells (21). EGF and TGF-α also stimulate angiogenesis in animal models (22). EGF increases the amount of extracellular matrix deposited in subcutaneous wound chamber implants in animals probably by increasing the rate of synthesis of extracellular matrix per cell and increasing the number of cells (23).

TGF-α is made in high levels by normal basal keratinocytes and is a potent keratinocyte mitogen (24). This has led to the concept that TGF-α is an important autocrine stimulator of mitosis of basal keratinocytes. In situ hybridization revealed the expression of EGF receptor and TGF-α messenger RNAs (mRNAs) increased dramatically in the epithelial cells adjacent to partial-thickness injuries created in pig skin within one day after injury (25). The elevated levels of TGF-α mRNA steadily decreased over 17 days until reaching the lower levels detected in unwounded skin. Levels of EGF receptor mRNA remained more highly elevated for the first 5 days then also decreased to the lower levels detected in unwounded skin on day 9. Similar results were found with EGF receptor distribution in burn wounds (26). In the early post-burn period (day 2 to 4), prominent immunostaining was detected in basal keratinocytes and epithelial cells lining hair follicles, sweat ducts, and sebaceous glands. During the late post-burn period (5 to 16 days), EGF receptor immunostaining decreased in migrating epithelial cells but remained intense in hypertrophic epidermis and all skin appendages. Eosinophils (27) and activated macrophages (28, 29) also synthesize and secrete TGF-α, which suggests that TGF-α is an important growth factor produced by macrophages during wound healing. Macrophages and their products play crucial roles in wound healing as demonstrated by the impaired healing of skin incisions that occurs when rats were made deficient in macrophages by administration of antimonocyte antibodies (30).

One experimental approach to evaluate the roles of EGF or TGF-α in wound healing is to create mice that are deficient in the growth factor and then analyze their process of wound healing. TGF-α–deficient mice were created using gene knockout technology. In addition, mice that are spontaneously deficient in TGF-α were identified and designated the wav-1 strain due to their peculiar wavy hair. Skin injuries created in both the wav-1 and TGF-α gene knockout mice healed normally (31, 32). This suggests that either TGF-α does not play a key role in healing skin injuries or that other growth factors in the EGF family such as HB-EGF compensated for the lack of TGF-α. Evidence suggests that the latter explanation is probably more correct. Recently, the levels of HB-EGF mRNA and protein were found to increase dramatically in biopsies and fluids collected 2 days after partial-thickness injuries were made to pig skin (33).

Effects of Exogenously Applied EGF Family Proteins in Wound Healing

The ability of EGF and TGF-α to stimulate processes in vitro that are important in wound healing such as migration, mitosis, angiogenesis, and ECM deposition suggested that exogenously applied EGF or TGF-α might enhance healing of wounds in vivo. EGF and other members of the EGF family were first evaluated for their effects on enhancing healing of wounds in animal models. Topical application of EGF accelerated the rate of epidermal regeneration of partial-thickness burns or dermatome wounds created on pigs (34–37). EGF was also reported to increase tensile strength of surgical skin incisions during the early period of healing in normal rats (38) and to increase formation of granulation tissue in subcutaneous sponges in rats when applied in a slow release vehicle (23). EGF also increased deposition of collagen in cylinders implanted subcutaneously in rats treated with streptozocin to impair healing (39).

In the first clinical trial of a peptide growth factor, recombinant human EGF accelerated epidermal regeneration of paired dermatome wounds in patients requiring skin grafting (40). Paired donor sites were created in 12 patients who required skin grafting for burns or reconstructive surgery. One donor site of each patient was treated daily with vehicle (silver sulfadiazine cream) containing recombinant human EGF (10 μg/ml) while the other donor site was treated with the vehicle. Treatment with EGF significantly decreased the average length of time to 50% healing by 1 day and decreased the average time to complete healing by 1.5 days ($p = .02$).

The eye is another organ that has been studied extensively for the effects of growth factors on wound healing (41–44). EGF is a mitogen in vitro for all three types of corneal cells—epithelial cells, stromal fibroblasts, and endothelial cells—and stimulates chemotactic migration of all three cell types in Boyden chambers (20). Topical eye drops of EGF have been reported to accelerate the rate of corneal epithelial regeneration in rabbits, rats, and primates, and in patients with a variety of epithelial wounds (45–47). EGF also increased the tensile strength of corneal incisions in rabbits (48) and increased central endothelial cell density of primates corneas (49) and cat corneas (50, 51) following injury to the endothelium.

Two prospective, randomized, double-blind, placebo-controlled clinical trials have evaluated topical eye drops of mouse EGF for treatment of traumatic corneal epithelial injuries (52, 53). In both studies, EGF treatment significantly accelerated the rate of epithelial regeneration. In 1992 Pastor and Calonge (52) reported the results of 47 patients treated with mEGF eye drops five times daily at 10 μg/ml compared with healing of 57 patients treated with vehicle. Epithelial defects were detected by fluorescein staining, and healing was considered complete when no staining was observed. Mean epithelial healing time was significantly decreased for the EGF-treated group (44.17 hours) compared with the placebo-treated group (61.05 hours) ($p < .01$). The number of epithelial defects healed completely at 24, 48, and 72 hours after onset of treatment was significantly greater in the EGF-treated group.

In 1993 Scardovi and colleagues (53) reported results of 20 patients treated with two drops of mouse EGF (10 μg/ml) four times daily and 20 patients treated with vehicle until healing occurred or for 7 days. Epithelial defects were detected by fluorescein staining using a slit lamp biomicroscope and covered at least 20% of the entire corneal surface. On day 4 of treatment, all EGF-treated ulcers were healed while 85% of vehicle-treated ulcers were healed ($p < .05$). On day 6 all placebo-treated ulcers were healed. No adverse reactions were detected in either clinical trial.

Although EGF and TGF-α consistently stimulate the processes in vitro that are required for wound healing, topical treatment with the growth factors in acute and chronic human wounds in vivo has not been as consistent. For example, recombinant human EGF was used to topically treat chronic venous stasis ulcers in a prospective, randomized, double-blind, placebo-controlled study (54). In this study of 35 patients (17 h-EGF and 18 placebo), ulcers with a median baseline size of 18.5 cm^2 were treated twice a day with an aqueous solution of EGF (10 μg/ml) for a maximum of 10 weeks. Ulcers were evaluated weekly for size and granulation tissue suitable for grafting. By study end, six (35%) of the EGF treated ulcers had healed and two (11%) of the placebo group had healed completely ($p = .10$). The median ulcer size reduction per week was 7% for EGF and 3% for placebo ($p = .32$); total healing was 73% versus 33% at the end of the study ($p = .32$). EGF treatment was safe but the level of healing enhanced by EGF treatment was not statistically significant at the $p = .05$ level.

EGF has also failed to improve healing in corneal wound healing studies. Kandarakis and colleagues (49) evaluated the efficacy of mouse EGF eye drops on epithelial healing after penetrating keratoplasty. All patients had 7.5-mm grafts placed in 8-mm beds. The epithelium of the donor cornea was removed, antibiotics were given, and the eye was pressure-patched. Eight patients were treated four times a day on the day of surgery and twice a day for the next two days with one drop of mouse EGF at 2 mg/ml solution. Eight patients received placebo eye drops. Eyes were stained with fluorescein, photographed twice a day for 2 days after surgery, and the area of epithelial defect was measured by planimetry. No difference in the percent of epithelial defect area was found between the two treatment groups. In a second study, nine patients were treated with one drop of mouse EGF at 1 mg/ml and 10 patients received a placebo dose eight times a day beginning 1 day before surgery and continuing until epithelial healing occurred. No difference in the percent of epithelial defect area was found between the two treatment groups. Intraocular pressures were normal in all patients during the course of the study and there was no evidence of toxicity by slit lamp biomicroscopy. The mixed success of EGF treatment of human wounds suggests that the molecular environment is much more complex than was initially thought. This concept led us to biochemically characterize the molecular environment of acute and chronic wounds to better understand what factors may influence the effect of growth factor treatment of human wounds.

Biochemical Differences in Environments of Healing and Chronic Wounds

Cytokine Levels

Our concept of normal wound healing is based on the model that wound healing is regulated by the sequential, balanced action of cytokines, proteases, and growth factors. A corollary to this concept is our hypothesis that elevated levels of cytokines induce excessive levels of proteases that impair wound healing by degrading ECM proteins, growth factors, and their receptors. If this concept is true, then therapies that reestablish an environment in chronic wounds that permit growth factors to function normally should lead to healing of chronic wounds. To investigate this hypothesis, we collected fluids from human wounds that represent the extreme ends of the spectrum of wound healing: acute, healing mastectomy incisions and chronic, nonhealing skin ulcers.

Cytokine Levels in Acute Human Wound Fluids

The initial component of our hypothesis of the molecular pathogenesis of chronic human skin wounds states that levels of proinflammatory cytokines are chronically elevated. Our initial analysis of cytokines in 21 samples of acute wound fluid collected from five patients during their postsurgery period and five samples of chronic wound fluid are shown in Figure 12.2. TNF-α levels peaked on days 2 and 4 after surgery (50 pg/ml) and returned to near baseline values on days 5, 6, and 7 after surgery. Levels of IL-1β (25 pg/ml) and IL-6 (35 pg/ml) were highest on day 1 after surgery and progressively decreased to baseline levels from days 2 to 7. Levels of IL-8 (5,000 pg/ml) and interferon-γ (INF-γ) (4 pg/ml) were relatively constant across the time from days 1 to 8 after surgery.

In addition to regulation at the level of transcription, the activities of TNF-α and IL-1β can be modulated posttranslationally by naturally occurring proteins that can bind to the cytokine or its receptor. A soluble form of the TNF-α receptor protein, p55, binds TNF-α much like a

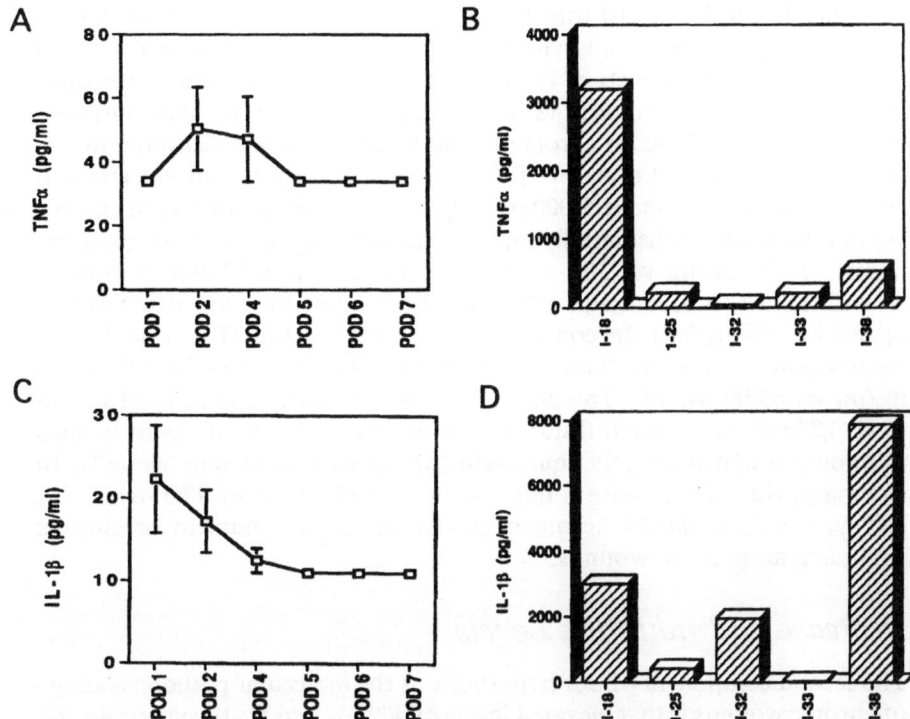

FIGURE 12.2. Cytokine levels in acute and chronic wound fluids. A. Concentrations of TNF-α in mastectomy fluids. B. Concentrations of TNF-α in chronic wound fluids. C. Concentrations of IL-1β in mastectomy fluids. D. Concentrations of IL-1β in chronic wound fluids. POD, postoperative day in mastectomy fluids; I, chronic wound fluids from various samples.

neutralizing antibody and inhibits TNF-α activity. Levels of p55 were approximately 300 pg/ml in acute wound fluid samples collected during the 8 days following mastectomy. Thus, the ratio of p55/TNF-α in acute wound fluids is about 6 to 1 in favor of p55 to TNF-α (300 pg/ml vs. 50 pg/ml). Levels of IL-1ra, the natural inhibitor of IL-1α and IL-1β, were approximately 8,000 pg/ml in the 21 acute wound fluid samples. The ratio of IL-1ra to IL-1β in acute wound fluids was about 320 to 1 in favor of the IL-1ra (8,000 pg/ml vs. 25 pg/ml). In summary, the ratios of antagonist/inflammatory cytokines for TNF-α and IL-1β in the molecular environment of acute wounds strongly favor the inhibitors, indicating that the effects of TNF-α and IL-1β are finely regulated.

Cytokine Levels in Chronic Human Wound Fluids

In chronic wound fluids, the levels of TNF-α and IL-1β were higher and more variable than in acute wound fluids (Fig. 12.2). TNF-α levels averaged

500 pg/ml, which was 10-fold higher than in acute wound fluids. IL-1β levels averaged 2,500 pg/ml, which was about 100-fold higher than levels in acute wound fluids. Levels of INF-γ were about threefold higher in chronic wounds than acute wounds (4 vs. 15 pg/ml). Levels of IL-6 (30 pg/ml) were two- to fourfold higher in chronic wounds than the levels measured in late acute wound fluids. Levels of IL-8 were low and similar in chronic and acute wound fluids (about 5,000 pg/ml). While the levels of p55 in chronic wound fluids were substantially higher than in acute wound fluids (approximately 1,700 pg/ml vs. 300 pg/ml), the ratio of p55/TNF-α in chronic wound fluids had decreased twofold to about 3 to 1 in favor of p55 (1,700 pg/ml vs. 500 pg/ml). In contrast, the average level of IL-1ra in chronic wound fluids was lower than in acute wound fluids (approximately 3,000 pg/ml vs. 8,000 pg/ml). The decrease in IL-1ra caused the ratio of IL-1ra to IL-1β in chronic wound fluids to decrease from 320 to 1 in acute wounds to about an approximately equal ratio of 1.2 to 1 in chronic wounds. In summary, these data indicate that the biological effects of TNF-α, IL-1β, INF-γ, and IL-6 should be much greater in the environment of chronic wounds than in acute wounds.

Protease and Inhibitor Levels

The second component of our hypothesis of the molecular pathophysiology of chronic wounds is that elevated levels of TNF-α and IL-1β synergistically increase levels of MMPs and decrease levels of TIMPs in chronic wounds. The elevated protease activities degrade components in the wound environment that are essential for healing, including extracellular matrix proteins, growth factors, and their receptors. In addition, the fragments of ECM components, such as fibronectin, generated by the proteases act as chemotactic factors for inflammatory cells. This further increases the number of inflammatory cells drawn into the wound and creates a self-amplifying cycle that elevates protease levels. We have analyzed a substantial number of fluids from acute and chronic human wounds for several proteases and inhibitors using a number of different assays. These include gelatin zymography, casein zymography, Azocoll proteolysis assay, Azocasein proteolysis assay, growth factor degradation assay, neutrophil elastase assay, neutrophil elastase inhibitor assay, and cathepsin G assay. The results of these assays consistently demonstrate elevated levels of proteases and reduced levels of inhibitors in chronic wound fluids compared with acute wound fluids.

Azocoll Assay of Acute, Chronic, and Sequential Wound Fluids

Our initial data indicate there are major differences in the levels of protease activity between acute and chronic wound fluids. The average level of protease activity in 20 different acute wound fluids collected from mastectomy incisions, determined using Azocoll as the substrate (55), is low (0.75 μg collagenase equivalents/ml), with a range of 0.1 to 1.3 μg collagenase equivalents/ml. Also, the average levels do not change substantially during the first 7 days after surgery. In addition, the levels of TIMP-1 determined using an enzyme-linked immunosorbent assay (ELISA) in three acute wound fluids is 38 ± 6 μg/ml (Fig. 12.3A). The ELISA detects both free TIMP-1 and TIMP-1/MMP complexes, although not with the same efficiency as free TIMP-1. This suggests that protease activity is tightly controlled during the early phase of wound healing.

In contrast, the range of Azocoll protease activity in chronic wound fluids collected before clinical treatments had begun is quite large, ranging from 5 to 584 μg collagenase equivalents/ml. The average level of protease activity in 32 different chronic wound fluids was 87 ± 24 μg collagenase equivalents/ml, which is 116-fold higher ($p < .05$) than in mastectomy fluids. Furthermore, addition of the MMP inhibitor Galardin to chronic wound fluids reduced hydrolysis of Azocoll by an average of 90%. This indicates that the majority of proteases in these chronic wound fluids that degrade Azocoll are MMPs (Fig. 12.3B). In addition, the levels of TIMP-1 measured in five of these chronic wounds was inversely related to the level of Azocoll hydrolysis activity. As shown in Figure 12.3A, samples I-33 and I-25 had low levels of Azocoll hydrolysis and had high levels of TIMP-1. In contrast, chronic wound fluids I-24, I-29, and I-42 had low levels of TIMP-1 that were 50- to 100-fold lower than levels in acute wound fluids that had low levels of Azocoll hydrolysis. Similar results were found for neutrophil elastase and its inhibitor and cathepsin G.

We also analyzed an initial series of sequential wound fluids collected from 10 patients with venous stasis ulcers before beginning treatments and collected again after 2 weeks of treatment when the ulcers typically are about 30% healed. Our hypothesis predicts that the levels of MMPs should decrease in chronic wound fluids as healing progresses. To standardize the collection process, these patients were hospitalized the night before beginning treatment and had no fluids after midnight. At 8 A.M. the next morning, they drank 1 L of water, and the ulcer was covered with occlusive dressing and placed in a dependent position. After 1 hour the fluid that had spontaneously collected was removed and analyzed.

The average level of Azocoll hydrolysis was quite high in the 10 samples collected before therapy began (52 ± 12 μg collagenase equivalents/ml). After 2 weeks of treatment, the levels of Azocoll hydrolysis decreased in 8 of 10 of the patients to an average level of 15 ± 6 μg collagenase/ml. Overall, this is a 3.4-fold decrease in protease levels of the 10 patients. We also assessed the effects of addition of the MMP inhibitor Galardin on the Azocoll hydrolysis by the sequential wound fluids. Galardin inhibited almost all the Azocoll hydrolysis activity in the sequential wound fluids. For example, Galardin decreased the average Azocoll hydrolysis activity by

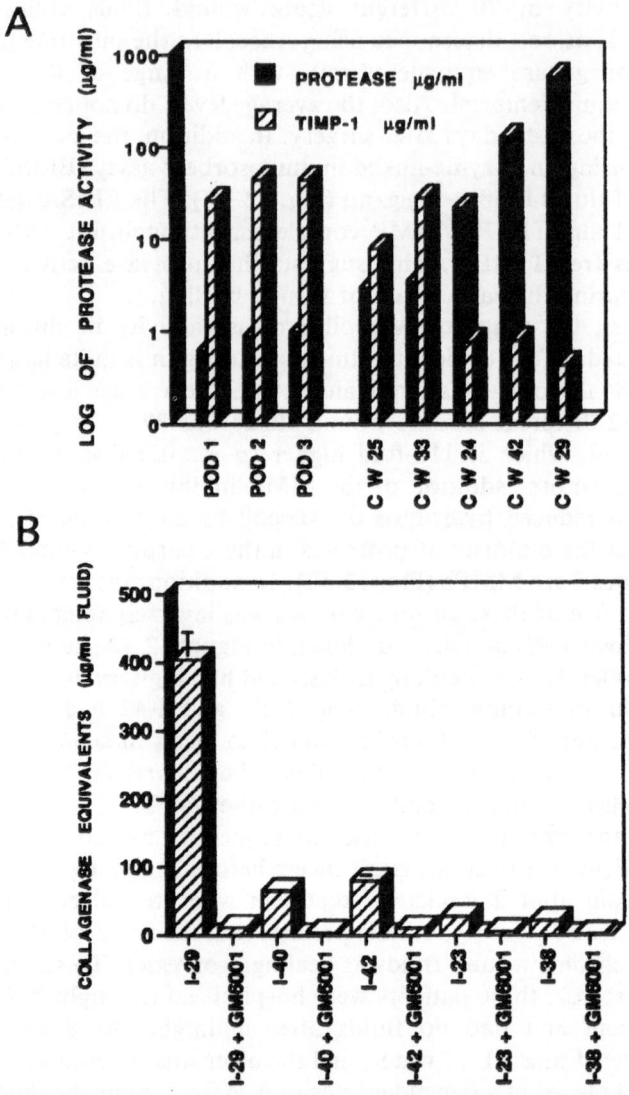

FIGURE 12.3. Determination of protease and inhibitor levels in wound fluids. A. Protease levels in mastectomy and chronic wound fluids were determined by Azocoll assay. TIMP-1 levels in wound fluids were determined by ELISA. B. Determination of protease levels in chronic wound fluids with Azocoll and inhibition by Galardin.

99.2% from 52 μg collagenase/ml to 0.4 μg/ml in the samples collected before treatment began. Galardin also effectively decreased protease activity in fluids collected 2 weeks after treatment began from 15 μg collagenase/ml to 0.4 μg/ml.

Gelatin and Casein Zymography of Acute, Chronic, and Sequential Wound Fluids

Results of the Azocoll assay and Galardin inhibition indicated that the wound fluids contained activated MMPs. To help identify which MMPs might be present and activated, we performed gelatin and casein zymograms of acute and chronic wound fluids (56). As shown in Figure 12.4, analysis of three acute wound fluids collected on postoperative days 1, 2, and 3 revealed the presence of one major band of molecular weight 92 kd and two minor bands at molecular weights of approximately 130 kd and 200 kd. Based on migration of purified samples of MMPs, we identified these bands as the pro-MMP-9 (92-kd gelatinase, gelatinase B) and complexes of MMP-9 with other proteins. The activated forms of MMP-9 and MMP-2 migrated as slightly lower molecular weight bands. There was an extremely faint band migrating at 89 kd in acute fluid POD-1, which is probably activated MMP-9, consistent with the results of the Azocoll assay that showed very low levels of protease activity.

The gelatin zymogram of five chronic wound samples showed dramatically different patterns of bands from the acute wound fluids. The samples 1 through 5 (Fig. 12.4) had a large range of protease activity determined by the Azocoll assay of 3, 3.5, 22, 584, and 130 μg/ml, respectively. The band pattern for sample 2 was very similar to the acute wound fluid with three

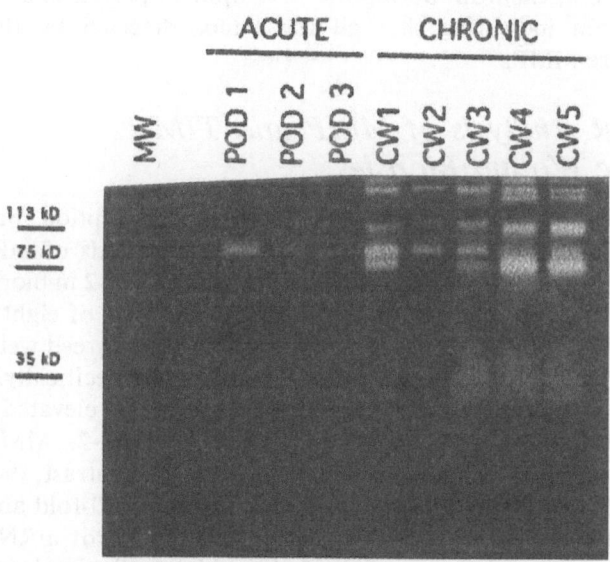

FIGURE 12.4. Gelatin zymography of wound fluids. Visualization of gelatinolytic proteinases in acute and chronic wound fluids.

major bands, but the higher molecular weight bands were more intense and there was a faint diffuse band at a molecular weight range of 35 to 55 kd. Chronic wound sample 1 had an intense band at 85 kd and the diffuse band at 35 to 55 kd. Samples 3, 4, and 5 all had multiple, intense bands especially at 85 kd (activated MMP-9), 68 kd (probably activated MMP-2), and 35 to 55 kd (probably MMP-3). MMP-1, or collagenase, is not readily detected by gelatin zymography since it makes a single cut in native collagen. Thus, gelatin zymograms of acute and chronic wound fluids support the quantitative measurements of protease activity made with the Azocoll assay and indicate the presence of several active MMPs in chronic wound fluids.

We also analyzed the sequential wound fluids using gelatin and casein zymography. The patterns of the fluids collected from 10 patients with chronic venous stasis ulcers before they began conventional compression therapy had six intense bands at approximate molecular weights of >200 kd, 150 kd, 100 kd, 85 kd, 65 kd, and 45 kd. These patterns were more intense in the sample collected from each patient before treatment began compared with the second sample collected after 2 weeks of treatment. This is particularly apparent in a pair of samples where the initial sample collected before treatment had very intense bands especially at the three higher molecular weights (>200 kd, 150 kd, 100 kd) and faint bands at <45 kd. In contrast, the bands generated by the second sample collected 2 weeks after treatment began were much less intense and no activated MMP-9 (92-kd gelatinase B) was detected. Incubation of an identical gel in buffer containing Galardin during the development period totally blocked band formation indicating that all the bands detected by the gelatin zymogens were MMPs.

Q-RT-PCR Analysis of MMP and TIMP of Chronic Wound Biopsies

Using competition-based quantitative reverse transcription polymerase chain reaction (Q-RT-PCR), we also measured the levels of mRNAs for MMP-1, MMP-2, MMP-3, MMP-9, TIMP-1, and TIMP-2 in biopsies from normal skin, the edge of each ulcer, and from the base of eight different chronic wounds (Fig. 12.5) (57). The levels of mRNAs agreed well with the levels of proteins measured in chronic wound fluids. Specifically, levels of mRNAs in the biopsies from the base of the wounds were elevated 300-fold, 200-fold, 100-fold, and 450-fold for MMP-1, MMP-2, MMP-3, and MMP-9, respectively, compared with normal skin. In contrast, the levels of mRNAs for TIMP-1 and TIMP-2 were only increased 30-fold and 15-fold in the wound tissue compared with normal skin. Levels of mRNAs at the edge of the wound tended to be about half as high as the levels in the base of the ulcers. Thus, the levels of mRNAs for MMPs were consistently elevated several hundred-fold in chronic wounds compared with levels in normal skin, whereas mRNAs for TIMPs were increased substantially less.

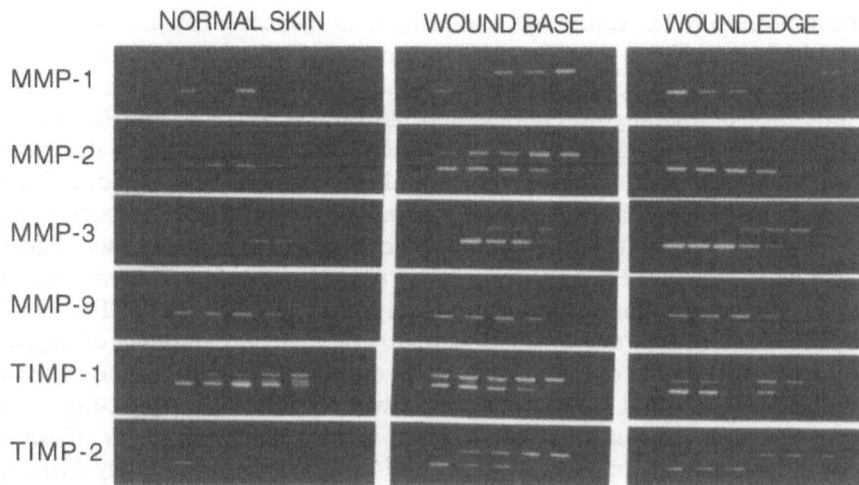

FIGURE 12.5. Quantitative RT-PCR measurement of mRNA levels for MMPs and TIMPs.

In summary, these data indicate that the environment of acute wounds have low levels of active MMPs and high levels of TIMP-1 proteins. In contrast, most chronic wound fluids contain high levels of activated MMPs and low levels of TIMP-1. Levels of mRNAs measured by Q-RT-PCR agree with the trend seen in the protease measurements. The physiologic implications of these data are that MMP activity is tightly controlled in acute wounds due to the presence of TIMPs (and to low levels of TNF-α and IL-1β and elevated levels of p55 and IL-1ra). In chronic wounds, however, levels of active MMPs are elevated and levels of TIMPs are decreased (presumably induced by high levels of TNF-α and IL-1β and by low levels of p55 and IL-1ra). These data support our hypothesis that the elevated inflammatory cytokines induce synthesis of MMPs in chronic wounds. In the next section, we examine what biologic effects the elevated levels of proteases may have on the biologic activities of essential ECM proteins, growth factors, and receptors.

Growth Factor Degradation

Our hypothesis of the molecular pathophysiology of chronic wounds predicts that elevated levels of proteases in chronic wound fluids destroy essential ECM, growth factors, and their receptors, which prevent wounds from healing. To assess if growth factors are stable or are destroyed in acute and chronic wound fluids, we added iodinated EGF, PDGF, and IGF-I to samples of acute and chronic wound fluid and measured their stability by precipitation with trichloroacetic acid (TCA). These growth factors are insoluble in 15% TCA, whereas small fragments generated by proteolysis are soluble in 15% TCA. As shown in Figure 12.6, the results were essentially the same as we found using Azocoll as the substrate. Only 2 of 20 mastectomy fluids caused any measurable destruction (0.05%) of the added EGF (0.15 ± 0.01 μg EGF degraded/ml wound fluid/24 hours) while all 14 different chronic wound fluids caused substantial destruction of the added EGF (average of 16.72 ± 6.07 μg EGF degraded/ml wound fluid/24 hours, 60% of the added EGF). Addition of Galardin or ethylenediaminetetraacetic acid (EDTA) prevented the destruction of EGF to the low levels measured in acute wound fluids. Similar results were obtained for PDGF and IGF-I using samples of our acute and chronic wound. The different amounts of degradation of growth factors in acute and chronic wound fluids are not due to higher levels of total proteins in acute wound fluids simply acting as a "protease sink" and sparing the growth factors since the levels of total proteins in acute and chronic wound fluids are both approximately 6 to 8 g per 100 ml. In addition, the pH and osmolarity of chronic wound fluids were not significantly different from normal serum: the average pH was 7.26 ± 0.16 and the average osmolarity was 312 ± 13 mOsm.

Our hypothesis predicts that the levels of biologically active growth factors should be high in acute wound fluids while levels in chronic wound fluids should be low. Our initial analyses of growth factors in acute and chronic wound fluids support this general concept. Mastectomy fluids contained physiologically significant levels of four growth factors (TGF-α, EGF, TGF-β, and IGF-I) at concentrations that can stimulate mitosis and migration of cells in culture as well as induce or suppress transcription of

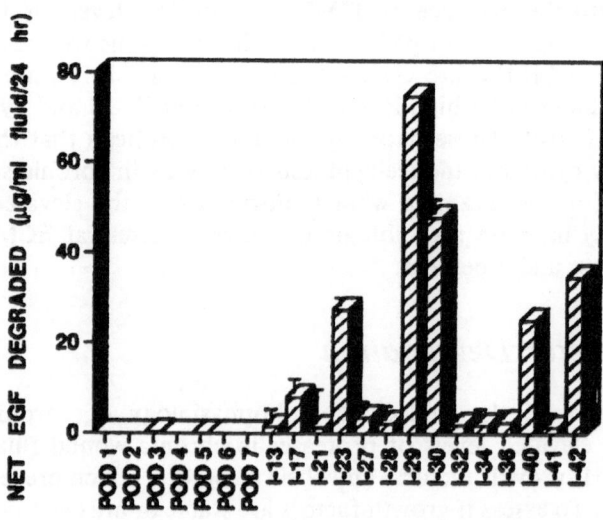

FIGURE 12.6. Degradation of EGF by wound fluids. Radiolabeled EGF was incubated with samples of acute and chronic wound fluids and degradation determined by measurement of TCA precipitable counts.

genes in vitro. Also, the levels of EGF and IGF-I are lower in chronic wound fluids compared with acute wound fluids. However, average levels of TGF-α and TGF-β are slightly elevated in chronic wound fluids. This may be due to the detection of proteolytic fragments of TGF-α in wound fluids by the RIA.

Growth Factor Receptor Degradation

Receptor proteins are another class of proteins that are necessary for growth factors and cytokines to function in wound healing. In an initial experiment investigating the stability of EGF receptors incubated with acute and chronic wound fluids, we found that the EGF receptor was indeed stable in acute wound fluids but not in chronic wound fluids. Preincubation of human placental microvilli membranes (a very rich source of EGF receptors) with two mastectomy fluids for 2 hours did not reduce binding of ^{125}I-EGF to receptors. In contrast, preincubation of the placental membranes with two chronic wound fluids reduced EGF binding by 40% and 60%. Addition of EDTA or Galardin prevented the destruction of EGF-R by chronic wound fluids, indicating that MMPs were responsible for the inactivation of the EGF-R. Thus, proteases in chronic wound fluids can degrade EGF receptors and may impede wound healing in vivo by degrading both growth factors and their receptors.

Biological Effects of Acute and Chronic Wound Fluids on Wound Cells

The final stage of our hypothesis of chronic wounds predicts that fluids from acute wounds should stimulate essential processes of wound healing such as DNA synthesis of wound cells, while chronic wound fluids would not. We evaluated the ability of a series of acute and chronic wound fluids to influence DNA synthesis of the three major types of wound cells: fibroblasts, keratinocytes, and vascular endothelial cells.

Addition of mastectomy fluids to serum-free chemically defined medium stimulated high levels of DNA synthesis by cultures of human foreskin fibroblasts. As seen in Figure 12.7A, mastectomy fluids collected during days 1 and 2 after surgery stimulated DNA synthesis to levels slightly higher than addition of 10% calf serum, while fluids collected during days 4, 5, and 7 after surgery stimulated levels slightly below 10% serum. In marked contrast, 13 of 14 fluids collected from chronic wounds decreased DNA synthesis of fibroblast cultures when added to serum-free medium (Fig. 12.7B). Similar effects were found when acute and chronic wound fluids were added to cultures of human umbilical vein endothelial cells held in low serum (2%). Mastectomy fluids collected on days 1, 2, 3, and 5 after surgery

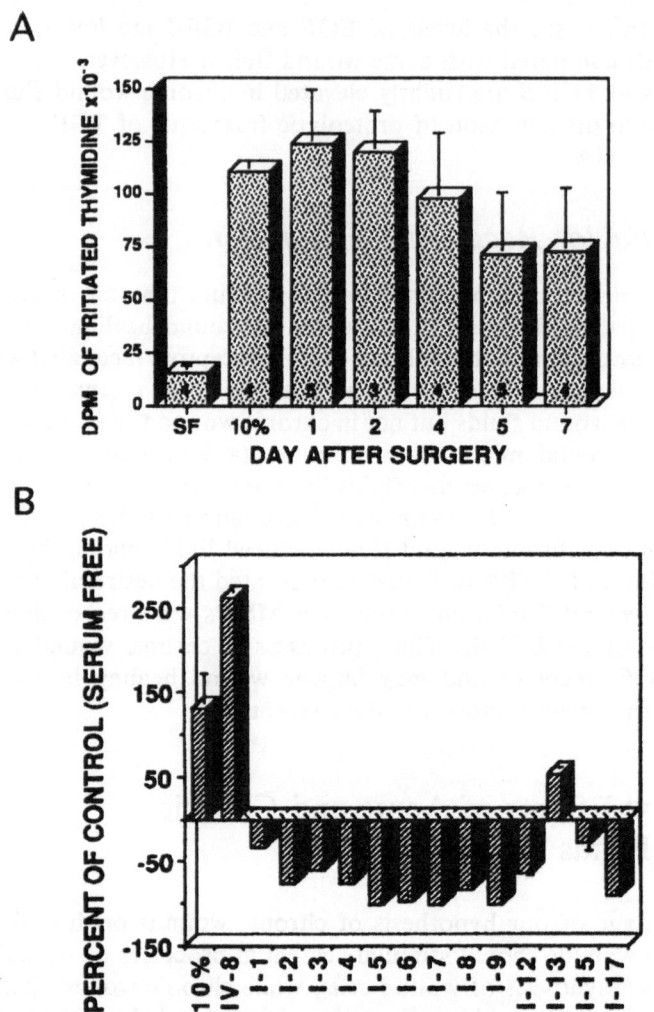

FIGURE 12.7. Effects of wound fluids on DNA synthesis. A. Effect of mastectomy fluids on wound fibroblasts tritiated thymidine incorporation. B. Effect of chronic wound fluids on wound fibroblast tritiated thymidine incorporation.

increased DNA synthesis approximately twofold above low serum, while four of five chronic wound samples substantially decreased DNA synthesis. Wound fluids produced similar effects on keratinocyte cultures. Acute wound fluids collected from five patients on days 1, 2, 3, 4, 5, and 7 supported DNA synthesis, while fluids from 8 of 12 chronic wounds reduced DNA synthesis an average of 55%. Thus, fluids from acute wounds promote DNA synthesis while fluids from chronic wounds impair DNA synthesis.

Future Concepts for the Treatment of Chronic Wounds

Our biochemical analyses of the molecular environments of acute and chronic human wounds support our hypothesis that chronic wounds fail to heal because the environment degrades essential ECM proteins, growth factors, and receptors. It is reasonable to propose that new treatment strategies for chronic, nonhealing wounds can be developed that reestablish the balance between cytokines and proteases with their inhibitors, ECM, growth factors, and receptors found in acute, healing wounds.

Identification of the active proteases in wound fluids is essential to designing strategies to reduce the elevated levels. Our data clearly indicate that a high percentage of the protease activity in chronic wound fluids is attributable to the metalloproteinase class as defined by inhibition by nonspecific chelators of zinc such as EDTA. Of particular interest is our result that Galardin, a specific inhibitor of MMP activity, is also very effective in reducing proteolysis of Azocoll, EGF, and the EGF receptor by chronic wound fluids. The inhibition of a high percent of total protease activity in chronic wound fluids by Galardin would justify using MMP inhibitors for the treatment of chronic wounds. In data not presented, we also have recently found that Galardin and doxycycline both inhibit the specific metalloproteinase that processes TNF-α from its inactive, membrane-bound precursor form to the active secreted molecule. Since Galardin and doxycycline block both MMPs and TNF-α processing enzyme in vitro, treatment of chronic wounds with Galardin or doxycycline may have a double beneficial effect by blocking secretion of TNF-α and blocking activity of MMPs. Finally, serious consideration should be given to combination therapies for chronic wound treatment based on the molecular pathophysiology of chronic wounds. Specifically, inhibitors of MMPs and TNF-α processing enzyme in combination with growth factors might well act synergistically to promote healing. Combination therapies of EGF and protease inhibitors have proven to be superior to single agent treatments in a variety of animal models of wound healing in the eye (58) and in the skin. Understanding the molecular pathophysiology of chronic human wounds should lead to more logical design of treatment strategies that will promote healing of these difficult wounds.

Acknowledgments. Results reported in this chapter were supported by U.S. Army Contract DAMD17-91-C-1905 and National Institutes of Health grant EY05587.

References

1. Bennett NT, Schultz GS. Growth factors and wound healing: biochemical properties of growth factors and their receptors. Am J Surg 1993;165:728–37.

2. Bennett NT, Schultz GS. Growth factors and wound healing: Part II. Role in normal and chronic wound healing. Am J Surg 1993;166:74–81.
3. Pierce GF, Mustoe TA, Altrock BW, Deuel TF, Thomason A. Role of platelet-derived growth factor in wound healing. J Cell Biochem 1991;45:319–26.
4. Karey KP, Sirbaska DA. Human platelet-derived mitogens, II. Subcellular localization of insulin-like growth factor I to the a-granule and release in response to thrombin. Blood 1989;74:1092–100.
5. Carpenter G, Cohen S. Epidermal growth factor. J Biol Chem 1990;265:7709–12.
6. Border WA, Noble NA. Transforming growth factor β in tissue fibrosis. N Engl J Med 1994;10:1286–92.
7. Gadek JE, Fells GA, Wright DG, Crystal RG. Human neutrophil elastase functions as a type III collagen "collagenase." Biochem Biophys Res Commun 1980;95:1815–22.
8. Morel F, Berthier S, Guillot M, et al. Human neutrophil gelatinase is a collagenase type IV. Biochem Biophys Res Commun 1993;191:269–74.
9. Hibbs MS, Hasty KA, Seyer JM, Kang AH, Mainardi CL. Biochemical and immunological characterization of the secreted forms of human neutrophil gelatinase. J Biol Chem 1985;260:2493–500.
10. Ross R. The fibroblast and wound repair. Biol Rev 1968;43:51–96.
11. Kronke M, Schutze S, Scheurich P, Pfizenmaier K. In: Affarwal BB, Vilcek J, eds. Tumor necrosis factor: structure, function, and mechanism of action. New York: Marcel Dekker, 1995.
12. Vilcek J, Lee TH. Tumor necrosis factor. J Biol Chem 1991;266:7313–6.
13. Ito A, Sato T, Iga T, Mori Y. Tumor necrosis factor bifunctionally regulates matrix metalloproteinases and tissue inhibitor of metalloproteinases (TIMP) production by human fibroblasts. Fed Exp Biol Sci 1990;269:93–5.
14. So T, Ito A, Sato T, Mori Y, Hirakawa S. Tumor necrosis factor-α stimulates the biosynthesis of matrix metalloproteinases and plasminogen activator in cultured human chorionic cells. Biol Rep 1992;46:772–8.
15. Massague J. Transfroming growth factor-α. J Biol Chem 1990;265:21393–6.
16. Shoyab M, Plowman GD, McDonald VL, Bradley GJ, Todaro GJ. Structure and function of human amphiregulin: a member of the epidermal growth factor family. Science 1989;243:1074–6.
17. Higashiyama S, Abraham JA, Miller J, Fiddes JC, Klagsbrun M. A heparin-binding growth factor secreted by macrophage-like cells that is related to EGF. Science 1991;251:936–9.
18. Ando Y, Jensen PJ. Epidermal growth factor and insulin-like growth factor I enhance keratinocyte migration. J Invest Dermatol 1993;100:633–9.
19. Ju WD, Schiller JT, Kazempour MK, Lowy DR. TGF-alpha enhances locomotion of cultured human keratinocytes. J Invest Dermatol 1993;100:628–32.
20. Grant MB, Khaw PT, Schultz GS, Adams JL, Shimizu RW. Effects of epidermal growth factor, fibroblast growth factor and transforming growth factor-β on corneal cell chemotaxis. Invest Ophthalmol Vis Sci 1992; 33:3292–301.
21. Grotendorst GR, Soma Y, Takehara K, Charette M. EGF and TGF-alpha are potent chemoattractants for endothelial cells and EGF-like peptides are present at sites of tissue regeneration. J Cell Physiol 1989;139:617–23.
22. Schreiber AB, Winkler ME, Derynck R. Transforming growth factor-α: a more

potent angiogenic mediator than epidermal growth factor. Science 1986; 232:1250-3.

23. Buckley A, Davidson JM, Kamerath CD, Wolt TB, Woodward SC. Sustained release of epidermal growth factor accelerates wound repair. Proc Natl Acad Sci USA 1985;82:7340-4.

24. Coffey RJ, Derynck R, Wilcox JN, et al. Production and auto-induction of transforming growth factor-α in human keratinocytes. Nature 1987;328: 817-20.

25. Antoniades HN, Galanopoulos T, Neville-Golden J, Kiritsy CP, Lynch SE. Expression of growth factor and receptor mRNAs in skin epithelial cells following acute cutaneous injury. Am J Pathol 1993;142:1099-110.

26. Wenczak BA, Lynch JB, Nanney LB. Epidermal growth factor receptor distribution in burn wounds. J Clin Invest 1990;90:2392-401.

27. Todd R, Donoff BR, Chiang T, et al. Rapid communication: the eosinophil as a cellular source of transforming growth factor alpha in healing cutaneous wounds. Am J Pathol 1991;138:1307-13.

28. Madtes DK, Raines EW, Sakariassen KS, et al. Induction of transforming growth factor-α in activated human alveolar macrophages. Cell 1988;53:285-93.

29. Rappolee DA, Mark D, Banda MJ, Werb Z. Wound macrophages express TGF-α and other growth factors in vivo: analysis by mRNA phenotyping. Science 1988;241:708-12.

30. Leibovich SJ, Ross R. The role of the macrophage in wound repair. Am J Pathol 1975;78:71-100.

31. Mann GB, Fowler KJ, Gabriel A, Nice EC, Williams RL, Dunn AR. Mice with a null mutation of the TGF-α gene have abnormal skin architecture, wavy hair, and curly whiskers and often develop corneal inflammation. Cell 1993; 73:249-61.

32. Luetteke NC, Qiu TH, Peiffer RL, Oliver P, Smithies O, Lee DC. TGF-alpha deficiency results in hair follicle and eye abnormalities in targeted and waved-1 mice. Cell 1993;73:263-78.

33. Marikovsky M, Breuing K, Liu PY, et al. Appearance of heparin-binding EGF-like growth factor in wound fluid as a response to injury. Proc Natl Acad Sci USA 1993;90:3889-93.

34. Brown GB, Curtsinger L, Brightwell JR, et al. Enhancement of epidermal regeneration by biosynthetic epidermal growth factor. J Exp Med 1986; 163:1319-24.

35. Nanney LB. Epidermal and dermal effects of epidermal growth factor during wound repair. J Invest Dermatol 1990;94:624-9.

36. Lynch SE, Nixon JC, Colvins RB, Antoniades HN. Role of platelet-derived growth factor in wound healing: synergistic effects with other growth factors. Proc Natl Acad Sci USA 1987;84:7696-700.

37. Lynch SE, Colvin RB, Antoniades HN. Growth factors in wound healing: single and synergistic effects on partial thickness porcine skin wounds. J Clin Invest 1989;84:640-6.

38. Brown GL, Curtsinger LJ, White M, et al. Acceleration of tensile strength of incisions treated with EGF and TGF-beta. Ann Surg 1988;208:788-94.

39. Hennessey PJ, Black CT, Andrassy RJ. Epidermal growth factor and insulin act synergistically during diabetic healing. Arch Surg 1990;125:926-39.

40. Brown GL, Nanney LB, Griffen J, et al. Enhancement of wound healing by topical treatment with epidermal growth factor. N Engl J Med 1989;321:76-9.
41. Schultz GS, Chegini N, Grant MB, Khaw PT, MacKay S. Effects of growth factors on corneal wound healing. Acta Ophthalmol 1992;70:60-6.
42. Schultz GS, Khaw PT, Oxford K, Macauley S, Van Setten G, Chegini N. Growth factors and ocular wound healing. Eye 1994;8:184-7.
43. Schultz GS, Rotatori SD, Clark W. EGF and TGF-α in wound healing and repair. J Cell Biochem 1991;45:346-52.
44. Schultz GS, Grant MB. Neovascular growth factors. Eye 1991;5:170-80.
45. Leibowitz HM, Morello S, Stern M, Kupferman A. Effect of topically administered epidermal growth factor on corneal wound strength. Arch Ophthalmol 1990;108:734-7.
46. Brightwell JR, Riddle SL, Eiferman RA, et al. Biosynthetic human EGF accelerates healing on neodecadron-treated primate corneas. Invest Ophthalmol Vis Sci 1985;26:105-10.
47. Brazzell RK, Stern ME, Aquavella JV, Beuerman RW, Baird L. Human recombinant epidermal growth factor in experimental corneal wound healing. Invest Ophthalmol Vis Sci 1991;32:336-40.
48. Woost PG, Brightwell J, Eiferman RA, Schultz GS. Effect of growth factors with dexamethasone on healing of rabbit corneal stromal incisions. Exp Eye Res 1985;40:47-60.
49. Kandarakis AS, Page C, Kaufman HE. The effect of epidermal growth factor on epithelial healing after penetrating keratoplasty in human eyes. Am J Ophthalmol 1984;98:411-5.
50. Rich LF, Hatfield JM, Louiselle, I. The influence of epidermal growth factor on cat corneal endothelial wound healing. Curr Eye Res 1991;10:823-30.
51. Raphael B, Kerr NC, Shimizu RW, et al. Enhanced healing of cat corneal endothelial wounds by epidermal growth factor. Invest Ophthalmol Vis Sci 1993;34:2305-12.
52. Pastor JC, Calonge M. Epidermal growth factor and corneal wound healing: a multicenter study. Cornea 1992;11:311-4.
53. Scardovi C, De Felice GP, Gazzaniga A. Epidermal growth factor in the topical treatment of traumatic corneal ulcers. Ophthalmologica 1993;206:119-24.
54. Falanga V, Eaglestein WH, Bucalo B, Katz MH, Harris B, Carson P. Topical use of human recombinant epidermal growth factor (h-EGF) in venous ulcers. Phlebology 1992;18:604-6.
55. Chavira RJ, Burnett TJ, Hageman JH. Assaying proteinases with azocoll. Anal Biochem 1984;136:446-50.
56. Birkedal-Hansen H, Taylor RE. Detergent-activation of latent collagenase and resolution of its component molecules. Biochem Biophys Res Commun 1982;107:1173-8.
57. Tarnuzzer RW, Macauley SP, Farmerie WG, et al. Competitive RNA templates for detection and quantitation of growth factors, cytokines, extracellular matrix components and matrix metalloproteinases by RT-PCR. Biotechniques, in press.
58. Schultz GS, Strelow S, Stern GA, et al. Treatment of alkali-injured rabbit corneas with a synthetic inhibitor of matrix metalloproteinases. Invest Ophthalmol Vis Sci 1992;33:3325-31.

Part IV

Clinical Application of Growth Hormone and IGF-I Therapy

Part IV

Clinical Application of Growth Hormone and IGF-I Therapy

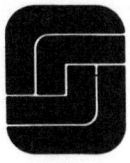

13

Growth Hormone Therapy in Human Burn Injury

DAVID N. HERNDON, EDGAR J. PIERRE, J. KEITH ROSE,
KARINA N. STOKES, AND ROBERT E. BARROW

Improvements in burn care have lowered mortality rates significantly over the last 40 years. Survival rates of 50% are now evident in children with 98% total body surface area (TBSA) burns, while in the 1950s children with at most 49% TBSA burns were the only ones accorded such favorable odds (Table 13.1). Advances in fluid resuscitation, infection control, and techniques designed to achieve early wound closure all contribute to improved survival rates; strategies for supporting the metabolic responses to burn injuries have been of particular importance. Burn injuries covering more than 40% TBSA prompt a stress response accompanied by a release of catabolic hormones, which increase metabolic rate by 50% to 150% above basal levels. This hypermetabolic response contributes to increases in oxygen consumption, fat and protein wasting, cardiac output, elevated body temperature, and immunologic compromise as well as impaired wound healing. During prolonged periods of burn induced catabolism, loss of lean muscle mass and lipolysis result in peripheral muscle wasting and hepatic fat deposition. Improvements in resuscitation, wound treatment, antibiotic therapies, and nutritional support are often unable to prevent the devastating effects of this hypermetabolic response to burn injury. This catabolic state can endure long after wound closure is achieved, up to 180 days after injury in cases of massive thermal injury. Pediatric burned patients often display significant growth arrests for up to 3 years after injury (1).

An inflammatory response to trauma or sepsis is a physiologic survival mechanism; however, when this response becomes overwhelming, it can initiate a self-destructive sequence that can result in multiple organ failure and death (2). After thermal injury, counterregulatory hormones such as catecholamines and cortisol exhibit significant increases, while levels of anabolic hormones such as insulin, growth hormone (GH), and insulin-like growth factor-I (IGF-I) are decreased. These initial hormonal changes

TABLE 13.1. Percent of the total body surface area (TBSA) burned for an expected 50% mortality in 1952 and 1993.

Age	1952	1993*
0–14	49%TBSA	98%TBSA
15–44	46%TBSA	72%TBSA
45–64	27%TBSA	51%TBSA
>65	10%TBSA	25%TBSA

*Galveston Burn Unit.
From Herndon et al. (62), with permission.

produce increases in metabolic rate, oxygen consumption, and cardiac output, and they cause concomitant rises in serum glucose, free fatty acids, and lactate. Persistently elevated levels of cortisol and catecholamines characterize the hypermetabolic response to burn injury, and can result in gluconeogenesis, hyperglycemia, glycogenolysis, skeletal muscle proteolysis, and lipolysis. The erosion of body protein that is produced by the catabolic response is associated with increased infection rates, delayed tissue repair, reduced wound healing, and diminished skeletal muscle function. Chronically elevated levels of catecholamines produce pathologic conditions such as cardiomyopathy as well as increases in heart rate and contractility (3), which can lead to heart failure. Catecholamines also promote fat and protein catabolism, which result in peripheral muscle wasting and a redistribution of subcutaneous fat (especially to the liver) (4, 5). Liver size often increases to two or three times normal and can impair respiration due to restricted diaphragmatic excursion. As the hypermetabolic response continues, patients with larger burns lose skeletal muscle mass to the point of becoming feeble. This delays independence and self care. While total body weight can be maintained with generous caloric intakes supplemented with protein and other nutrients, parenteral caloric intakes above maximally tolerated enteral nutrition can lower the immune response and, according to randomized prospective studies, heighten risk of mortality (6). Early enteral feeding (within a few hours of an injury) prevents protein-caloric malnutrition, reduces gastric atrophy, and limits bacterial translocation and sepsis (7–9). Weeks after a burn injury, GH and IGF-I concentrations are still decreased, while glucagon, catecholamines, and cortisol levels remain elevated. Prolongation or exaggeration of the hypermetabolic response can result in added morbidity and increased incidence of mortality in severe thermal injury.

While the exact mechanisms of postburn hypermetabolism are not fully understood, it is thought to begin with a bacterial toxin as the stimulus. Monocytes and macrophages secrete prostaglandins (especially thromboxane and PGE_2, which inhibits lymphocyte activation) and incite the production of inflammatory cytokines, especially tumor necrosis factor

(TNF). Many metabolic alterations seen with burn injuries can be attributed to upregulations of TNF, thromboxane, and PGE_2 (10). TNF receptors can be found on nearly all somatic tissues except for erythrocytes (11). Animal studies suggest that TNF, which is cytotoxic for damaged cells and active in host defense (12), may cause body wasting which is seen in some chronic diseases. The sera of septic, thermally injured patients exhibit elevated levels of TNF (13), and animals that have been treated with TNF antibodies can survive subsequent lethal injections of endotoxin (14). TNF acts in a synergistic manner with epidermal growth factor (EGF), platelet-derived growth factor (PDGF), and insulin to produce a mitogenic effect in several cell lines (15). Upon encountering bacterial products, macrophages secrete monokines such as TNF and interleukin-1. These factors interact with others and create a cascade of events that serves to mediate the body's response to shock by increasing concentrations of epinephrine, norepinephrine, and glucagon. In sepsis, thromboxanes are increased and contribute to tissue damage, while cytokines, such as interleukin-1 (IL-1), interleukin-2 (IL-2), interleukin-6 (IL-6), and tumor necrosis factor-α (TNF-α), act as intermediaries in bringing about immunologic depression and catabolism (16, 17). Cytokines and prostanoids prompt the hypothalamus to reset the core body temperature to about 2° higher than normal. A typical compensation mechanism of a burned patient is to increase his resting energy expenditure (REE). Maintaining environmental temperatures at 30° to 32°C can reduce a patient's REE and relieve stress. Septic patients are especially vulnerable to environmental temperatures as they cannot respond to cold stress by appropriately elevating REE, and their core temperatures drop when they are exposed to cold. Sepsis may limit a patient's ability to raise REE or may inhibit mediators or cellular functions that usually respond to cold stress. Metabolic derangements and infections that threaten such basic regulations are critical to survival.

In addition to the typical complications of severe thermal injuries, pediatric patients frequently experience growth delays after severe burn injuries without subsequent growth compensation. In a review by Herndon et al. (18) of 80 patients sustaining 40% or greater TBSA burns, the catabolic processes that lead to growth delays are not averted by early wound excision and coverage (within 72 hours) combined with aggressive nutritional supplementation designed to maintain weight. In spite of this support and treatment, along with maximum exercise, these pediatric patients display profound growth arrests during the first year after their burn injuries. These children do not return to near normal growth rates until 3 years postinjury. Possibly, the hypermetabolic response consumes energy resources that would otherwise contribute to anabolic growth. These profound growth delays and muscle wasting with a concomitant lower production of GH and IGF-I suggest that exogenous administration of growth hormone could be advantageous for severely burned pediatric patients.

The Role of Growth Hormones in Burn
Wounds and Hypermetabolism

Burn wounds themselves prompt neural pain impulses, thromboxane release, and the production of cytokines such as IL-1, IL-2, IL-6, and TNF. Lymphocytes produce interleukins, TGF-β, TNF, and interferons, all of which play important roles in the local inflammatory response process. Normally, an orderly release of chemicals follows specific stimuli in a controlled manner so as to coordinate the wound healing process. A platelet plug forms, and fibroblasts, neutrophils, and macrophages follow after and prompt the appearance of collagen fibers and other matrix components. Granulation tissue macrophages clean damaged areas; fibroblasts deposit collagen in order to seal rifts, and endothelial cells provide resources for growing dermal tissue by way of neovessels (19). Growth factors and cytokines influence the formulation of granulation tissue involved in wound healing. Initially, growth factors congregate near wound sites and, when sufficiently elevated concentrations are attained, they repress chemotaxis and activate mitogenesis or matrix production. Some growth factors promote cell division and others enhance DNA synthesis. While some T lymphocytes enhance the processes involved in wound healing, others have the opposite effect (20). Fibroblasts, endothelia, and keratinocytes promote local tissue repair and can enhance the function of white cells, but with time they cause generalized immunosuppression. Animal studies and clinical trials demonstrate that growth hormones, growth factors, and interleukin-4 (21) and interleukin-8 (22) may ease some the devastating effects of the hypermetabolic response and improve wound healing.

The radical metabolic changes and hormonal shifts seen in burned patients are exceptionally difficult to control because of complicated interactions within an interconnected network of chemical messengers. Mediators are produced in wounds and carried by the circulation to distant organs and tissues that secrete growth factors. Cytokines such as IL-6, IL-1, and TNF; growth factors; prostaglandins; and thromboxanes A_2 and B_2 move to target tissues. These mediators cause changes in permeability, decrease circulating plasma volume, and result in hypovolemia. Thromboxanes A_2, catecholamines, and superoxide ions prompt systemic vasoconstriction and increased cardiac rate. Thromboxanes can cause gastrointestinal vasoconstriction, which, along with hypovolemia, can cause damage to the mucosal barrier of the bowel and thereby permit bacterial translocation into the circulatory and lymphatic systems. Arachidonic acid, a dietary polyunsaturated fatty acid, is a precursor from which thromboxanes and prostaglandins are produced. Prostacyclin (PGE_2 in particular) can provide some benefit to burned patients by causing vasodilation, and by attracting neutrophils (23–25); it can also amplify vascular permeability, which results in wound edema, erythema, and pain. Damaged tissues release proteases that can be harmful, and many of the proteins released during the acute phase in response to an injury act to inhibit such proteases.

Growth factors appear to govern the production and dissemination of cells into and away from wound sites so as to coordinate the processes of coagulation, inflammation, and repair. PDGF promotes chemotaxis in fibroblasts, endothelia, and inflammatory cells (26). Monocytes and neutrophils can be activated by low levels of PDGF. This growth factor increases fibroblast and inflammatory cell infiltration as well as the production of collagen and granulation tissue (27). PDGF gathers and degranulates neutrophils and augments their ability to produce superoxide and lysosomal enzymes (28). Animal studies show that PDGF expedites healing for partial-thickness (29), full-thickness (30), and incisional wounds (31). The presence of additional growth factors may be necessary in order for PDGF to act. Macrophages secrete large quantities of PDGF, transforming growth factors, fibroblast growth factor (FGF), and interleukins. Fibroblasts and endothelia are then able to produce autocrine growth factors such as endothelins and insulin-like growth factors. The most significant function of FGF probably involves the stimulation of angioneogenesis where injury occurs or repair is needed (32, 33). Further, FGF stimulates endothelial cells to proliferate, and secrete proteases that lyse the basement membranes of vessel walls (34–37). Endothelial cells form capillary sprouts and then capillary tubes that run parallel to one another and perpendicular to the wound surface. The newly formed vessels create arched loops that conjoin. If these newly formed endothelial junctions leak, edema can result (38). FGF prompts new vessel growth, and in vitro studies suggest that it stimulates the multiplication and migration of endothelia as well as tube formation. Transforming growth factor-β (TGF-β), PDGF, and IGF influence the creation of collagen, which is an essential product of fibroblasts and provides tensile strength in healing skin.

The hypermetabolic response to traumatic injury is driven by many hormonal changes, and a treatment aimed at hormonal modulation is apt to be complex. β-blockade mitigates some of the consequences of hypermetabolism; it reduces free fatty acid levels, cardiac rate, basal metabolic rate, and blood pressure (39). Unfortunately, when catecholamine-induced lipolysis is reduced, proteolysis sometimes increases because the process of gluconeogenesis requires fuel. β_1-blockers, which influence cardiovascular function but leave protein and fat kinetics untouched, show some success in preliminary clinical trials (40). Additionally, β_2-agonists (e.g., clenbuterol) can stimulate protein synthesis so that, in combination with β_1-blockers, the harmful effects of catecholamines can be thwarted without causing damaging side effects. Efforts to block prolific mediators, to stimulate insufficient factors, or to replace lost biologic mechanisms, however, could result in an unexpected cascade.

Growth hormone is an anabolic agent that stimulates cell proliferation, fat mobilization, skeletal growth, and amino acid entry into cells for protein synthesis. One of the detrimental effects of the hypermetabolic response to traumatic injury, loss of nitrogen, can be abated or even reversed by recombinant human growth hormone. Early studies of Liljadahl et al. (41), Soroff et al. (42), Roe and Kinney (43), and others (44–46) show that rhGH reduces nitrogen losses and up-regulates protein metabolism in traumatically injured patients. Administration of rhGH can improve nitrogen balance by 2 to 4 g per day (143 to 246 mmol per day). Early investigations suggest that rhGH acts to increase oxygen utilization, promote nitrogen retention, enhance electrolyte storage, and increase levels of circulating insulin-like growth factor-I (IGF-I) (47). Furthermore, rhGH can promote a positive nitrogen balance, reduce protein oxidation, increase lipolysis, and produce a positive mineral and trace element balance even with hypocaloric nutritional support. Growth hormones are necessary for cell repair and development and also have the capacity to cause cellular migration; they organize cellular proliferation.

Recombinant human growth hormone is noted for its ability to reverse protein catabolism by increasing cellular uptake of amino acids and stimulating translation and transcription of nucleic acid. It prompts adipose tissue to release fatty acids that are transformed in the liver into acetyl coenzyme A; fat is a preferred energy source. Growth hormone enhances wound healing by increasing epithelial cell mitosis, the rate of collagen deposition, and tensile strength. Histologic studies of skin biopsies of patients who received exogenous rhGH for 7 days demonstrate that growth hormone upregulates IGF-I surface receptors, increases levels of types IV and VII collagen, and improves the formation of basal lamina at chosen donor harvest sites. Clinical studies suggest that protein synthesis is greatly augmented in burn wounds and becomes significant in the course of the healing process compared with protein synthesis rates in the rest of the body (48).

GH can produce deleterious side effects such as insulin resistance and hyperglycemia. Hyperinsulinemic euglycemic clamp studies demonstrated that administration of exogenous rhGH may reduce peripheral protein wasting in severely injured patients via a mechanism that is similar to that of insulin (49). A group of severely burned patients treated with 0.2 mg/kg/day of rhGH were given an infusion of insulin to maintain serum concentrations at 500 μU/ml. A primed constant infusion of N15 lysine was administered before and after the clamp procedure in order to measure protein synthesis rate. Patients treated with rhGH showed protein synthesis rates three times above those of placebo-treated patients; however, no additional protein synthesis increases were noted during the clamp procedure. Like rhGH, insulin produces anabolic effects on protein kinetics; recent studies by Sakurai et al. (50) on the effects of long-term administration of insulin on protein and glucose kinetics in burned patients indicate that insulin levels maintained at 250 to 500 μU/ml markedly stimulate protein synthesis and also increase protein breakdown, with protein synthesis in muscle mass increased by 352% above basal value. The combination of rhGH and insulin does not cause significant improvement over administration of either one alone, and the effect of insulin on muscle protein synthesis is as large as that of GH at these doses. Fleming et al. (51) examined the effects of rhGH on circulating levels of catabolic hormones in pediatric burned patients. Patients with burns greater than 40% TBSA were randomly assigned to receive placebo or 0.2 mg/kg/day rhGH throughout their hospitalization. The rhGH-treated group showed a significant increase in plasma levels of IGF-I, total catecholamines, norepinephrine, insulin, glucagon, and free fatty acids compared with the placebo group.

IGF-I alone can produce significant reductions in hypermetabolic responses; it can decrease oxygen consumption and promote weight retention in thermally injured animals (52). IGF-I, an anabolic agent synthesized primarily in the liver, encourages body weight and height gains and increases organ tissue weights. IGF-I acts to increase peripheral glucose uptake and reduce protein breakdown and circulating amino acid levels (53). Growth hormone stimulates production of IGF-I. It is hypothesized that rhGH enhances wound healing by stimulating hepatic and local production of IGF-I. In a 40% TBSA scald rat model (54), a combination treatment with GH and IGF-I shows a significant increase in epithelialization rate, body weight retention, and attenuation of hypermetabolism. Rats receiving 2.5 mg/kg/day rhGH and 5.0 mg/kg/day IGF-I are compared with those receiving rhGH alone (Fig. 13.1). Insulin-like growth factor

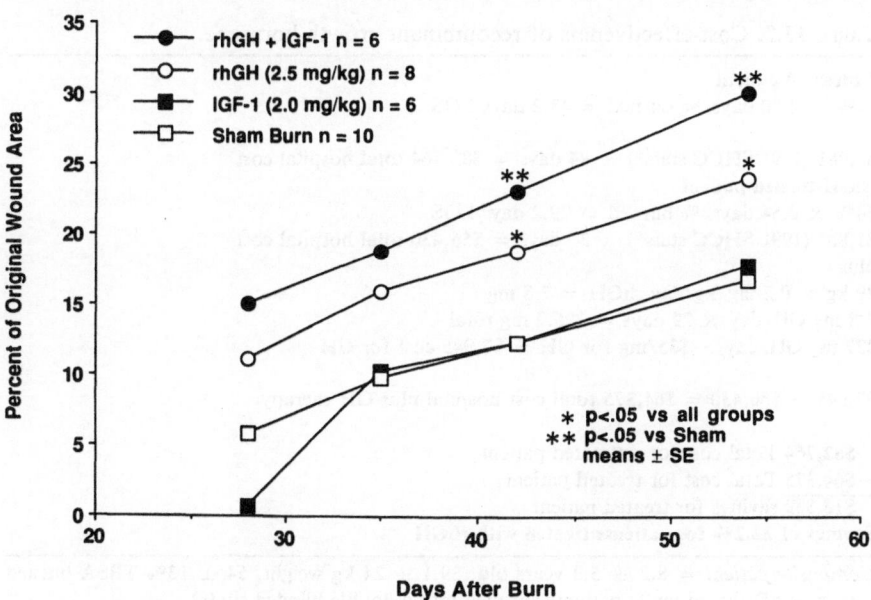

FIGURE 13.1. Epitheliazation rates for rats with 40% TBSA burns treated with rhGH, IGF-I, both or placebo.

reduces stress related responses to traumatic injury, accelerates wound healing rates, and increases tensile strength.

Growth Hormone Improves Donor Site Healing Rates

Administration of rhGH accelerates the healing rates of skin graft donor sites by 25% in children with burns covering an average of 60% of TBSA. Thus, severely burned children treated with rhGH can tolerate repeated skin grafting procedures in which donor sites are reharvested on an average of 2 days earlier than those not treated. Exogenous rhGH treatment is expensive, but it is cost-effective for patients with burns greater than 40% TBSA because it significantly decreases the time required for wound closure and thereby decreases the overall length of hospital stay (Table 13.2). Patients with burns greater than 50% TBSA are completely dependent on donor site re-epithelialization for achievement of wound coverage, and rhGH therapy is particularly beneficial for them.

Forty-six children with burns covering 53% ± 19% TBSA participated in a double blind, randomized study to receive 0.2 mg/kg/day of rhGH from the time of admission until complete wound coverage. Donor sites were harvested at 0.006 to 0.010 inches in depth and dressed with Scarlet Red impregnated fine mesh gauze (Sherwood Medical, St. Louis , MO). Donor site healing time was recorded as the day when the gauze could be removed

TABLE 13.2. Cost-effectiveness of recombinant growth hormone.

Untreated patient
54% × 0.80 days/% burned = 43.2 days LOS

$1,881 (1991 SHCC stats*) × 44 days = $82,764 total hospital cost
rhGH-treated patient
54% × 0.54 days/% burned = 29.2 days LOS
$1,881 (1991 SHCC stats*) × 30 days = $56,430 total hospital cost
plus
39 kg × 0.2 mg/kg/day rhGH = 7.8 mg
7.8 mg GH/day × 29 days = 226.2 mg total
227 mg GH/day × $35/mg for GH = $7,945 cost for GH

$7,945 + $56,430 = $64,375 total cost hospital plus GH therapy

 $82,764 Total cost for untreated patient
−$64,375 Total cost for treated patient
 $18,389 savings for treated patient
Savings of 22.2% for patients treated with rhGH

Composite patient = 8.2 ± 5.3 years old, 39.1 ± 24 kg weight, 54 ± 13% TBSA burned (Mean ± SD, based on 24 patients enrolled into a double-blinded study).
LOS, length of stay in hospital.
*Based on all patients admitted to the Shriners Burn Institute in Galveston.
From Pierre et al. (63), with permission.

without any trauma to the healed site (55). Two forms of growth hormone were tested in this study: 18 patients received Protropin, 20 received Nutropin, and 26 received placebo. Donor site healing times for these groups were 6.0, 6.8, and 8.5 days, respectively. Length of hospital stay decreased concomitantly with healing times so that rhGH treated patients stayed 0.76 ± 0.04 days per % TBSA of third-degree burn as compared with 1.01 ± 0.07 days per % TBSA of third-degree burn for untreated patients. Therapeutic growth hormone was administered in conjunction with morning feedings, although the optimal timing has not yet been determined. While the precise mechanisms at work in growth hormone therapy in burned patients have not been fully understood, it appeared that GH exerted a direct influence on wound healing as well as improving protein synthesis (56–58).

Recently, nine patients with full-thickness burns covering greater than 40% of their TBSAs were selected for a study to determine the wound healing effects of growth hormone (59). Levels of IGF-I and IGF-I receptors, laminin, collagen, and cytokeratin systemically and locally in wound sites were the focus of the study. The patients, whose ages ranged from 6 to 30 years, were resuscitated with a standard formula and their urinary outputs were maintained at 0.5 to 1.0 ml per kg per hour. Fluids were supplemented with electrolytes, and nutritional support was provided enterally to deliver 1500 Kcal per m^2 of TBSA plus 1500 Kcal per m^2 of TBSA burned per day (60). Two surgeons were alternately responsible for excising and grafting burn wounds (except for the face and perineum) within 48 hours of admission. Two evaluators, blinded to the treatments, alternately examined donor sites beginning on the third day after surgery. Harvested donor sites were dressed with a Scarlet Red impregnated fine mesh gauze. Forceps were used to gently lift the corners of the gauze via sterile technique to assess the adherence of the dressing to the underlying tissue, and any detached dressing was trimmed away. Daily repetitions of this procedure continued until the Scarlet Red gauze no longer adhered to the wound. The number of days until achievement of atraumatic removal of the Scarlet Red gauze constituted the healing time.

At the time of the second split-thickness skin harvest, treated patients began rhGH therapy via subcutaneous injection of 0.2 mg per kg of body weight per day, and control patients received placebo. A biopsy of the second donor site was performed 7 days later for the patients receiving rhGH therapy and for those receiving placebo. Skin biopsies were evaluated via immunohistochemical assay. The results of the study showed that the therapy caused a threefold increase in IGF-I serum concentrations and a decrease in healing time for donor sites by about 1.5 days. Growth hormone therapy also caused more extensive basal lamina formation (28% $\pm$ 14% for placebo as compared with 73% $\pm$ 15% for rhGH therapy), produced increased expression of cytokeratin (CK14) in the keratinocytes of the middle layer of the epidermis (0.7 + 0.3 for placebo and 2.3 $\pm$ 0.06 for

TABLE 13.3. Means and standard deviation of staining intensities for laminin, cytokeratin 14, IGF-I receptors, collagen IV, and collagen VII with placebo and rhGH.

	Laminin	Cytokeratin 14	IGF-1 receptors	Collagen IV	Collagen VII
Placebo	0.2 ± 0.3	0.7 ± 0.3	0.8 ± 0.3	0.4 ± 0.5	0.6 ± 0.5
rhGH	2.8 ± 2.0	2.3 ± 0.6	2.3 ± 0.6	2.3 ± 1.5	2.3 ± 1.5

From Herndon et al. (59), with permission.

rhGH therapy on a scale of 0 to 4 in staining intensity), and prompted a significant increase in IGF-I receptors present in keratinocyte cytoplasm, in type IV collagen, and in type VII collagen along the dermal-epidermal junction (Table 13.3).

This study was the first to quantitatively investigate the structural effects of growth hormone therapy on wound healing in human patients. Previous work on sheep tracheal epithelium (61) coupled with the recognized effects of growth hormone led to the hypothesis that growth hormone therapy would activate mitosis and proliferation of epidermal cells and would prompt earlier and more complete reformation of structures that were needed for dermal-epidermal attachment and growth. Various components of the basement membrane were quantified. Laminin and type IV collagen were known to be principle components of the basal lamina. Cytokeratin 14 was understood to be a keratin species associated with epidermal basal cells, and collagen type VII was known as the principle component of anchoring fibrils that extend from the hemidesmosomes into the dermis. Growth hormone's action may have directly stimulated cell division or protein synthesis via its own surface receptors or it may have stimulated its intermediary, IGF-I, to be released from the liver into the circulation or to be produced at wound sites. IGF-I was known to be mitogenic for cultured human keratinocytes, and IGF-I receptors have been found in human epidermis where they were altered in the presence of increased keratinocyte proliferation. The study measured completeness of newly formed basal lamina, levels of protein components of basal lamina (laminin and collagen type IV), and presence of the major component of anchoring fibrils (type VII collagen) with and without growth hormone treatment. The study determined that growth hormone enhanced re-epithelialization in healing donor site wounds either directly or indirectly.

Conclusion

Wound healing and the hypermetabolic response to a burn injury are regulated by an interconnected network of chemical messengers. Mediators produced at the wound site are carried by the circulation to distant tissues and organs that secrete growth factors targeted at other tissues. Traumatic injuries and severe infections cause metabolic changes and hormonal shifts that cannot be pharmacologically controlled unless they are better understood. Growth hormones and growth factors that are intimately involved in the hypermetabolic response to burn injury may hold the key to controlling and alleviating the devastating sequelae of severe burn injuries.

Evidence suggests that rhGH increases concentrations of IGF-I and its receptors at wound sites. Growth hormone therapy has the capacity to improve body mass composition and weight retention, and it has been shown to improve healing rates for burn wounds and donor sites. Further, rhGH can stimulate cell mitosis and increase the synthesis of laminin, collagen types IV and VII, and cytokeratin 14. In combination with IGF-I, GH therapy is especially effective in attenuating the hypermetabolic response to burn injury and in accelerating the processes of wound healing.

Administered subcutaneously, rhGH improves donor site healing rates by about 2 days and can shorten the overall length of hospital stay for burned patients by nearly 25%. Treatment with GH and IGF-I has been shown to improve body mass composition, weight retention, and re-epithelization rates at both burn wound and donor sites more than GH therapy alone. The combination of these anabolic hormones may produce an even more marked improvement. Future studies of treatment with GH in combination with insulin or with IGF-I are warranted.

References

1. Rutan RL, Herndon DN. Growth delay in postburn pediatric patients. Arch Surg 1990;125:392–5.
2. Baue AE. Progress in trauma care through understanding the cell biology of injury. In: Faist E, Meakins JL, Schildberg FW, eds. Host defense dysfunction in trauma, shock and sepsis: mechanisms and therapeutic approaches. New York: Springer-Verlag 1993:3–14.
3. Joshi VV. Effects of burns on the heart. JAMA 1970;211:2130–4.
4. Wilmore DW, Aulick LH. Metabolic changes in burned patients. Surg Clin North Am 1978;58:1173–87.
5. Wilmore DW. Hormone responses and their effect on metabolism. Surg Clin North Am 1976;56:999–1018.
6. Waymack JP. The effect of ibuprofen on postburn metabolism and immunologic function. J Surg Res 1989;46:172–6.
7. Herndon DN, Zeigler ST. Bacterial translocation after thermal injury. Crit Care Med 1993;21(2):S50–4.
8. Hildreth MA, Herndon DN, Desai MH, Duke MA. Calorie needs of adolescent patients with burns. J Burn Care Rehab 1989;10(6):523–6.
9. Hildreth MA, Herndon DN, Desai MH, Broemling LD. Current treatment reduces calories required to maintain weight in pediatric patients with burns. J Burn Care Rehab 1990;11(5):405–9.
10. Mannick JA. Trauma, sepsis and immune defects. In: Faist E, Meakins JL,

Schildberg FW, eds. Host defense dysfunction in trauma, shock and sepsis: mechanisms and therapeutic approaches. New York: Springer-Verlag, 1993: 15–21.

11. Beutler B, Cerami A. The common mediator of shock, cachexia and tumor necrosis. Adv Immunol 1988;42:213–31.

12. Balkwill FR. Tumor necrosis factor and lymphotoxin. In: Balkwill FR, ed. Cytokines in cancer therapy. Oxford: Oxford University Press, 1989:54–87.

13. Marano M, Fong Y, Moldawer LL, et al. Cachectin/TNF in the serum of ICU and burn patients. Am Burn Assoc Ann Proc 1988;20:18.

14. Beutler B, Milsark IW, Cerami A. Passive immunization against cachectin/ tumor necrosis factor protects mice from lethal effect of endotoxin. Science 1985;229:869–71.

15. Vilcek J, Palombella VJ, Zhang Y, Lin JX, Feinman R, Reis LF, Le J. Mechanisms and significance of the mitogenic and antiviral actions of TNF. Ann Inst Pasteur Immunol 1988;139:307–11.

16. Nguyen TT, Cox CS, Traber DL, Gasser H, Redl H, Schlag G, Herndon DN. Free radical activity and loss of plasma antioxidants, vitamin E, and sulfhydryl groups in patients with burn. J Burn Care Rehabil 1993;14:602–9.

17. Drost AC, Burleson DG, Cioffi WG, Jordan BS, Mason AD, Pruitt BA. Plasma cytokines following thermal injury and their relationship with patient mortality, burn size, and time postburn. J Trauma 1993;35:335–9.

18. Herndon DN, Barrow RE, Kunkle KR, Broemeling LD, Rutan RL. Effects of recombinant human growth hormone on donor site healing in severely burned children. Am Surg 1990;212:424–31.

19. Linares HA. Pathophysiology of the burn scar. In: Herndon DN, ed. Total burn care. London: WB Saunders, in press.

20. Barbul A. Role of T-cell dependent immune system in wound healing. In: Barbul A, Pines E, Calwell M, Hunt TK, eds. Growth factors and other aspects of wound healing: biological and clinical implications. Progress in clinical and biological research series, vol. 266. New York: Alan R. Liss, 1987:19.

21. Lee JD, Swisher SG, Minehart EH, McBride WH, Golub SH, Economou JS. Interleukin-4: a potent inhibitor of IL-6, TNF, IFN, IL-1 production. Surg Forum 1990;61:441–4.

22. Hechtman DH, Cybulsky MI, Baker JB, Gimbrone MA. Intravenous interleukin-8 reduces neutrophil accumulation at intradermal sites of inflammation. Surg Forum 1990;61:96–8.

23. Demling RH, Lalonde C. Topical ibuprofen decreases early postburn edema. Surgery 1987;5:857–61.

24. Haung YS, Li A, Yang ZC. Roles of thromboxane and its inhibitor anisodamine in burn shock. Burns 1990;4:249–53.

25. Herndon DN, Abston S, Stein MD. Increased thromboxane B2 levels in the plasma of burned and septic patients. Surg Gynecol Obstet 1984;159:210–13.

26. Grotendorst GR, Seppa HEJ, Kleinman HK, Martin GR. Attachment of smooth muscle cells to collagen and their migration toward platelet-derived growth factor. Proc Natl Acad Sci USA 1981;78:3669–72.

27. Bauer EA, Cooper TW, Huang SJ, Altman J, Deuel TF. Stimulation of in vitro human skin collagenase expression by platelet-derived growth factor. Proc Natl Acad Sci USA 1985;82:4132–6.

28. Tzeng DY, Deuel TF, Huang JS, Senior RM, Boxer LA, Baehner RL.

Platelet-derived growth factor promotes polymorphonuclear leukocyte activation. Blood 1984;64:1123-8.

29. Lynch SE, Colvin RB, Antoniades HN. Growth factors in wound healing. Single and synergistic effects on partial thickness porcine skin wounds. J Clin Invest 1989;84:640-6.

30. Greenhaulgh DG, Sprugel KH, Murray MJ, Ross R. PDGF and FGF stimulate wound healing in the genetically diabetic mouse. Am J Pathol 1990; 136:1235-46.

31. Pierce GF, Mustoe TA, Senior RM, et al. In vivo incisional wound healing augmented by platelet-derived growth factor and recombinant c-sis gene homodimeric proteins. J Exp Med 1988;167:974-87.

32. Shing Y, Folkman J, Haudenschild C, Lund D, Crum R, Klagsbrun M. Angiogenesis is stimulated by tumor derived endothelial cell growth factor. J Cell Biochem 1985;29:275-87.

33. Lobb RR, Alderman EM, Fett JW. Introduction of angiogenesis by bovine brain derived class I heparin binding growth factor. Biochemistry 1985; 24:4969-73.

34. Gross JL, Moscatelli D, Jaffe EA, Rifkin DB. Plasminogen activator and collagenase production by cultured capillary endothelial cells. J Cell Biol 1982;95:974-81.

35. Gross JL, Moscatelli D, Rifkin DB. Increased capillary endothelial cell protease activity in response to angiogenic stimuli in vivo. Proc Natl Acad Sci USA 1983;80:2623-7.

36. Saksela O, Moscatelli D, Rifkin DB. The opposing effects of basic fibroblast growth factor and transforming growth factor beta on the regulation of plasminogen activator activity in capillary endothelial cells. J Cell Biol 1987; 105:957-63.

37. Mignatti P, Tsuboi R, Robbins E, Rifkin DB. In vitro angiogenesis on the human amniotic membrane: requirement for basic fibroblast growth factor-induced proteinases. J Cell Biol 1989;108:671-82.

38. Schoefl GI. Studies of inflammation. III. Growing capillaries: their structure and permeability. Virchows Arch Pathol Anat 1963;337:97-104.

39. Wilmore DW, Long JM, Mason AD, Skreen RW, Pruitt BA Jr. Catecholamines: mediators of the hypermetabolic response to thermal injury. Ann Surg 1974;18(4):653-69.

40. Maggi SP, Biolo G, Muller MJ, Barrow RE, Wolfe RR, Herndon DN. Beta-1 blockade decreases cardiac work without affecting protein breakdown or lipolysis in severely burned patients. Surg Forum 1993;75:1081.

41. Liljadahl SO, Gemzell CA, Plantin LO, Birke G. Effect of human growth hormone in patients with severe burns. Acta Chir Scand 1961;122:1-14.

42. Soroff HS, Rozin RR, Mooty J, Lister J, Raben MS. Role of human growth hormone in the response to trauma: 1. Metabolic effects following burns. Ann Surg 1967;166:739-52.

43. Roe CF, Kinney J. The influence of human growth hormone on energy sources in convalescence. Surg Forum 1962;13:369-71.

44. Johnston IDA, Hadden DR. Effect of human growth hormone on the metabolic response to surgical trauma. Lancet 1963;1:584-6.

45. Henneman PH, Forbes AP, Moldawer M, Dempsey EF, Carroll EL. Effects of human growth hormone in man. J Clin Invest 1960;39:1223-38.

46. Raben MS. Growth hormone: II. Clinical use of human growth hormone. N Engl J Med 1962;266:82.
47. Wilmore DW, Moylan JA Jr, Bristow BF, Mason AD Jr, Pruitt BA Jr. Anabolic effects of growth hormone and high caloric feedings following thermal injury. Surg Gynecol Obstet 1974;138:875–84.
48. Gilpin DA, Herndon DN. Acute metabolic response to skin injury following burn and the potential use of growth hormone. In: Update in Intensive Care. Berlin: Springer-Produktions-Gellschaft, in press;157–69.
49. Gore DC, Honeycutt D, Jahoor F, Wolfe RR, Herndon DN. Effect of exogenous growth hormone on whole-body and isolated-limb protein kinetics in burned patients. Arch Surg 1991;126(1):38–43.
50. Sakurai Y, Aarsland A, Herndon DN, et al. Stimulation of muscle protein synthesis by long-term insulin infusion in severely-burned patients. Ann Surg (in press).
51. Fleming RYD, Rutan RL, Jahoor F, Barrow RE, Wolfe RR, Herndon DN. Effect of recombinant human growth hormone on catabolic hormones and free fatty acids following thermal injury. J Trauma 1992;32:698–703.
52. Strock LL, Singh H, Abdulla A, Miller JA, Herndon DN. The effect of insulin-like growth factor I on postburn metabolism. Surgery 1990;108:161–4.
53. Jacob R, Barrette E, Plewe G, Fagin KD, Sherwin RS. Acute effects of insulin-like growth factor I on glucose and amino acid metabolism in the awake, fasted rat. J Clin Invest 1989;83:1717–23.
54. Meyer NA, Barrow RE, Pierre EJ, Herndon DN. Effects of growth hormone and insulin like growth factor-1 on burn wound healing: a dose response. Proc Am Burn Assoc 1995;27:(in press).
55. Gilpin DA, Barrow RE, Rutan RL, Broemeling L, Herndon DN. Recombinant human growth hormone accelerates wound healing in children with large cutaneous burns. Ann Surg 1994;220(1):19–24.
56. Fraser R. Endocrine disorders and insulin action. Br Med Bull 1960;16:242–6.
57. MacGorman LR, Rizza R, Gerich JE. Physiological concentrations of growth hormone exert insulin like and insulin antagonist effects on both hepatic and extrahepatic tissues in man. J Clin Endocrinol Metab 1981;53(3):556–9.
58. Wolf RF, Pearlstone DB, Newman E, et al. Growth hormone and insulin net whole-body and skeletal muscle protein catabolism in cancer patients. Ann Surg 1992;216(3):280–90.
59. Herndon DN, Hawkins HK, Nguyen TT, Pierre EJ, Cox R, Barrow RE. Characterization of growth hormone enhanced donor site healing in patients with large cutaneous burns. Ann Surg 1995;221(6):649–59.
60. Hildreth MA, Herndon DN, Desai MH, Broemeling LD. Current treatment reduces calories required to maintain weight in pediatric patients with burns. J Burn Care Rehabil 1990;11:405–9.
61. Barrow RE, Wang CZ, Evans MJ, Herndon DN. Growth factors accelerate tracheal epithelial repair in sheep. Lung 1993;171:335–44.
62. Herndon, Muller, Blakeney. Teamwork for total burn care. In Herndon DN, ed. Total burn care. London: W. B. Saunders, 1995.
63. Pierre EJ, Herndon DN, Barrow RE. Growth hormone therapy in the treatment of burns. In: Torosian MH, ed. Growth hormone in critical illness. In press.

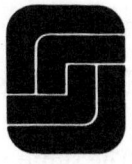

14

Effects of Exogenous Growth Hormone in Postoperative Immune Function and Other Clinical Outcomes

RAFAEL VARA-THORBECK, ESTRELLA RUIZ-REQUENA, AND
JOSÉ ANTONIO GUERRERO

The use of human growth hormone (hGH) in humans as a means of inducing nitrogen storage is attractive to the surgeon, since he or she is continually confronted with patients who could regain their health if only a means were found to heal their wounds and reverse their protein malnutrition. This can be done by providing an adequate intake of nitrogen and by activating an endocrine mechanism that would reverse catabolic predominance.

In 1974 Wilmore et al. (1) suggested that adequate nutritional intake was necessary for hGH to have a nitrogen-saving effect. In 1986 Phillips (2) demonstrated that hGH stimulates hepatic production of somatomedin-C [insulin-like growth factor (IGF-I)], whose action promotes diverse anabolic processes such as the synthesis of RNA, DNA, proteins, proteoglycans, and so on. Poor nutrition, on the other hand, stimulates the production of somatomedin inhibitors, which leads to a decrease in somatomedin activity. In previous papers (3–5) we have shown that the administration of hGH in patients receiving total parenteral nutrition (TPN) following major gastrointestinal surgery and in those receiving hypocaloric parenteral nutrition (HPN) following moderate surgical trauma produces an increase in protein synthesis in the postoperative period.

To our knowledge, until 1993 no clinical study had dealt with the immune function after surgery and exogenous growth hormone administration, and only the experimental studies in rats undertaken by Saito et al. (6) have dealt with the issue.

The purpose of our study was thus to determine whether the administering of hGH could improve the systemic host defenses and promote wound healing, thereby reducing the risk of infection.

Materials and Methods

The subjects in this placebo-controlled randomized double-blind trial were 180 patients suffering from cholecystitis/cholelithiasis with or without choledocholithiasis requiring cholecystectomy with or without choledocho-duodenostomy.

All the patients satisfied the following eligibility criteria:

- They were between the ages of 45 and 60.
- They were not obese; body mass index (BMI) $\leq$ 30.
- They showed no evidence of diabetes mellitus or other chronic disease.
- They had no evidence of sepsis or malignant disease.
- Their hepatic and renal function was normal; this was determined by means of standard clinical and biochemical tests.

Design of the Study

The patients were admitted to the hospital 3 days before the date scheduled for operation. On the day immediately before the operation urine was collected from each patient and a sample was analyzed for urea, creatinine, electrolytes, and glucose. A venous blood sample was also analyzed for glucose, BUN, electrolytes (Na^+, K^+, Cl^-) creatinine, insulin, GOT, glutamic pyruvic transaminase (GPT), cholesterol, total bilirubin, prealbumin, transferrin, retinol-binding protein (RBP), albumin, total proteins, immunoglobulins (IgG, IgM, IgA) growth hormone, and somatomedin-C (IGF-1).

All patients were operated on under general anaesthesia, with tracheal intubation, and a standard cholecystectomy with or without choledocho-duodenostomy was performed.

After the operation all patients were given HPN using a PE-900 Kabi-Pfrimmer nutrition solution (40 ml/kg/day). The diet provided 1 to 1.5 g of protein/kg body weight/day and 900 kcal/day; that is, approximately 40% of energy requirements. The energy was only provided in carbohydrate form (120 to 150 g/day).

Hypocaloric nutrition was administered in a peripheral vein for 6 days and the patients were not allowed to eat until the 6th postoperative day.

hGH (8.IU GRORM-Serono) or placebo (saline serum) was given subcutaneously for 1 week, at 9:30 A.M. daily.

During the postoperative period, urine was collected every 24 hours, and a sample was analyzed for urea, creatinine, electrolytes (Na^+, K^+, Cl^-), and glucose. A venous blood sample was also analyzed daily for BUN, glucose, creatinine, and electrolytes (Na^+, K^+, Cl^-).

On the day before the operation, as we mentioned above, and on the 5th and 12th day after the operation blood was measured using a standard hospital autoanalyzer for GOT, GPT, total bilirubin, cholesterol, alkaline phosphatase, albumin, and total proteins.

We also performed a nephelometric-assay using an ARRAY Protein system (Beckman) to measure prealbumin, transferrin, and RBP. Growth hormone was measured using an hGH radioimmunoassay kit (Sorin Biomedica, 13040 Saluggia, Italy) and IGF-I using the SM-C radioimmunoassay kit (Nichols Institute, San Juan de Capistrano, California). Insulin was also determined by means of a radioimmunoassay kit Insi-5 (Sorin Biomedica).

The host defense mechanism was also tested. This was determined on the day before the operation and on the 5th and 12th postoperative days using radioimmunoassay techniques (Nephelometric Immunsera Behring). Immunoglobulins (IgG, IgM, and IgA) were measured to provide a rough check on the humoral response, or B-cell function.

We performed the skin antigen test (Multitest IMC, Institut Mérieux, Lyon, France) to obtain an approximate estimate of the cell-mediated response. This test was applied on the surface of the volar forearms 3 days before the operation and on the 3rd and 10th days after it. The skin response was examined after 24 and 48 hours, this last measurement being the significant one.

According to the Institut Mérieux, the skin test can be considered positive (that is, the patient can be considered normoergic) when the diameter of induration (at a 48-hour reading) is >10 mm in men and >5 mm in women. Male hypoergic patients show results ranging from 2 to 10 mm, while in women the range is from 2 to 5 mm. The patient is considered anergic if the diameter is < 2 mm. Finally, we also checked wound infection and average hospitalization time.

Results

Wound Infections and Clinical Outcome

Wound infection was found in 16 patients of the control group (17.2%), but in only 3 patients of the hGH-treated group (3.4%) (Fig. 14.1). Total hospitalization averaged 12.5 ± 7.1 days for patients in the control group, whereas those in the hGH-treated group remained in hospital an average of 9.6 ± 3.6 days. In fact, if we discount the 3 hospitalization days before the date scheduled for operation, which were necessary to ensure a reliable design for this study, mean hospitalization was 9.5 ± 7.1 days for patients in the placebo-control group and 6.6 ± 3.6 days for patients in the hGH-treated group.

In modern clinical practice it is difficult to understand the extraordinarily high infection rate (17.2%) observed in the placebo-control group, but we should note that in our social milieu in the South of Spain 30% of patients

A   **Postoperatory infections**

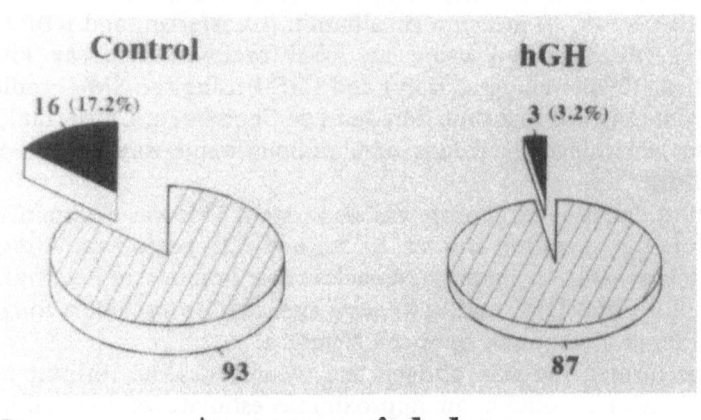

B   **Average sick leave**

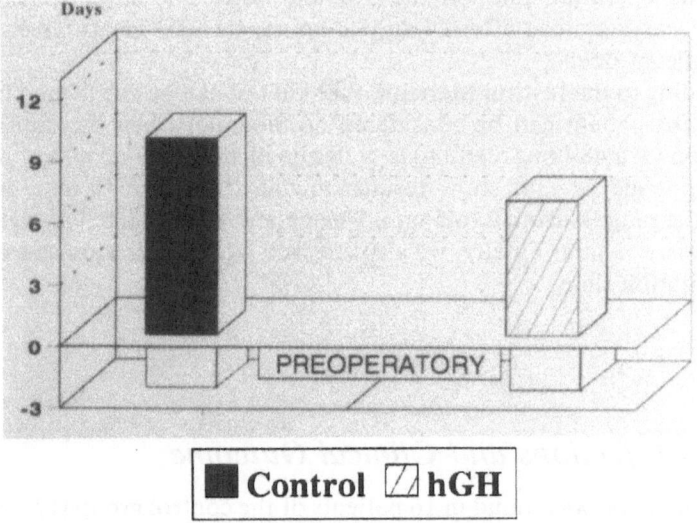

FIGURE 14.1. Postoperative infections (A) and average sick leave (B). Control group and hGH treated.

are hypoergic or anergic preoperatively and, as is well known, after the operation the number of normoergic patients decreases significantly due to the posttraumatic systemic immunosuppressive state (7, 8). These deficiencies in the host defense mechanism, together with the frequently prolonged hospital stay, may explain the high rate of wound infection.

In Spain (especially in the South), there are no private patients in university hospitals since hospital expenses are covered by the Social Security (Health

Service). The insured patient thus tends to exercise his "rights" and declines any release from hospital until all sutures have been removed.

Mechanisms Involved in the Low Infection Rate in the hGH-Treated Group

Maintenance of the B-Cell Function or Humoral Immune Function after Surgery (Fig. 14.2)

Our study shows that on the 5th day after the operation no significant changes were observed in serum levels of immunoglobulins (IgG, IgM, IgA) in the hGH-treated group compared with the preoperative basal levels.

On the other hand, in the placebo-control group immunoglobulin levels in serum fell significantly on this day. These results agree with those obtained by Gebhardt et al. (9), who demonstrated in humans that pulmonary resection resulted in a statistically significant decrease in IgG, IgM, and IgA.

Increase in the Cell-Mediated Host Defense Mechanism (Fig. 14.3)

In our study we performed the skin antigen test (Institut Mérieux score) to obtain an estimate of the cell-mediated response, since delayed hypersensitivity skin testing appears to be a useful and simple method of checking the cell-mediated host defense mechanisms.

We found the following:

- Placebo-control group: After the operation the number of normoergic patients fell from 56 (60%) to 40 (43%), whereas the number of hypoergic patients rose from 26 (27.6%) to 42 (45%). The number of anergic patients remained constant (11 patients).
- hGH-treated group: Here the opposite was the case: the number of normoergic patients increased from 59 (67.8%) to 81 (93.1%), whereas the number of hypoergic patients fell from 25 (28.7%) to 6 (6.9%). The number of anergic patients fell from 3 to 0.

Our conclusion is that our study (5) demonstrates that administering hGH can improve the systemic host defenses, both cellular and humoral.

Promotion of Wound Healing

Wound healing is a dynamic process involving complex mechanisms that manifest themselves in various stages: from blood clotting through inflammation, cellular proliferation, new blood vessel and lymphatic formation, and reconstitution of extracellular matrix.

Some of the key steps in the healing processes are affected by the metabolic changes induced by surgical stress. However, it should be emphasized that the problems of wound healing and wound infection are

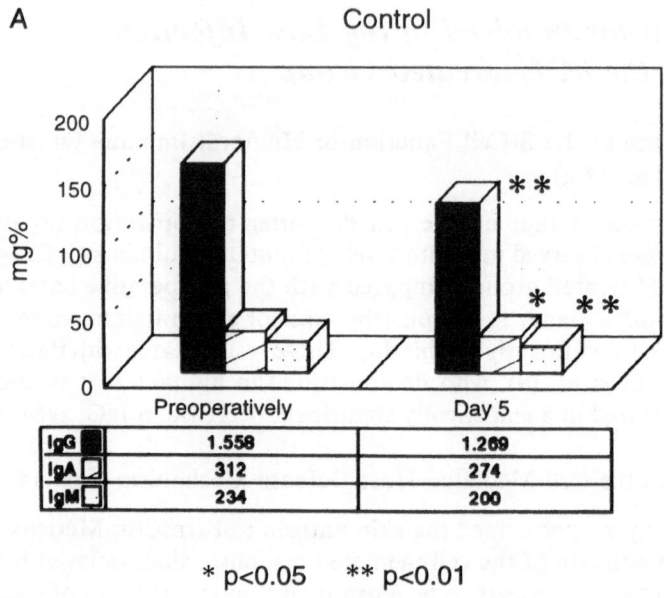

* p<0.05   ** p<0.01

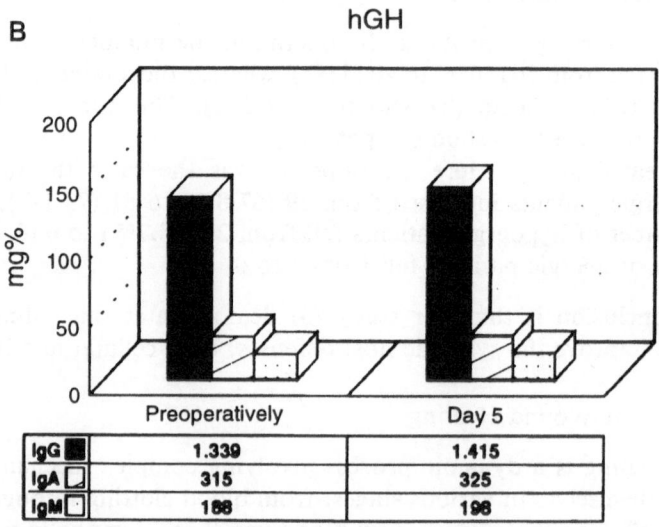

FIGURE 14.2. Immunoglobulins (mg/dl) measured preoperatively (A) and by post-operative day 5 (B).

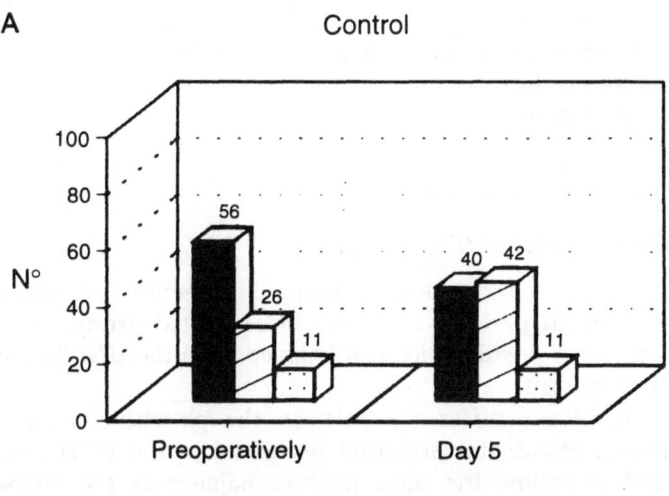

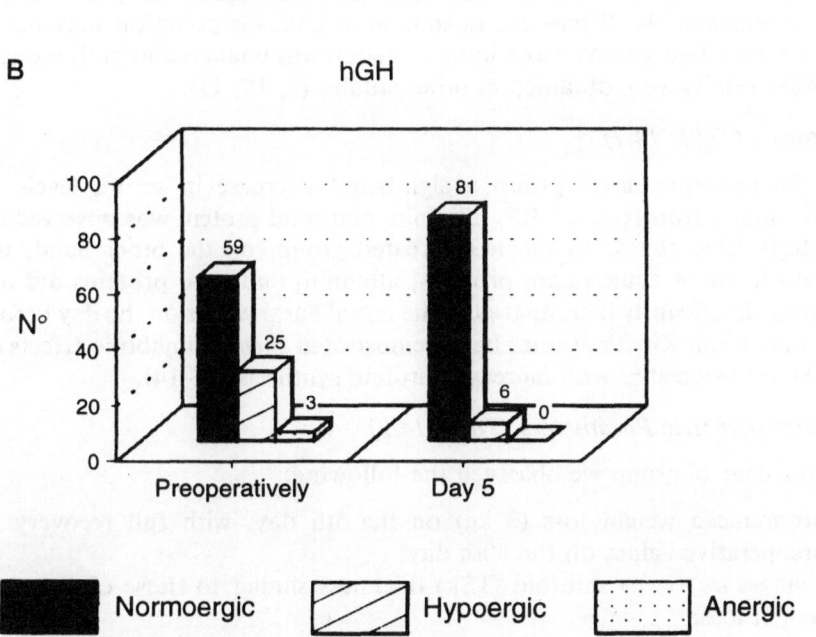

FIGURE 14.3. Immunocompetence index (Institut Mérieux scores). Control group (A) and hGH-treated group (B).

interrelated and when wound healing is impaired, infection is a frequent complication, and vice versa: when wound infection is present, healing is delayed.

Thus, if the systemic catabolic response after surgical trauma can be restrained, wound healing will be promoted and the risk of infection will be reduced. This was done by administering exogenous growth hormone. In our studies we have checked the following functions after cholecystectomy:

- nitrogen and mineral kinetics
- some acute-phase proteins, albumin, and total proteins
- anthropometric parameters
- carbohydrate metabolism
- fat metabolism.

We obtained the following results:

Nitrogen and Mineral Kinetics (Fig. 14.4)

While on fixed nitrogen and caloric intake, a reduction of nitrogen excretion occurred in all patients from the hGH-treated group. In this group, then, there was a positive nitrogen balance from the first 24 hours after the operation onward.

There was a significant difference between the placebo-control and hGH-treated groups. Potassium excretion decreased in the hGH-treated group and tended to follow the same positive balance as the nitrogen measurements. No differences in sodium or chloride excretion were noted between the two groups. Creatinine excretion was unaltered in both groups. Similar results were obtained in other studies (1, 10, 11).

Proteins (Table 14.1)

In the placebo-control group a significant decrease in serum levels of prealbumin, transferrin, RBP, albumin, and total protein was observed on postoperative day 5. In the hGH-treated group, on the other hand, the serum levels of acute-phase proteins, albumin, and total proteins did not change significantly if compared to the initial basal values on the day before the operation. Kinetic studies have demostrated that the anabolic effects of hGH are associated with increased protein synthesis (12–14).

Anthropometric Parameters (Table 14.2)

In the control group we observed the following:

- pronounced weight loss (3 kg) on the 5th day, with full recovery to preoperative values on the 30th day;
- changes in triceps skinfold (TSk) thickness similar to those observed in weight loss;
- arm muscle circumference decreased significantly from preoperative values to those registered on the 5th and 30th days after the operation.

In the hGH-treated group we observed the following:

- a slight decrease in body weight (1 kg) on the 5th day, and weight continued to drop until the 30th postoperative day (mean weight loss = 4.7 kg);
- slight but continuous reduction in TSk thickness;
- arm muscle circumference did not change significantly during the postoperative period.

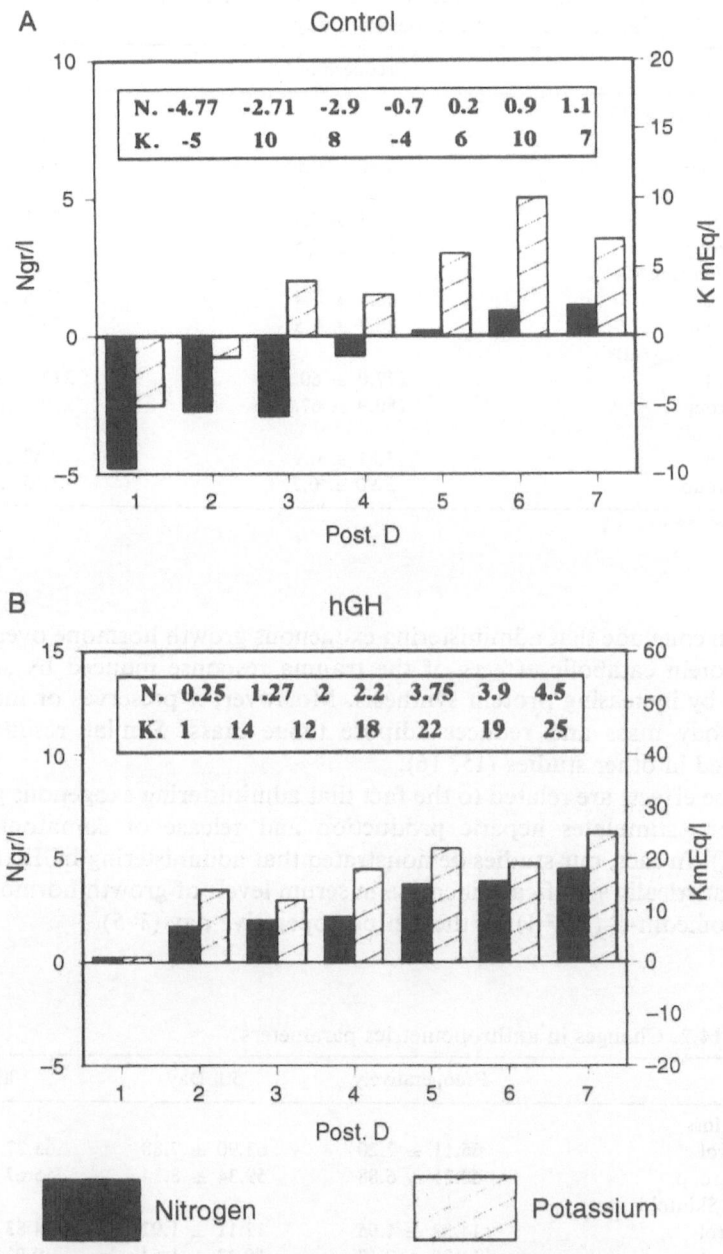

FIGURE 14.4. Nitrogen and potassium balance. Control group (A) and hGH-treated group (B).

TABLE 14.1. Serum levels of total proteins (g/dl), albumin (g/dl), prealbumin (mg/dl), transferrin (mg/dl), retinol-binding protein (RBP) (mg/dl) preoperatively and on the 5th postoperative day.

Test	Preoperatively	Day 5
Total proteins (g/dl)		
Control	7.18 ± 0.5	6.61 ± 0.7*
GH group	6.96 ± 0.05	6.80 ± 0.5
Albumin (g/dl)		
Control	4.03 ± 0.7	3.41 ± 0.5**
GH group	3.93 ± 0.5	3.77 ± 0.5
Prealbumin (mg/dl)		
Control	26.9 ± 7.4	17.8 ± 5.5**
GH group	26.7 ± 8.5	25.2 ± 7.3
Transferrin (mg/dl)		
Control	277.0 ± 60.1	212.6 ± 49.0**
GH group	280.9 ± 67.2	270.3 ± 56.6
RBP (mg/dl)		
Control	3.81 ± 0.9	2.32 ± 0.7**
GH group	3.90 ± 0.7	3.65 ± 0.7

$*p < .05; **p < .01.$

We can conclude that administering exogenous growth hormone overcomes the protein catabolic effects of the trauma response induced by surgical stress, by increasing protein synthesis. Moreover, it preserves or increases lean body mass and reduces adipose tissue mass. Similar results were obtained in other studies (15, 16).

These effects are related to the fact that administering exogenous growth hormone stimulates hepatic production and release of somatomedin-C (IGF-I). In fact, our studies demonstrated that administering hGH resulted in a statistically significant increase in serum levels of growth hormone and somatomedin-C (IGF-I) by the 5th postoperative day (3–5).

TABLE 14.2. Changes in anthropometrics parameters.

Test	Preoperatively	5th Day	30th Day
Weight loss			
Control	66.11 ± 7.20	63.90 ± 7.88	65.27 ± 4.21
GH group	60.31 ± 6.88	59.34 ± 8.34	55.67 ± 2.85
Triceps Skinfold			
Control	14.33 ± 1.95	12.11 ± 1.97	14.83 ± 1.90
GH group	11.25 ± 2.13	10.42 ± 1.54	9.92 ± 0.89
Arm muscle circulation			
Control	24.12 ± 3.58	21.85 ± 2.75	23.15 ± 2.88*
GH group	22.87 ± 2.95	22.35 ± 3.15	22.12 ± 3.45

$*p < .01.$

Glucose and Insulin (Fig. 14.5)

As is well known (7, 8), low insulin serum levels are associated with trauma and infection. In our placebo-control group of patients who had suffered moderate surgical stress (cholecystectomy) the initial basal levels of insulin concentration had fallen significantly by postoperative day 5, whereas there was no change in glucose serum levels.

In the hGH-treated group insulin levels on postoperative day 5 had greatly increased in relation to preoperative levels and in comparison with the values obtained in the control group. Thus exogenous growth hormone administration was associated with hyperinsulinemia.

Given that insulin is more effective in promoting glucose uptake than IGF-1, exogenous growth hormone–induced increases in serum insulin concentration might be expected to enhance glucose delivery to injured tissue, thereby providing improved nutrient delivery for wound repair.

Although glucose serum concentration increased in the hGH-treated group, this rise occurred without the normal inversely proportional relationship with the level of insulin. It seems, as other authors have pointed out, that the marked insulin resistance induced by growth hormone administration may be due to a deficiency in glucose transport (17).

In our patients no hyperglucemia (plasma glucose levels 250 mg/dl) or glycosuria was observed, perhaps due to the small amount of glucose present in the hypocaloric diets (120 to 150 g/day).

Cholesterol Metabolism (Fig. 14.6)

It has been shown (18, 19) that 24 hours after a surgical stress the serum levels of cholesterol decrease, and in our study the lower values of cholesterol were reached on day 2 after the operation. Thereafter cholesterol showed a tendency toward more or less complete normalization, which occurred between the 5th and 10th postoperative days, depending on the severity of the surgical trauma.

In our placebo-control group cholesterol values on the 5th postoperative day were lower than those registered preoperatively, but this decrease was not statistically significant. In the hGH-treated group the decrease of cholesterol levels in serum were statistically significant, if compared to the preoperative values and those registered in the placebo-control group. The cholesterol loss in both groups was mainly due to a decrease in β-lipoproteins [low-density lipoproteins (LDL)]. Our results agree with those obtained by other authors (19–21).

We can speculate, along with Aufenanger et al. (19), that the shortened half-lives of LDL in serum favor lipoprotein delivery to the traumatized tissue for the formation of water-insoluble membranes and, more generally, for the purpose of wound healing.

A

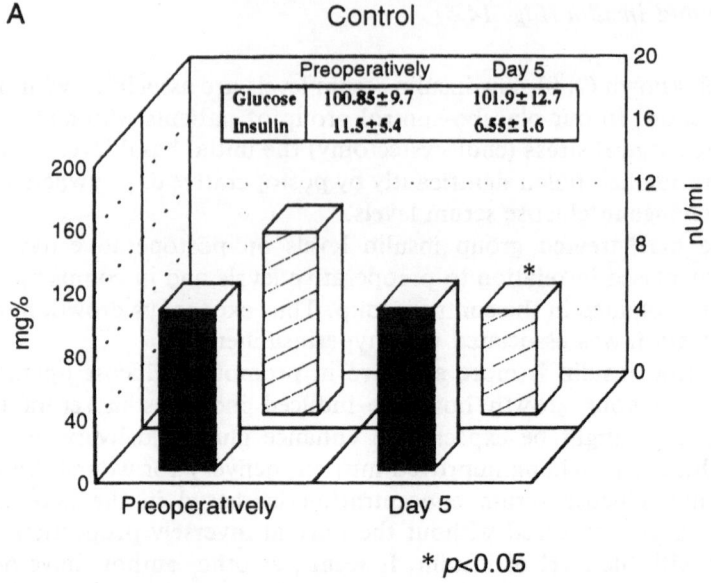

* p<0.05

B

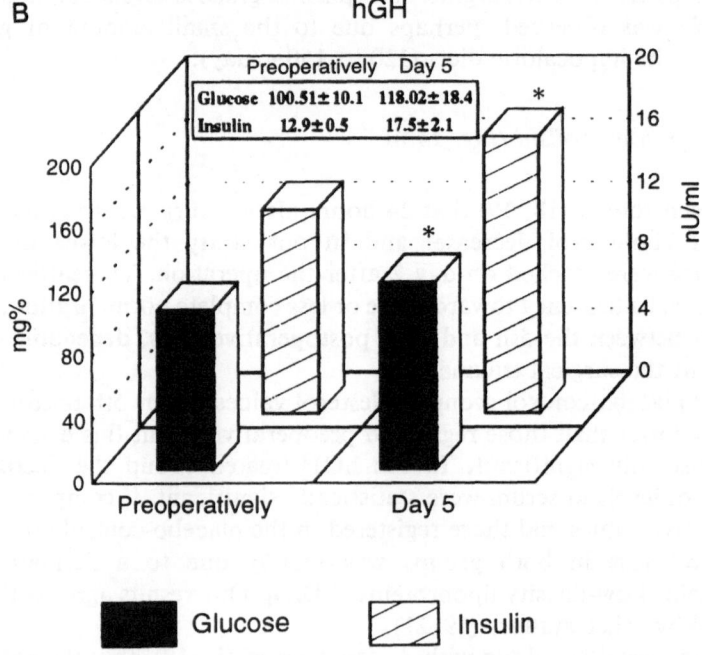

FIGURE 14.5. Modifications in serum levels of glucose and insulin. Control group (A) and hGH-treated group (B).

A   Control

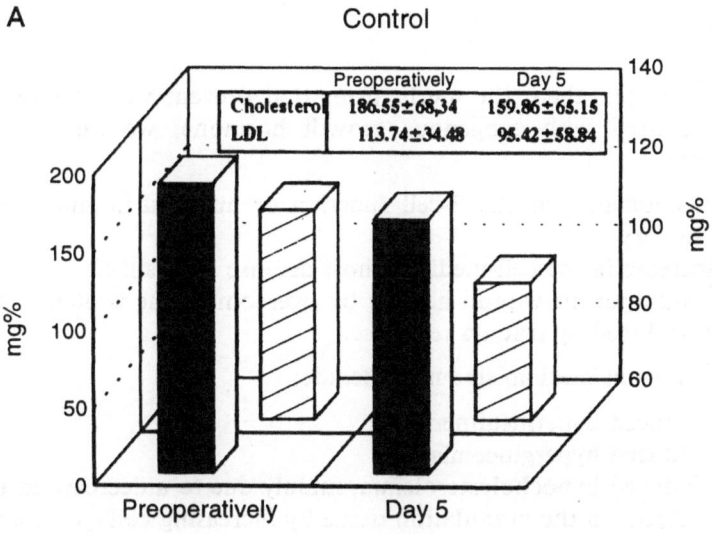

	Preoperatively	Day 5
Cholesterol	186.55±68,34	159.86±65.15
LDL	113.74±34.48	95.42±58.84

B   hGH

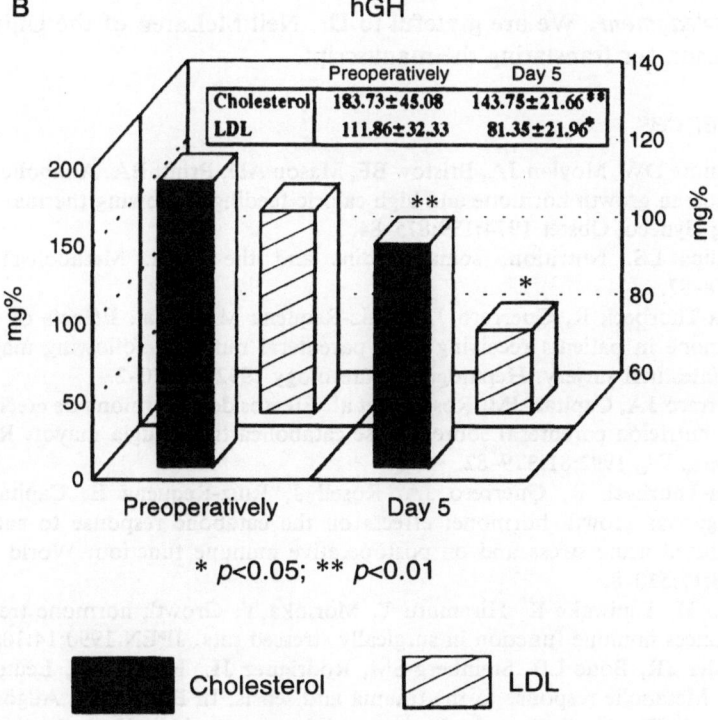

	Preoperatively	Day 5
Cholesterol	183.73±45.08	143.75±21.66**
LDL	111.86±32.33	81.35±21.96*

* $p<0.05$; ** $p<0.01$

■ Cholesterol   ▨ LDL

FIGURE 14.6. Modifications of cholesterol (A) and β-lipoproteins (LDL) (B) in serum levels.

Summary

If we reconsider, then, the mechanisms that prevent wound infection in patients treated with exogenous growth hormone, we can report the following:

1. The maintenance of the B-cell function or humoral immune function after surgery.
2. The increase in the cell-mediated host defense mechanism.
3. The promotion of wound healing by overcoming the protein catabolic effects induced by trauma response.

Other relevant mechanisms may include:

1. hGH-induced hyperinsulinemia
2. hGH-induced hyperglucemia
3. hGH-induced hypocholesterolemia, mainly due to a decrease in LDL
4. hGH effects on the granulation tissue by increasing collagen content or by inducing the liberation of other growth factors in the wound (22).

Acknowledgment. We are grateful to Dr. Neil McLaren of the University of Granada for translating the manuscript.

References

1. Wilmore DW, Moylan JA, Bristow BF, Mason AD, Printt BA. Anabolic effects of human growth hormone and high caloric feedings following thermal injury. Surg Gynecol Obstet 1974;139:875–84.
2. Phillips LS. Nutrition, somatomedins and the brain. Metabolism 1986; 35:78–87.
3. Vara-Thorbeck R, Guerrero JA, Ruiz-Requena ME, et al. Effects of growth hormone in patients receiving total parenteral nutrition following major gastrointestinal surjery. Hepatogastroenterology 1992;39:270–2.
4. Guerrero JA, Capitán JM, Rosell J, et al. Efectos de la hormona de crecimiento y la nutrición parenteral sobre la fase catabólica tras cirugía mayor. Rev Esp Enferm Dig 1992;81:379–82.
5. Vara-Thorbeck R, Guerrero JA, Rosell J, Ruiz-Requena E, Capitán JM. Exogenous growth hormone: effects on the catabolic response to surgically produced acute stress and on postoperative immune function. World J Surg 1993;17:530–8.
6. Saito H, Taniwaka K, Hiramutu T, Morioka Y. Growth hormone treatment enhances immune function in surgically stressed rats. JPEN 1990;14:10S.
7. Border JR, Bone LB, Steinberg SM, Rodriguez JL, Hasset JM, Leutenegger AF. Metabolic response to the trauma and sepsis. In Border JR, Allgöwer M, Hansen ST, Rüedi Th, eds. Blunt multiple trauma. New York-Basel: Marcel Dekker, 1990:191–258.
8. Ross RJ, Miell JP. Avoiding autocannibalism. Br Med J 1991;303:1147–8.
9. Gebhardt F, Malzinzig M, Vogel P, Lenz J, Brückner UB, Hartel W. Pathobiochemie und Immunologie der direkten Lungengewebsverletzung. Langen-

becks Arch Chir Suppl Chir Forum 1992 f. experiment. u. klinische Forschung. Gall/Berger/Ungehuer, eds. Berlin-Heidelberg, Springer, 1992:321–5.

10. Manson JMcK, Wilmore DW. Positive nitrogen balance with human growth hormone and hypocaloric intravenous feeding. Surgery 1986;100:188–97.

11. Ponting GA, Halliday D, Teale JD, Sim AJW. Postoperative nitrogen balance with intravenous hyponutrition and growth hormone. Lancet 1988;1:438–40.

12. Jiang Z, He GZ, Zhang SY, Wang XR, Jang NF, Zhu Y, Wilmore DW. Low dose growth hormone and hypocaloric nutrition attenuate the protein-catabolic response after major operation. Ann Surg 1989;210:513–25.

13. Ziegler TR, Young LS, Manson JMcK, Wilmore DW. Metabolic effects of recombinant human growth hormone in patients receiving parenteral nutrition. Ann Surg 1988;208:6–16.

14. Ward HC, Halliday D, Sim AJW. Protein and energy metabolism with biosynthetic human growth hormone after gastrointestinal surgery. Ann Surg 1987;206:56–61.

15. Wolf RF, Heslin MG, Newman P, Pearlstone DV, Gonenne A, Brennam MF. Growth hormone and insulin combine to improve whole-body and skeletal muscle protein kinetics. Surgery 1992;112:284–92.

16. Byrne TA, Morrissey ThB, Gatzen C, et al. Anabolic therapy with growth hormone accelerates protein gain in surgical patients who require nutritional rehabilitation. Ann Surg 1993;218:400–18.

17. Gore DC, Honeycutt D, Hahoor F, Rutan T, Wolfe RR, Herndon DN. Effect on exogenous growth-hormone on glucose utilization in burn patients. J Surg Res 1991;51:518–23.

18. Symbas PN, Abbot OA, Ende N. Surgical stress and its effects on serum cholesterol. Surgery 1967;61:221–7.

19. Aufenanger J, Walter H, Kattermann R. Untersuchungen zum Lipid-und Lipoprotein stoffwechsel beim Menschen nach operative Eingriffen. Langenbecks Arch Chir 1993;378:41–8.

20. Oscarsson J, Otorsson M, Wiklund O, et al. Low-dose continuously infused growth hormone results in increase lipoprotein and decrease low density lipoprotein cholesterol concentration in middle-age men. Clin Endocrinol 1994;41:109–16.

21. Russell-Jones DL, Wastt GF, Weissbergel A, Naoumova R, Myers J, Thompson JR. The effect of growth hormone replacement on serum lipids, lipoproteins, apolipoproteins and cholesterol precursors in adults growth deficient patients. Clin Endocrinol 1994;41:345–50.

22. Revhaug A, Mjaaland M. Growth hormone and surgery. Horm Res 1993; 40:99–101.

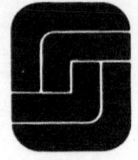

15

Effect of Growth Hormone Administration on Colonic Healing and Repair

HENRIK CHRISTENSEN

The understanding of anastomotic healing and wound management is fundamental in surgery because leakage of a colorectal anastomosis increases threefold the postoperative morbidity and remains the most important mortality factor in gastrointestinal surgery (1, 2). Rates of clinically manifest leaks of colonic anastomoses have been reported to reach 14%, and x-ray inspection of extraperitoneal anastomoses has revealed leakage rates of up to 51% (3, 4).

Recent decades have seen improvements of surgical techniques, preoperative bowel preparation, antimicrobial agents, advances in anesthesia, and better facilities for intensive postoperative care. Cuthbertson's (5) classic studies from the 1930s established that the body's response to surgery involves both a local healing process and a systemic metabolic response, followed by a greatly increased catabolic rate and a negative nitrogen balance. Because catabolism and depletion of protein inhibit normal healing, nutrition has been proposed to promote anabolism and prevent postoperative catabolism. However, postoperative and severely ill patients remain in negative nitrogen balance for a long period despite enteral and parenteral nutrition (6).

Growth hormone (GH), with its promotion of lipolysis, muscle synthesis, and retention of nitrogen, is another choice for improving the nitrogen balance of a critically ill patient (7). Several recent studies have shown that GH treatment improves patient outcome after injury and major surgery (8–12). These observations have now replaced the traditional adoption of GH as a "growth-mediator" promoting linear growth in childhood with knowledge about a much more complex action of the hormone throughout life, for example, as a potent anabolic regulator of body metabolism, an important stress hormone, and an agent stimulating healing.

Normal intestinal healing may be influenced by complex, clinically indeterminable interactions between growth, nutritional, and local or systemic supportive elements (13). Most studies of gastrointestinal healing have therefore been performed on rats.

GH and the Gastrointestinal Tract: Background

Several endogenous and exogenous factors reportedly influence the growth of the gastrointestinal tract (14–16). There is growing evidence of a symbiosis between intraluminal growth factors from the stools such as epidermal growth factor (EGF), transforming growth factor-α, glutamine, and short-chain fatty acids (17–19) and endogenous growth factors such as GH, insulin-like growth factor-I (IGF-I), and somatostatin (20, 21). GH is a 191 amino acid, 22-kd polypeptide secreted from the anterior lobe of the pituitary gland. Secretion of GH (somatotropin) is controlled by two hypothalamic hormones: the inhibitory somatostatin and the stimulatory growth hormone–releasing factor (GRF). Moreover, this release is regulated by peptides, e.g., vasoactive intestinal peptide (VIP), and by stimulatory glucocorticoids and inhibitory thyrotropin-releasing hormone (TRH) (22, 23).

Leblond and Carriere (24) in 1955 were the first to ascertain a local effect of GH on the gastrointestinal tract by reporting its effect on mitosis in the crypts of Lieberkühn in the duodenum of hypophysectomized rats. Hypophysectomy of rats was later shown to lead to atrophy of the small intestine with reduced intestinal length and mucosal weight and a decrease in the height of the villi (25, 26), changes that were reversed after GH treatment (27, 28). Others have shown an effect of GH on the weight and length of the small and large intestine, so that GH may have a trophic effect on intact gastrointestinal tissues (29, 30). In addition, GH reportedly has an effect on gastrointestinal physiology, including the regulation of electrolyte and fluid transportation, the effect of vitamin D–dependent calcium-binding protein synthesis and calcium absorption, and the ventral release of somatostatin and gastrin (31–34).

Early studies on the effect of GH were hampered by the limited commercial availability of GH and were often performed in hypophysectomized rats that therefore contained other pituitary hormones than GH itself. The amino acid sequence of GH was deduced in 1971 and biosynthetic GH (bGH) was approved for human use in 1985. Manufacturing of bGH by means of modern DNA technology has now improved the economy and availability of the hormone, which has prompted studies of the hormone in clinical situations other than those in which patients are GH deficient.

How to Elicit GH's Effects

A target cell's responsiveness to a hormone is regulated by the concentration of circulating hormone and by the availability and affinity of the receptors with which the hormone can interact. GH actions also depend on age, sex, species, steroids, estrogens, testosterone, pregnancy, insulin, thyroid hormones, IGF-I, sleep, and nutritional state. The somatomedin hypothesis predicts that GH acts via stimulation of synthesis and release of somatomedins (IGFs) from the liver (35). IGF-I acts on specific intestinal IGF-I receptors and stimulates the gastrointestinal tract (36, 37). Salub et al. (38) found that GH administration stimulates IGF-I expression in the gastrointestinal tract of hypophysectomized rats. GH transgenetic mice reportedly have a significantly increased jejunal, ileal, and colonic length, mucosal weight, and villus height compared with normal controls (29, 30). Their jejunal and colonic IGF-I messenger ribonucleic acid (mRNA) levels are also significantly higher and their mucosa weighs more because the mucosal cells live longer, not because GH spurs mucosal cell proliferation (29, 30). Studying transgenetic mice with an overproduction of GH, Lund et al. (20) proposed that GH is a promoter of intestinal adaption via mediation of IGF-I action. The observation of a direct stimulating effect of GH on cartilage explants and incubated muscle preparations in vitro (39) was followed by demonstration of specific local GH receptors in a variety of different organs (40). According to Lobie et al. (41), specific GH-receptors are localized throughout the rat's gastrointestinal tract, and the most intense immunoreactivity appears in the intestinal mucosa. These findings confirm that GH partly acts directly on specific GH receptors in the gastrointestinal tract, and that the effect may be synergistic with IGF-I. Furthermore, GH has recently been shown to stimulate the intestinal uptake of glutamine, which is the preferred substrate for small intestine, fibroblasts, macrophages, and lymphocytes (42).

Healing of Colon: The Repair Process

The healing cascade primarily ensures recovery of the mechanical strength of the cut gut and secondarily reestablishment of normal intestinal function and the complicated and complex structure of the intestinal wall. An electron micrograph of a through-cut of a normal rat's left colon (Fig. 15.1) shows that the strength-bearing submucosal collagen fiber is composed of bundles of collagen fibrils.

The fibroblasts, and to a lesser extent the smooth muscle cells, are believed to be responsible for the formation and remodeling of new collagen in a healing anastomosis and the fibroblast has been shown to be stimulated by GH in vitro (43). Fibroblasts appear at the edges of an anastomosis

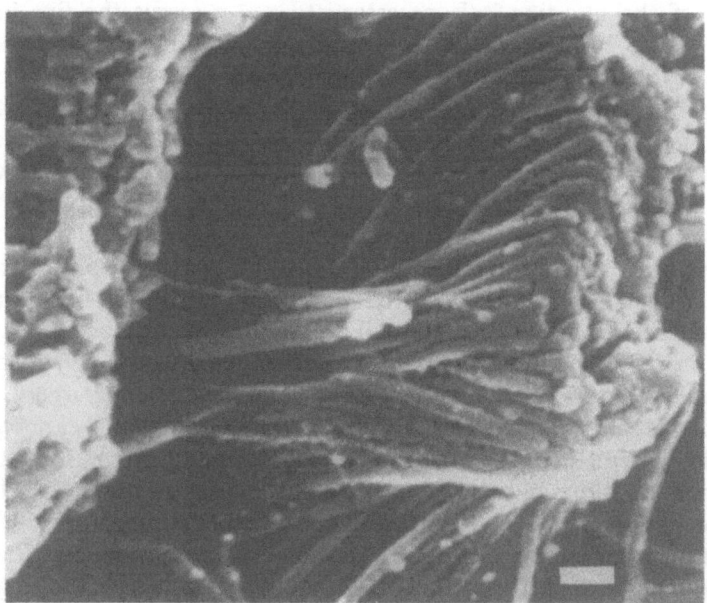

FIGURE 15.1. Scanning electron micrograph of a through-cut rat colon representing a part of a collagen fiber from submucosa composed of bundles of collagen fibrils. ($\times$ 42,000, bar = 100 nm).

already within the first 24 hours after surgery, and collagen synthesis is accelerated as early as 12 hours after anastomosis is performed (44). The number of fibroblasts peaks 3 to 5 days after surgery. Together with the invasion of inflammatory cells starting the reparative process, the fibroblasts start to proliferate and synthesis of collagen begins. In the ground substance proteoglycans and glycosaminoglycans play specific roles in the extracellular maturation of collagen, the regulation of the development of collagen fibrils, and the intestinal growth regulation (45). The submucosal remodeling ends with the simultaneous reestablishment of the mechanical strength of the intestine and re-epithelialization at the anastomotic interface by crypt cell mitosis, and ultimately migration ends the healing process. Studies on the healing of colonic anastomoses have therefore focused on two main processes: the anastomotic strength and the anastomotic collagen metabolism.

GH and Anastomotic Strength

Background

Almost 200 years ago Larrey (46), surgeon to the Élite Guard of Napoleon, described the seminal principles of intestinal anastomosis: "In suturing wounds of the intestine it is necessary to . . . preserve the lips in exact contact . . . to include within the points of the suture the least possible portion of the intestinal tube . . . to keep in view that union is effected by the bowel's own vessels." Still, although the intervening period has seen consistent progress in surgical techniques and an ensuing drop in leakage rates, anastomotic leakage remains a substantial clinical problem with an unsatisfactory high mortality rate, and attention has therefore spread to other factors that may also affect the healing process.

In 1958 and 1968 Prudden et al. (47) and Kowalewski and Yong (48) suggested that bovine GH injected intraperitoneally or subcutaneously could increase wound tensile strength and hydroxyproline accumulation in dermal skin wounds in rats. In 1966 Meffert and Liebow (49) reported a GH-stimulated development of collateral vessels after lung surgery. Later, Hollander et al. (50) and Pessa et al. (51) showed that treatment with synthetic GH enhances the incisional wound-breaking strength of the skin of normal and tumor-bearing rats, and the use of met-hGH did not augment tumor growth. Later studies have demonstrated that GH has a stimulating effect on the healing of incisional wounds and bone fractures, and on donor sites, postresectional mucosal hyperplasia following extensive intestinal resection, and the production of collagens in subcutaneously implanted cellulose sponges (52-56).

Biomechanical strength is an important criterion for the success of anastomotic repair. The strength of intestinal anastomoses reportedly is at its lowest point 2 to 3 days after surgery, which is when clinical leaks from colorectal surgery often happen (2). The early postoperative days are therefore, clinically, the most important and interesting period for studying healing.

The methods used for evaluating the strength of experimental colonic anastomosis have either been the bursting strength test or the breaking strength test. The former measures maximal intracolonic pressure at the burst of the anastomosed segment caused by inflation of liquid or air. The latter measures the uniaxial force required to break the anastomosis. Chlumsky (57) was the first to describe bursting strength, which he tested in a study of gastrointestinal healing by measuring the maximal intraluminal pressure at disruption following inflating of sodium chloride into the closed anastomosed segment. The bursting strength measures the weakest point of the anastomotic line in which a leakage occurs, a factor of obvious clinical significance (58, 59). In addition, this technique evenly distributes transmural pressure from which the actual bursting wall tension (BWT) can be calculated if the radius of the anastomosis is measured at burst. Furthermore, the test can be performed in vivo without disrupting vascular supply and with a minimum of manipulation of the anastomosis before the test procedure. Finally, the bursting pressure is a valid strength parameter because a burst takes place at the time of maximum intraluminal pressure (60). The breaking strength test has been preferred by several investigators

because it can provide complete load-deformation curves and thereby give
detailed information about the uniaxial biomechanical properties of a
wound or an anastomosis (61). Furthermore, breaking strength is more
specifically related to the strength of the suture line than to the entire
anastomosed segment as such. The in vivo bursting strength test with
sutures left in place allows minimal manipulation before the test procedure
and seems to be the most useful method for measuring anastomotic strength
until days 4 to 5. The in vitro breaking strength test then becomes the
method of choice since the anastomosis can be tested without sutures and
up to 3 to 4 weeks after surgery. In the following studies both tests have
been used.

bGH and the Strength of Left Colonic Anastomoses

The effect of exogenous administration of bGH was studied after 2, 4, and
6 days of healing of standardized left colonic anastomoses (the design of the
healing studies is shown in Fig. 15.2). Daily treatment with 2.0 mg
bGH·kg^{-1} raised bursting pressures twofold after 2 days and threefold
after 4 days of healing compared with controls when begun 7 days before
surgery (Fig. 15.3) (62). Initiation of bGH treatment at the time of surgery
yielded a 55% higher bursting pressure after 2 days compared with controls,

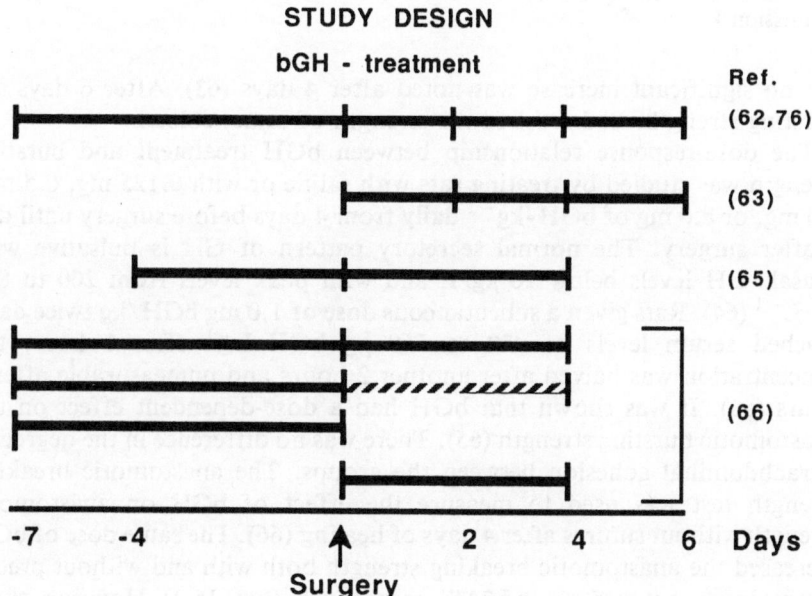

FIGURE 15.2. Design of the healing studies. Horizontal lines indicate bGH treatment
periods.

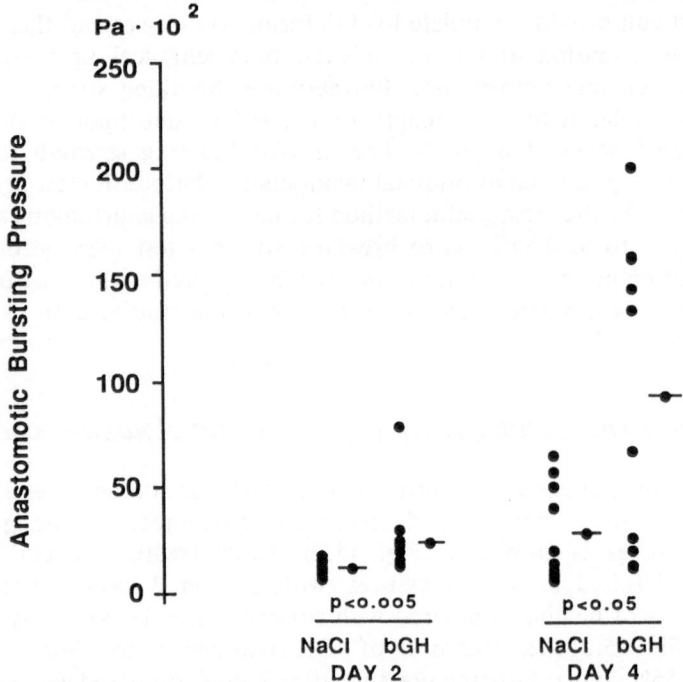

FIGURE 15.3. The effect of 2.0 mg bGH•kg^{-1}•day^{-1} on the anastomotic bursting pressure on postoperative day 2 and day 4. (Data derived from refs. 62 and 63, with permission.)

but no significant increase was noted after 4 days (63). After 6 days the bursting strengths had reached the strength of intact colons.

The dose-response relationship between bGH treatment and bursting strength was studied by treating rats with saline or with 0.125 mg, 0.5 mg, 2.0 mg, or 8.0 mg of bGH•kg^{-1} daily from 4 days before surgery until day 4 after surgery. The normal secretory pattern of GH is pulsative with "basal" GH levels below 10 μg/L and with peak levels from 200 to 800 μg•L^{-1} (64). Rats given a subcutaneous dose of 1.0 mg bGH/kg twice daily reached serum levels of 420 to 760 μg bGH•L^{-1} after 1 hour; the concentration was halved after another 2 hours and unmeasurable after 8 hours (53). It was shown that bGH had a dose-dependent effect on the anastomotic bursting strength (65). There was no difference in the degree of intraabdominal adhesion between the groups. The anastomotic breaking strength test was used to measure the effect of bGH on anastomotic strength without sutures after 4 days of healing (66). The same dose of bGH increased the anastomotic breaking strength both with and without preoperative treatment by 59% and 34%, respectively (Fig. 15.4). However, there was no difference in the anastomotic breaking strength on the same day between the groups if bGH was only given prior to surgery, and not in the healing period.

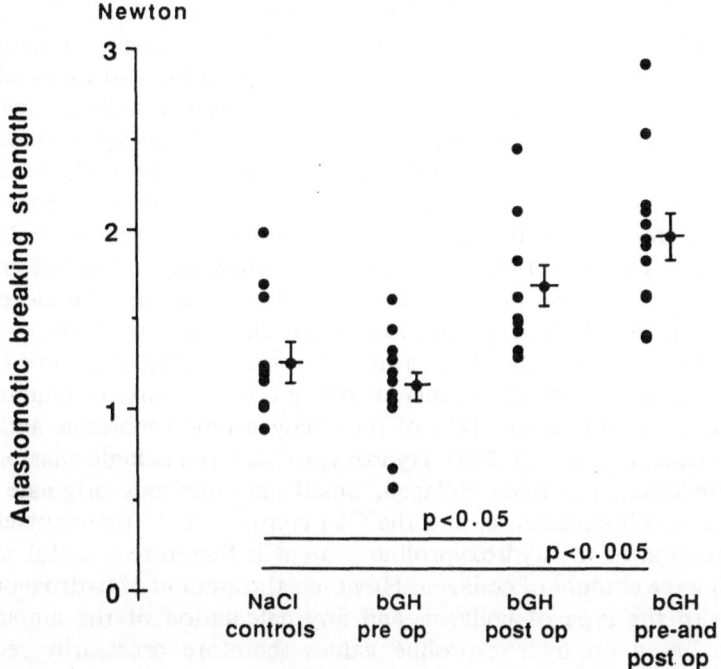

FIGURE 15.4. The effect of 2.0 mg $bGH \cdot kg^{-1} \cdot day^{-1}$ on the anastomotic breaking strength on postoperative day 4. (Data derived from ref. 66, with permission.)

The use of the bursting strength test requires that sutures are left in place. Removal of the sutures may weaken the anastomosis before testing, and a higher capacity for suture-binding could hence contribute to improve bursting strength. To test this assumption, rats were given bGH for 7 days before operation and the breaking strength of sutured anastomoses was then tested immediately after surgery. One week of preoperative bGH treatment did not alter the colon's ability to hold sutures (66), although it did accelerate the biosynthesis rate of the intact colon from 0.6% to 1.% per hour. Long-term bGH treatment also increased the strength of the intact colon (67).

GH and Anastomotic Collagen

Background

Reestablishment of intestinal anastomotic strength can only be achieved by deposition of collagen of sufficient quality in the healing zone. Anastomotic collagen changes massively during the first postoperative days (68, 69) mainly due to disturbances between the normal collagen degradation and formation. The early phase of colonic healing is characterized by lysis of mature collagen by collagenolytic enzymes and loss of tensile strength, and maximal collagenolysis occurs during the first 24 hours and predominates over collagen synthesis in the early days (70). When collagen synthesis surpasses collagen degradation, a net gain of the collagen content is obtained. It is generally accepted that synthesis of new collagen in the anastomotic line begins at the end of inflammatory phases 2 to 3 after operation. However, collagen synthesis begins much earlier according to Martens and Hendriks (44), who reported a much higher level of anastomotic collagen synthesis 12 hours after anastomosis than in the intact colon.

The amino acid hydroxyproline is a unique characteristic of the α-chains of collagen molecules, and it is formed by hydroxylation of proline before the α-chains are wrapped together, forming a triple helix. In mammalian tissues it is found in about 14% of the collagen type I molecule and, to a minor extent, in elastin (1–2%). Hydroxyproline from colonic anastomoses stems predominantly from collagen. Small amounts may originate from elastin, acetylcholinesterase, and the C1q component of the complement. Determination of the hydroxyproline content is therefore a useful way of measuring the amount of collagen. However, the amount of hydroxyproline varies with the type of collagen and any calculation of the amount of collagen based on hydroxyproline values therefore necessarily requires precise knowledge of the composition of the tissue in question. This is important also when intact colonic tissue is compared with healing anastomotic tissue, since the latter is relatively rich in type III collagen (45).

The hydroxyproline content is closely related to the strength of both intact tissues and healing wounds (68, 69), but the biomechanical strength is also influenced by the quality of the properties such as alterations in the number and quality of interfibrillar cross-links, changes in collagen fiber structure, and alterations in collagen types. Some studies have shown a decrease in the rate of cross-link stability in tail tendons of old hypophysectomized rats (71), and bGH treatment has contributed to raise the number of reducible collagen cross-links (72). Another study demonstrated that long-term treatment with bGH increased the quality of biomechanical properties of left colonic collagen in aged rats (73).

bGH and the Effect on Anastomotic Collagen

The administration of bGH to colon-operated rats at the time of surgery caused the hydroxyproline content of the anastomosed segment to rise on days 4 and 6 after the operation (63, 66). The effect on the deposition of anastomotic hydroxyproline was dose dependent up to a dose of 8.0 mg bGH per day (65). bGH had a similar dose-dependent effect on collagen deposition into subcutaneous implanted cellulose sponges (52). Garrel et al. found that stimulation of wound-breaking strength with GRF was accompanied by an accelerated maturation of wound collagen. Previous studies on the effect of GH on collagen metabolism have proposed that the GH effect results from both an increased de novo synthesis and an increased collagen degradation (72). Surgery with simultaneous bGH administration improved the anastomotic strength on day 2, at which time the amount of collagen was unchanged, a situation that is presumably due to a bGH-induced stimulation of the chemical stability of the anastomotic collagens, but also caused by the large amount of old collagen compared with newly synthesized collagen.

The identification and quantification of certain specific enzymes, e.g., collagenases, is still fraught with a number of methodological problems. The collagenases are involved in the collagen degradation process (70, 74). The effect of bGH on the newly formed anastomotic collagen was assessed by in vivo quantification of the synthesis by way of injection of ^{14}C-labeled proline and measurement of the production of ^{14}C-hydroxyproline per hour (66). To minimize reutilization of radioactive proline and to keep the specific radioactivity constant during the labeling period, we added a large flooding dose of "cold" proline and used a relatively short incorporation period (4 hours). Four days after surgery the collagen biosynthesis rate of the anastomosed segment of untreated rats was 4.4%. In rats receiving bGH at surgery, the collagen biosynthesis rate was increased to 9.0%, and to 12.9% when treatment was started 7 days before surgery and continued during the healing period (Fig. 15.5). Although the effect of bGH on the healing parameters was more pronounced when treatment was started before surgery, it was important from a clinical point of view that bGH was able to improve healing also when treatment was started at the time of surgery, since anastomotic dehiscence is most common in unplanned surgery.

Systematic studies aimed at visualizing the healing zone of healing anastomoses by means of light microscopy (75) have established that various staining methods can be used to specific visualization of collagen (Van Gieson). The use of a scanning electron microscope (magnification ×70,000) made it possible to morphometrically evaluate the collagens in the healing zone and hence paved the way for a study of the visualizability of collagen increases and strength parameters with bGH (76). After 4 days the healing zone in bGH rats was markedly different from that of controls. The normal anastomoses were characterized by relatively unorganized collagen fibrils, whereas the anastomoses from bGH-treated rats showed a much more structured network of collagen fibrils with early organization of the fibrils into new collagen fibers. After 6 days the bGH rats showed advanced healing with dense organization of collagen fibrils in the healing zone compared with controls. In this study it was not possible to quantify the number of vessels in the splanchnicus, but others have shown that exogenous GH stimulates the development of collateral vessels in the lung (49), a factor that may be important in the intestine also. In addition, somatostatin, which inhibits the secretion of GH from the pituitary gland, reportedly

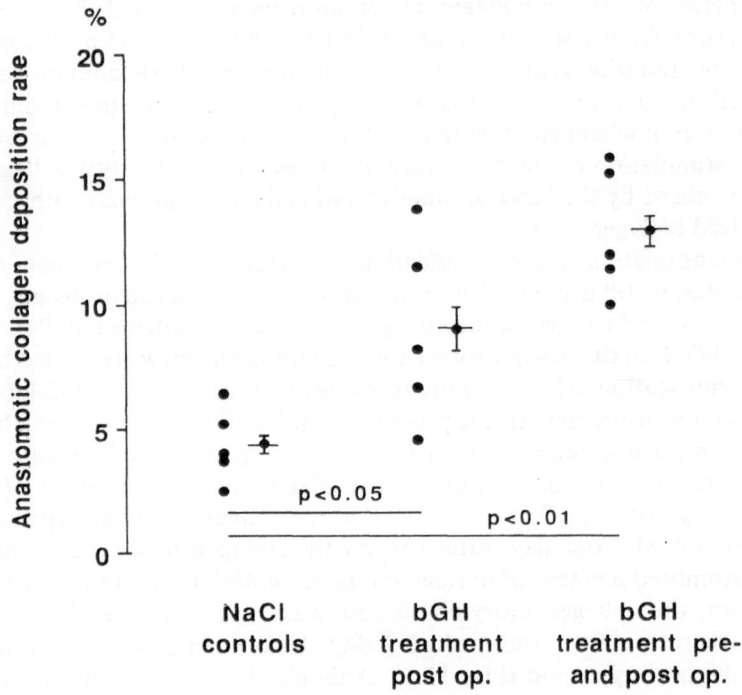

FIGURE 15.5. The effect of bGH on the anastomotic collagen deposition rate. (Data derived from ref. 66, with permission.)

decreases the mesenteric blood flow and increases mesenteric vascular resistance in a dose-dependent manner (77).

In conclusion, bGH seems to stimulate the reorganization of new collagen fibrils in the healing zone and accelerate the collagen biosynthesis rate, which leads to higher content of collagen of the anastomosed segment.

GH and Experimental Colitis

Background

In Crohn's disease the combination of colitis, diarrhea, small intestinal inflammation, malabsorption, and strictures contributes to chronic anorexia, malnutrition, weight loss, and failure of linear growth. Nutritional supplementation has been shown to diminish both symptoms and disease activity, and to lead to partial or full restoration of linear growth failure (78). Nutritional intake and GH are both important regulating factors of IGF-I, and serum IGF-I is considered a useful index of the nutritional status in critically ill patients (79). IGF-I is also reduced in serum from children and adolescents with chronic inflammatory bowel disease, and normalization of the IGF-I levels due to higher caloric intake has both improved growth velocity and reduced disease activity in patients with inflammatory bowel disease (80). The effect of bGH administration found on healing colonic anastomoses invites the question whether GH has an effect on the repair of another type of colonic damage, i.e., experimental colitis.

The ideal experimental colitis model should mirror the pathologic features and pathophysiologic mechanisms in human disease. Moreover, it should be reproducible and applicable in experiments with laboratory animals, e.g., rats. The serious limitations pertaining to any comparison between chemically induced experimental colitis in animal studies and the pathogenesis of ulcerative colitis and Crohn's disease in the colon of man have not discouraged the pursuit of experimental experience in induction of colitis in animals. One such well-described experimental colitis model consists in the instillation of trinitrobenzene (TNB) sulfonic acid into the intestinal lumen. This method is widely used since the inflammatory response after TNB instillation shows a transmural affection of the colonic wall, which has histopathologic similarities to Crohn's disease in man (81). The inflammatory activity can be determined by a macroscopical and microscopical evaluation, and by measuring the activity of myeloperoxidase (MPO) in colon. MPO is an enzyme contained in the azurophilic granules of the neutrophils. It is a suitable marker of these inflammation cells and has therefore been used in several studies of inflamed intestinal tissue (82).

bGH and Experimental Colitis

In an experimental study the effect of bGH was investigated in rats instillated with TNB (83). After 4 days the rats treated with bGH had lower macroscopical and microscopical damage scores than controls, which indicates that bGH attenuates the inflammatory response of chemical colitis. Also, the infiltration of neutrophils, measured as MPO activity, was lower in the rats given bGH (Fig. 15.6).

Patients with Crohn's disease are reported to have a higher collagenolytic activity level. This disturbance of collagen metabolism may be due to the stricturing process that precedes the gross pathologic changes in this disease (84). It therefore seemed relevant to test possible alterations of the biomechanical properties after induction of TNB-colitis, since migration of phagocytic inflammatory cells into the colon may be accompanied by increased collagenase activity, which could change the stability of the strength-bearing submucosal collagens (85). The breaking strength and energy absorption per unit length of colon from TNB-instilled control rats has been reported to decline, a deterioration that was attenuated by bGH (83).

The higher colonic damage score, MPO activity, and biomechanical properties induced by bGH were associated with a smaller fall in IGF-I

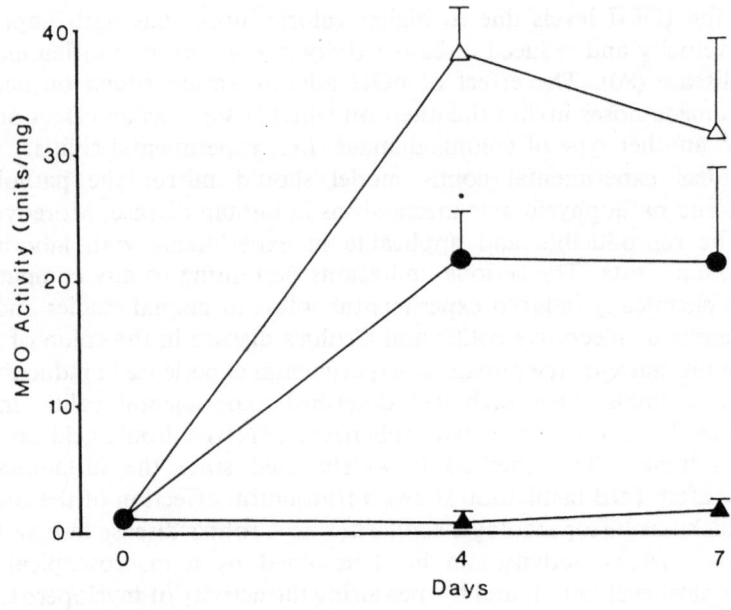

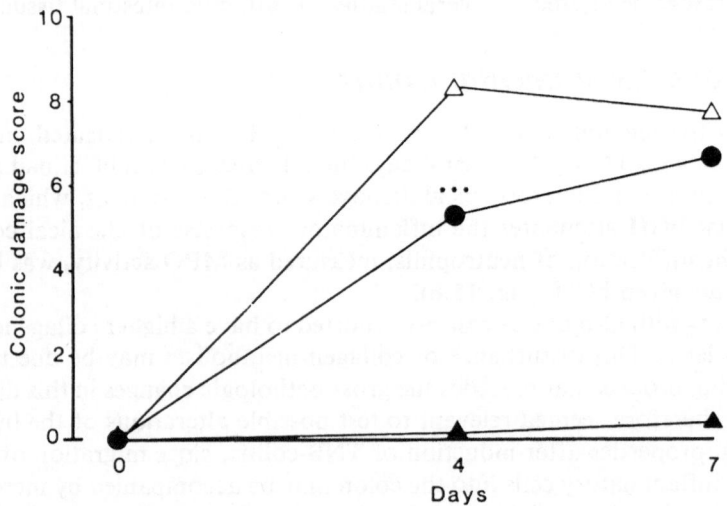

FIGURE 15.6. Colonic myeloperoxidases (MPO) activity and macroscopical colonic damage score (mean) 4 and 7 days after trinitrobenzene (TNB) sulfonic acid induced colitis in rats treated with either 2.0 mg bGH·kg^{-1}·day^{-1} (●), NaCl (△), and from intact colon of sham-instilled untreated rats (▲). *$p < .05$, **$p < .01$, ***$p < .005$, vs. TNB-controls. (Data derived from ref. 83, with permission.)

levels in serum from the bGH treated rats than in the TNB-instilled controls. The concerted dependence of IGF-I levels on GH stimulation and the patient's nutritional status (80, 86) and the local effect of bGH on the repair of inflamed colon may suggest that a combination of bGH and conventional treatment supplemented with parenteral and enteral nutrition represents a therapeutic potential in the treatment dependent not only on GH stimulation but also on the nutritional state of the patient (80, 86). These observations, together with the local effect of bGH on the repair of inflamed colon, suggest a potential therapeutic role for bGH in combination of conventional treatment and parenteral and enteral nutrition in the treatment of patients with inflammatory bowel disease. However, these suggestions call for further clinical studies.

Surgery, bGH, and Postoperative Weight Loss

The development in body weight (BW) after surgery reflects important parameters such as appetite, recovery, healing complications, and balance between catabolism and anabolism. In rats undergoing colon resection and anastomosis, and even in sham-operated rats, the BW decreased during the first postoperative days (66, 83). Colon-anastomosed control rats had a lower BW after 6 days than at surgery, whereas bGH-treated rats had regained their initial weight loss after 4 days (62, 63). bGH stimulation of the development of postoperative BW was dose dependent (65). Rats with experimentally induced colitis also experienced a decrease in BW, which remained continuously lower than the initial BW after 7 days. Inversely, bGH induction attenuated the fall in BW (83).

The BW of rats with experimental colitis was not higher than the BW of rats treated with bGH because they had had a higher daily food intake. However, the anastomosed rats treated with bGH did have a higher average daily food intake than the controls after 6 days, whereas there was no difference between bGH rats and controls 2 and 4 days after surgery. There is convincing evidence that the higher food intake of the bGH-treated rats stimulates the growth of intestinal mucosa, whereas the stimulation of other layers seems to happen also without food passage (87). It was demonstrated that bGH administration stimulated the mucosal weight (lamina epithelialis and muscularis mucosa) and the weight of muscularis externa of intact colon from rats of both sexes (88). The layers stimulated by bGH were the same as those in which specific GH receptors were found to be localized (41). The stimulating effect of bGH on normal colon may therefore be induced by a higher food intake (76) associated with a better passage of growth factors from the stools (19), but it remains unknown whether this also affects the repair of colon.

GH/IGF-I Axis in Rats and in Man

Operative procedures in the gastrointestinal tract increase the metabolic demands and may overwhelm the reparative process, and a negative nitrogen balance and malnutrition are both associated with diminished healing (89, 90). Clinical studies have demonstrated that patients improve when nutritional support is combined with GH treatment (10, 91, 92). GH may be useful in all patient groups with a negative nitrogen balance, such as inflammatory bowel disease with its complications in the form of chronic anorexia, malnutrition, weight loss, and failure of linear growth. Nutrition has been shown to diminish symptoms and disease activity, and it may lead to partial or full restoration of linear growth failure (78, 93). Administration of bGH to rats with colitis has been shown to reverse BW loss and attenuate the fall in IGF-I levels associated with a lower colonic inflammation (83).

GH secretion rises markedly in man in response to surgery (94) and may be an important stress hormone by increasing lipolysis and sparring carbohydrate and protein metabolism when nutrition is insufficient (95). The rise in pituitary GH secretion in response to stress has been reported to be proportional to the severity of the operation and to be relatively short-lived (96). In the rat, however, GH secretion is inhibited by stress (97). Both in humans and in rats the stress-induced alterations in GH secretion occur concomitantly with reductions in circulating IGF-I. This dissociation between GH levels and IGF-I levels in man implies resistance to endogenous GH secretion during stress, and it has been suggested that this is a mechanism by which it is possible to secure the preferential utilization of lipids due to the direct actions of GH without simultaneously expending precious nitrogen stores for growth. Improvement of this "normal" GH/IGF-I axis in severe catabolism by means of bGH treatment, perhaps in combination with nutrition, could elevate circulating IGF-I and thereby accelerate recovery. The lower GH levels in rats under stress may indicate that rats need smaller doses and may be easier to stimulate than man. In normal volunteers in negative nitrogen balance, a high dose of GH was shown to stimulate IGF-I and thereby improve nitrogen balance, and it was demonstrated that simultaneous use of GH and IGF-I treatment may further enhance the anabolic effect of both agents (98).

bGH could not raise serum IGF-I levels after colonic surgery nor after experimentally induced colitis, but the abrupt fall in IGF-I usually seen after operation was less pronounced with bGH treatment. The same effect of bGH on IGF-I levels has been shown in humans in negative nitrogen balance and in tumor-implanted rats with cachexia (99). The potential effect on colonic healing of IGF-I itself was shown by treating colon-operated rats with 500 μg IGF-I per day from surgery until test day 4. At this dose level IGF-I raised the anastomotic collagen content compared with controls, although the dose had no effect on the anastomotic strength parameters (100). Therefore, some of the healing effects induced by bGH treatment could be mediated by the higher IGF-I levels acting as a local growth factor on specific IGF-I receptors found throughout the gastrointestinal tract (36).

Future Directions: Can bGH Treatment Help Prevent Postoperative Complications?

It is known from clinical studies that an improved postoperative protein economy may shorten the convalescence period and hasten recovery. GH administration seems to have a beneficial effect in situations when the nitrogen balance is negative, e.g., during the catabolic phase after major surgery, burns, and in severely malnourished and ill patients with low IGF-I levels (8, 80, 101–103).

The use of bGH in the early postoperative period invites new questions. Of special interest from a surgical point of view is whether administration of bGH, alone or in combination with nutrition and growth factors such as IGF-I, may reduce the number of wound, fascial, and anastomotic leaks. It is expected to be particularly rewarding to conduct such studies on patients expected to have many postoperative healing complications, as after unplanned surgery (104) or on elderly malnutritioned patients (105). However, there is evidence that factors such as GH and IGF-I, which improve the healing process, also may lead to lower numbers of complications and may result in decreased mortality after colorectal surgery. Hence, GH and IGF-I may also reduce the number of complications and may decrease mortality after colorectal surgery.

References

1. Schrock TR, Deveney CW, Dunphy JE. Factors contributing to leakage of colonic anastomoses. Ann Surg 1973;177:513–8.
2. Fielding LP, Steward-Brown S, Blesovsky L, Kearney G. Anastomotic integrity after operations for large-bowel cancer: a multicenter study. Br Med J 1980;281:411–4.
3. Turunen MJ, Peltakallio P. Surgical results in 657 patients with colorectal cancer. Dis Colon Rectum 1983;26:606–12.
4. Goligher JC, Graham NG, De Dombal FT. Anastomatic dehiscence after anterior resection of rectum and sigmoid. Br J Surg 1970;57:109–18.
5. Cuthbertson DP. Observations on the disturbance of metabolism produced by injury to the limbs. Q J Med 1931;2:233–46.
6. Douglas RG, Shaw JHF. Metabolic response to sepsis and trauma. Br J Surg 1989;76:115–22.
7. Ross RJM, Miell JP. Avoiding autocannibalism. Consider growth hormone and insulin-like growth factor I. Br Med J 1991;303:1147–8.
8. Ward HC, Halliday D, Sim AJW. Protein and energy metabolism with biosynthetic human growth hormone after gastrointestinal surgery. Ann Surg 1987;206:56–60.
9. Ponting GA, Halliday D, Teale JD, Sim AJW. Postoperative positive nitrogen balance with intravenous hyponutrition and growth hormone. Lancet 1988;438–9.
10. Jiang ZM, He GZ, Zhang SY. Low-dose growth hormone and hypocaloric

nutrition attenuate the protein-caloric response after major operation. Ann Surg 1989;210:513–25.

11. Douglas RG, Humberstone DA, Heystead A. Metabolic effects of recombinant human growth hormone: isotopic studies in the postabsorptive state and during parenteral nutrition. Br J Surg 1990;77:785–90.

12. Koea JB, Douglas RG, Shaw JHF, Gluckman PD. Growth hormone therapy initiated before starvation ameliorates the catabolic state and enhances the protein-sparing effect of total parenteral nutrition. Br J Surg 1993;80:740–4.

13. Pessa ME, Bland KI, Copeland III EM. Growth factors and determinants of wound repair. J Surg Res 1987;42:207–17.

14. Johnson LR. Regulation of gastrointestinal growth. In: Johnson LR, ed. Physiology of the gastrointestinal tract. New York: Raven Press, 1987:301–3.

15. Burgess AW, Sizeland AM. Growth factors and the gut. J Gastroenterol Hepatol 1990;5:10–21.

16. Lemoine NR, Leung HY, Gullick WJ. Growth factors in the gastrointestinal tract. Gut 1992;33:1297–300.

17. Playford RJ, Woodman AC, Clark P, et al. Effect of luminal growth factor preservation on intestinal growth. Lancet 1993;341:843–8.

18. Sakata T, Engelhardt WV. Stimulatory effect of short chain fatty acids on the epithelial cell proliferation in rat large intestina. Comp Biochem Physiol 1983;74:459–62.

19. Stragand JJ, Hagemann RF. Effect of lumenal contents on colonic replacement. Am J Physiol 1977;233:E208–11.

20. Lund PK, Ulshen MH, Rountree DB, Selub SE, Buchan AM. Molecular biology of gastrointestinal peptides and growth factors: relevance to intestinal adaptation. Digestion 1990;46:66–73.

21. Rouiller D, Schusdziarra V, Conlon JM, Harris V, Unger RH. Release of somatostatin-like immunoreactivity from the lower gut. Gastroenterology 1979;77:700–3.

22. Denef C, Schramme C, Baes M. Stimulation of growth hormone release by vasoactive intestinal peptide and peptide PHI in rat anterior pituitary reaggregates. Neuroendocrinology 1985;40:88–91.

23. Wehrenberg WB, Janowski BA, Piering AW, Culler F, Jones KL. Glucocorticoids: potent inhibitors and stimulators of growth hormone secretion. Endocrinology 1990;126:3200–3.

24. Leblond CP, Carriere R. The effect of growth hormone and thyroxine on the mitotic rate of the intestinal mucosa of the rat. Endocrinology 1955;56:261–6.

25. Havivi Y, Havivi E, Levitan R. Histology and chemical composition of the small bowel of hypophysectomized rats. Am J Dig Dis 1968;13:735–42.

26. Schapiro H, Wruble LD, Brott LG. The effect of hypophysectomy on the gastrointestinal tract. Digest Dis 1970;15:1019–30.

27. Scow RO, Hagan SN. Effect of testosterone propionate and growth hormone on growth and chemical composition of muscle and other tissues in hypophysectomized male rats. Endocrinology 1965;77:852–8.

28. Jacobsen ED, Magnani TJ. Some effects of hypophysectomy on gastrointestinal function and structure. Gut 1964;5:473–9.

29. Dowling RH, Fuller R, Ulshen MH, Zimmermann E, Kay Lund P. Small and large bowel mRNA in the intestinal adaption of growth hormone transgenic mice. Gut 1991;32:1208 (abstr).

30. Ulshen MH, Dowling RH, Fuller CR, Zimmermann EM, Lund PK. Enhanced

growth of small bowel in transgenic mice overexpressing bovine growth hormone. Gastroenterology 1993;104:973–80.

31. Mainoya JR. Influence of ovine growth hormone on water and NaCl transport by the rat proximal jejunum and distal ileum. Comp Biochem Physiol 1982;71A:477–9.

32. Bruns MEH, Volmer SS, Bruns DE, Overpeck JG. Human growth hormone increases intestinal vitamin D–dependent calcium binding proteins in hypophysectomized rats. Endocrinology 1983;113:1387–92.

33. Finkelstein JD, Schacter D. Active transport of calcium by intestine: effects of hypophysectomy and growth hormone. Am J Physiol 1962;203:873.

34. Enochs MR, Johnson LR. Effect of hypophysectomy and growth hormone on serum and antral gastrin levels in the rat. Endocrinology 1976;70:727–32.

35. Daughaday WH. Growth hormone and the somatomedins. In: Daughaday WH, ed. Endocrine control of growth. New York: Elsevier, 1981:1–24.

36. Laburthe M, Rouyer-Fessard C, Gammeltoft S. Receptors for insulin-like growth factors I and II in rat gastrointestinal epithelium. Am J Physiol 1988;254:G457–62.

37. Lemmey AB, Martin AA, Read LC, Tomas FM, Owens PC, Ballard FJ. IGF-I and the truncated analogue des-(1-3)IGF-I enhance growth in rats after gut resection. Am J Physiol 1991;260:E213–19.

38. Salub SF, Ulshen MH, Lund PK. IGF-I mRNA disruption in rat gastrointestinal tract and growth hormone dependent expression. Abstract, Digestive Disease Week, New Orleans, May 19–22, 1991.

39. Kostyo JI, Isakson O. Growth hormone and regulation of somatic growth. In Int Rev Physiol Reprod Physiol 1977;13:255–74.

40. Isaksson OGP, Edén S, Jansson JO. Mode of actoin of pituitary growth hormone on target cells. Annu Rev Physiol 1985;47:483–99.

41. Lobie PE, Briepohl W, Waters MJ. Growth hormone receptor expression in the rat gastrointestinal tract. Endocrinology 1990;126:299–306.

42. Mjaaland M, Unneberg K, Jenssen TG, Reuhaug A. Experimental study to show that GH treatment before trauma increases glutamine uptake in the intestinal tract. Br J Surg 1995;82:1076–79.

43. Clemmons DR, Shaw PS. Purification and biologic properties of fibroblast somatomedin. J Biol Chem 1986;261:10294–8.

44. Martens MFWC, Hendriks T. Collagen synthesis in explants from rat intestine. Biochem Biophys Acta 1989;993:252–8.

45. Brasken P, Lehto M, Renvall S. Fibronectin, laminin, and collagen types I, III, IV and V in the healing rat colon anastomosis. Ann Chir Gynecol 1990;79:65–71.

46. Larrey J, Recueil de memoires de chirurgie (1821). Translated by John Revere. Baltimore, MD: 1823.

47. Prudden JF, Nishihara G, Ocampo L. The effect on wound tensile strength of marked postoperative anabolism induced with growth hormone. Surg Gynecol Obstet 1958;106:481–2.

48. Kowalewski K, Yong S. Effect of growth hormone and an anabolic steroid on hydroxyproline in healing dermal wounds in rats. Acta Endocrinol (Copenh) 1968;59:53–6.

49. Meffert W, Liebow AA. Hormonal control of collateral circulation. Circ Res 1966;18:228–33.

50. Hollander DM, Devereux DF, Marafino BJ, Hoppe H. Increased wound

breaking strength in rats following treatment with synthetic human growth hormone. Surg Forum 1984;35:612–4.

51. Pessa ME, Bland KI, Sitren HS, Miller GJ, Copeland EM. Improved wound healing in tumor-bearing rats treated with perioperative synthetic human growth hormone. Surg Forum 1985;36:6–8.

52. Jørgensen PH, Andreassen TT. Influence of biosynthetic human growth hormone on the biochemical properties of rat skin incisional wounds. Acta Chir Scand 1988;154:623–6.

53. Bak B, Jørgensen PH, Andreassen TT. The stimulating effect of growth hormone on fracture healing is dependent on onset and duration of administration. Clin Orthop 1991;264:295–301.

54. Jørgensen PH, Andreassen TT. A dose-response study of the effects of biosynthetic human growth hormone on formation and strength of granulation tissue. Endocrinology 1987;121:1637–41.

55. Hart MH, Phares CK, Erdman SH, Grandjean CJ, Park JHY, Vanderhoof JA. Augmentation of postresectional mucosal hyperplasia by plerocercoid growth factor (PGF). Analog of growth hormone. Dig Dis Sci 1987; 32:1275–80.

56. Herndon DN, Barrow RE, Kunkel KR, Broemeling L, Rutan RL. Effects of recombinant human growth hormone on donor-site healing in severely burned children. Ann Surg 1990;212:424–31.

57. Chlumsky V. Experimentelle Untersuchungen über dir verschiedenen Methoden der Darmvereinigung. Bruns' Beiträge zur Klinisch Chirurgie 1989; 25:539–600.

58. Peacock EE. Wound repair, 3rd ed. Philadelphia: W.B. Saunders, 1984.

59. Nelsen TS, Anders CJ. Dynamic aspects of small intestinal rupture with special considerations of anastomotic strength. ARch Surg 1966;93:309–14.

60. Christensen H, Langfeldt S, Laurberg S. Bursting strength of experimental intestinal anastomoses. A methodological study. Eur Surg Res 1993;25:38–45.

61. Gottrup F. Healing of incisional wounds in the stomach and duodenum. An experimental study. Thesis, University of Aarhus, 1983.

62. Christensen H, Oxlund H, Laurberg S. Growth hormone increases the bursting strength of colonic anastomoses. An experimental study in the rat. Int J Color Dis 1990;5:130–4.

63. Christensen H, Oxlund H, Laurberg S. Postoperative biosynthetic human growth hormone increases the strength and collagen deposition of experimental colonic anastomoses. Int J Color Dis 1991;6:133–8.

64. Edén S. Age- and sex-related differences in episodic growth hormone secretion in the rat. Endocrinology 1979;105:555–60.

65. Christensen H, Flyvbjerg A. Dose-dependent effect of human growth hormone on the strength and collagen deposition of colonic anastomoses in rats. Acta Endocrinol (Copenh) 1992;126:438–43.

66. Christensen H, Oxlund H. Growth hormone increases the collagen deposition rate and breaking strength of left colonic anastomoses in rats. Surgery 1994;116:550–6.

67. Christen H, Jørgensen PH, Oxlund H, Laurberg S. Growth hormone increases the mass, the collagenous proteins, and the strength of rat colon. Scand J Gastroenterol 1990;25:1137–43.

68. Jiborn H. Healing of left colonic anastomoses. An experimental study in the rat. Thesis, University of Lund, Malmö, 1978.

69. Hendriks T, Mastboom WJB. Healing of experimental intestinal anastomoses. Parameters for repair. Dis Colon Rectum 1990;33:891–901.
70. Stappen JWJ, Hendriks T, Boer HHM, Man BM, Pont JJHHM. Collagenolytic activity in experimental intestinal anastomoses. Int J Color Dis 1992;7: 95–101.
71. Delbridge L, Everitt AV. The effect of hypophysectomy and age on the stabilization of labile cross-links in collagen. Exp Gerontol 1972;7:413–5.
72. Oxlund H, Jørgensen PH, Ørtoft G, Andreassen TT. Alterations in the cross-links of skin collagen of rats treated with biosynthetic human growth hormone. Connect Tissue Res 1991;26:65–75.
73. Christensen H, Andreassen TT, Oxlund H. Increased mechanical strength of left colon in old rats treated with biosynthetic growth hormone. Gerontology 1992;38:245–51.
74. Chowcat NL, Savage FJ, Hembry RM, Boulos PB. Role of collagenase in colonic anastomoses: a reappraisal. Br J Surg 1988;75:330–4.
75. Houdart R, Lavergne A, Galian A, Hautefeuille P. Évolution anatomopathologique des anastomoses digestives bord a bord en un plan. Gastroenterol Clin Biol 1983;7:465–73.
76. Christensen H, Chemnitz J, Christensen BC, Oxlund H. Collagen structural organisation of healing colonic anastomoses and the effect of growth hormone treatment. Dis Colon Rectum 1995; in press.
77. Konturek SJ, Król R, Pawlik W, et al. Pharmacology of somatostatin. In: Bloom SR, ed. Gut hormones. Edinburgh: Churchill Livingstone, 1978:457–62.
78. Leyden T, Rosenberg J, Nemchausky B, Elson C, Rosenberg I. Reversal of growth arrest in adolescents with Crohn's disease after parenteral alimentation. Gastroenterology 1976;70:1017–21.
79. Underwood LE, Clemmons DR, Maes M, D'Ercole AJ, Ketelslegers J-M. Regulation of somatomedin C/insulin-like growth factor I by nutrients. Horm Res 1986;24:166–76.
80. Hawker FH, Steward PM, Baxter RC, et al. Relationship of somatomedin-C/insulin-like growth factor I levels to conventional nutritional indices in critically ill patients. Crit Care Med 1987;15:732–6.
81. Morris GP, Beck PL, Herridge MS, Depew WT, Szewczuk MR, Wallace JL. Hapten-induced model of chronic inflammation and ulceration in the rat colon. Gastroenterology 1989;96:795–803.
82. Krawisz JE, Sharon P, Stenson WF. Quantitative assay for acute intestinal inflammation based on myeloperoxidase activity. Gastroenterology 1984; 87:1344–50.
83. Christensen H, Flyvbjerg A, Ørskov H, Laurberg S. Effect of growth hormone on the inflammatory activity of experimental colitis in rats. Scand J Gastroenterol 1993;28:503–11.
84. Alexander AC, Irving MH. Accumulation and pepsin solubility of collagens in the bowel of patients with Crohn's disease. Dis Colon Rectum 1990;33:956–62.
85. Durdey P, Switala S, Williams NS. Collagenolytic activity in Crohn's colitis. Br J Surg 1987;74:527.
86. Thissen JP, Underwood LE, Maiter D, Maes M, Clemmons DR, Ketelslegers JM. Failure of insulin-like growth factor-I (IGF-I) infusion to promote growth in protein-restricted rats despite normalization of serum IGF-I concentrations. Endocrinology 1991;128:885–90.
87. Kissmeyer-Nielsen P, Christensen H, Laurberg S. Growth hormone treatment

of rats with chronic diverting colostomy. Different response on proximal functioning and distal atrophic colon. Eur J Endocrinol 1994;130:508-14.

88. Christensen H, Oxlund H, Laurberg S. Stimulating effect of biosynthetic human growth hormone on adult rat colon. Gastroenterol Int 1991;4:65-9.

89. Irvin TT. Effects of malnutrition and hyperalimentation on wound healing. Surg Gynecol Obstet 1978;146:33-7.

90. Spanheimer R, Zlatev T, Umpierrez G, DiGirolamo M. Collagen production in fasted and food-restricted rats: response to duration and severity of food-deprivation. J Nutr 1991;121:518-24.

91. Ziegler TR, Young LS, Manson JM, Wilmore DW. Metabolic effects of recombinant human growth hormone in patients receiving parenteral nutrition. Ann Surg 1988;208:6-16.

92. Zaizen Y, Ford EG, Costin G, Atkinson JB. The effect of perioperative exogenous growth hormone on wound bursting strength in normal and malnourished rats. J Pediatr Surg 1990;25:70-4.

93. Kelts DG, Grand RJ, Shen G, Watkins JB, Werlin SL, Boehme C. Nutritional basis of growth failure in children and adolescents with Crohn's disease. Gastroenterology 1979;76:720-7.

94. Desborough JP, Griffin RA, Moore CM, Burrin JM, Hall GM. Growth hormone secretion in response to surgery. Horm Metab Res 1993;25:640-3.

95. Manson J, Wilmore DW. Growth hormone in the surgical patient. In: Underwood LE, ed. Growth hormone. New York: Marcel Dekker, 1986:255-67.

96. Wright PD, Johnston IDA. The effect of surgical operation on growth hormone levels in plasma. Surgery 1975;77:479-86.

97. Arimura A, Smith WD, Schally AV. Blockade of the stress-induced decrease in blood GH by anti-somatostatin serum in rats. Endocrinology 1976;98:540-43.

98. Kupfer SR, Underwood LE, Baxter RC, Clemmons DR. Enhancement of the anabolic effects of growth hormone and insulin-like growth factor I by use of both agents simultaneously. J Clin Invest 1993;91:391-96.

99. Ng E-H, Rock CS, Lazarus D, et al. Impact of exogenous growth hormone on host preservation and tumor cell-cycle distribution in a rat sarcoma model. J Surg Res 1991;51:99-105.

100. Ingemann-Petersen T, Kissmeyer-Nielsen P, Flyvbjerg A, Laurberg S, Christensen H. The effects of insulin-like growth factor I on the healing of experimental colonic anastomoses. Int J Color Dis 1995; in press.

101. Ziegler TR, Young LS, Ferrari-Baliviera E, Demling RH, Wilmore DW. Use of growth hormone combined with nutritional support in a critical care unit. J Parenteral Enter Nutr 1990;14:574-81.

102. Lundeberg S, Belfrage M, Wernerman J, Decken Avd, Thunell S, Vinnars E. Growth hormone improves muscle protein metabolism and whole body nitrogen economy in man during a hyponitrogenous diet. Metabolism 1991; 40:315-22.

103. Clemmons DR, Underwood LE, Dickerson RO, et al. Use of plasma somato-medin C/insulin-like growth factor I measurements to monitor the response to nutritional repletion in malnourished patients. Am J Clin Nutr 1985; 41:191-98.

104. Irvin GL, Horsley JS, Caruana JA. The morbidity and mortality of emergency operations for colorectal disease. Ann Surg 1984;199:598-603.

105. Lewis AAM, Khoury GA. Resection for colorectal cancer in the very old: are the risks too high? Br Med J 1988;296:459-62.

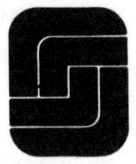

16

Modulation of IGF-I Therapy by IGFBP-3: Potential Utility in Wound Healing

David M. Rosen, Steven Adams, Jerome A. Moore, Christopher A. Maack, and Andreas Sommer

Insulin-like growth factor-I (IGF-I) is one of the most abundant growth factors in circulation (~200 ng/ml); however, very little of it exists in its free form. Normally, IGF-I is bound to one of its six known binding proteins designated as IGFBPs1–6 (1, 2). These IGFBPs exhibit variable tissue distributions and are believed to be involved in modulation of IGF activity (3–7). In circulation, IGF-I exists primarily as part of a ternary complex comprised of equimolar ratios of IGF-I, IGFBP-3, and a protein known as acid labile subunit (ALS) (1, 8). IGFBP-3 is by far the most abundant IGF binding protein and the only form that can bind to ALS to form the large 150-kd ternary complex. This complex found in serum greatly extends the circulating time of IGF-I and is believed to modulate the availability of free IGF-I (1, 9).

Local Tissue Repair

IGF-I is known to be present in wound fluid and platelet releasates (10, 11). Numerous groups have reported activities such as stimulation of cell proliferation and matrix production (12). We have demonstrated that local application of the IGF-I/IGFBP-3 complex can promote granulation tissue deposition in Schilling-Hunt wound chambers. In rats, local application of the IGF-I/IGFBP-3 complex appears to be more effective than free IGF-I in promoting granulation tissue in this model (Fig. 16.1). In this study, IGF-I (100 µg) was injected into the Schilling-Hunt chambers daily for 17 days either alone or complexed with an equimolar amount of IGFBP-3. IGF-I alone or complexed with IGFBP-3 resulted in an increase in deposition of collagen in the chambers. Treatment with an equimolar dose

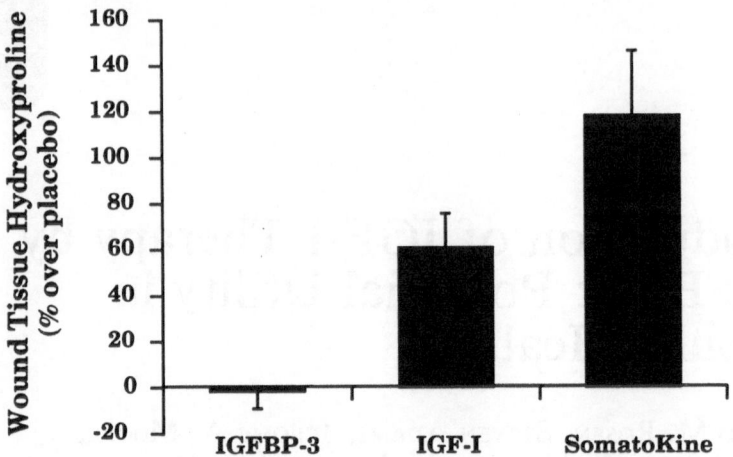

FIGURE 16.1. Comparison of equimolar doses of IGFBP-3 (64 μg), IGF-I (16 μg), and the IGF-I/IGFBP-3 complex (80 μg) on collagen accumulation in Schilling-Hunt chambers. Each component was injected daily for 17 days into wire mesh chambers (18 mm × 6 mm diameter). Chambers were implanted in subcutaneous pockets created on either side of midline incisions made on the backs of Sprague-Dawley rats (300–350 g). The cylinder contents were analyzed for hydroxyproline and DNA by standard methodology using the Chloromine T/perchloric acid and diphenylamine methods respectively. Data are expressed relative to placebo and are mean ± SEM for $n = 5$. (Adapted from ref. 24.)

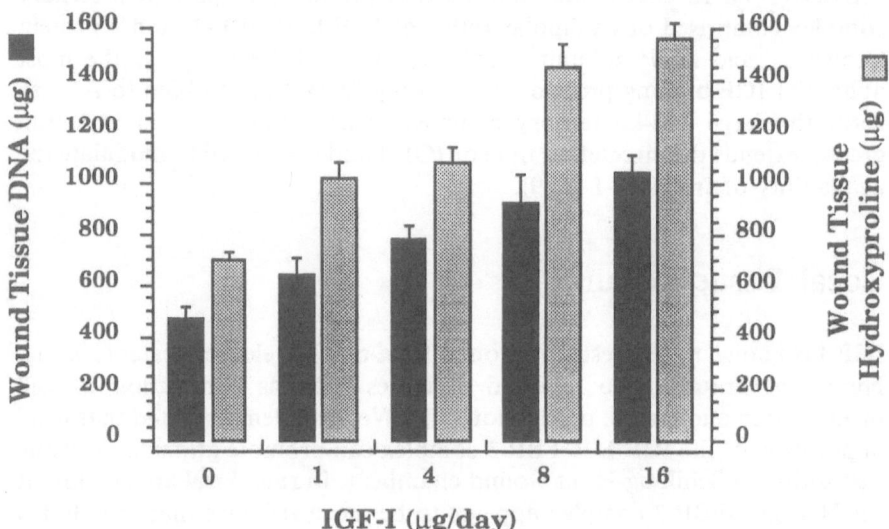

FIGURE 16.2. Effect of the IGF-I/IGFBP-3 complex on collagen accumulation in Schilling-Hunt chambers implanted in rats. The IGF-I/IGFBP-3 complex was injected daily for 17 days at the indicated doses of IGF-I (complexed with an equal molar amount of IGFBP-3) into wire mesh chambers as described for Figure 16.1. Wound chamber tissue was collected and analyzed as described for Figure 16.1. Data are expressed as mean ± SEM for $n = 5$. (Adapted from ref. 24.)

of IGFBP-3 alone at this dose did not have any significant effect on tissue deposition. One possible explanation for this might be that the complex may serve as a local slow release vehicle for IGF-I. In a subsequent study, various doses of the IGF-I/IGFBP-3 complex were evaluated and were found to increase DNA and collagen content of the enclosed tissue by more than twofold over a dose range of 1 to 6 μg/day (Fig. 16.2).

The ability of the IGFBP-3 to modulate the activity of IGF-I was further evaluated in the experiment summarized by Figure 16.3. In this experiment, addition of increasing doses of IGFBP-3 were able to inhibit normal tissue accumulation in the chambers. The high doses of IGFBP-3 may be sufficient to bind endogenously produced IGF-I and thereby limit the amount of available free IGF-I. Together, these studies are consistent with IGF's known activities on cell proliferation and matrix production as well as supporting the idea that the binding protein plays an important role in modulating the availability of free IGF-I.

The IGF-I/IGFBP-3 complex was also evaluated in partial-thickness wounds in pigs. In these studies, IGF-I $\pm$ IGFBP-3 was formulated in 3% methylcellulose and applied to dermal wounds. In Figure 16.4, an equimolar dose of IGF-I, IGFBP-3, or the complex was applied daily for 6 days. The data indicate that both IGF-I and the complex increased the extent of re-epithelialization after 6 days; however, application of the IGF-I/IGFBP-3

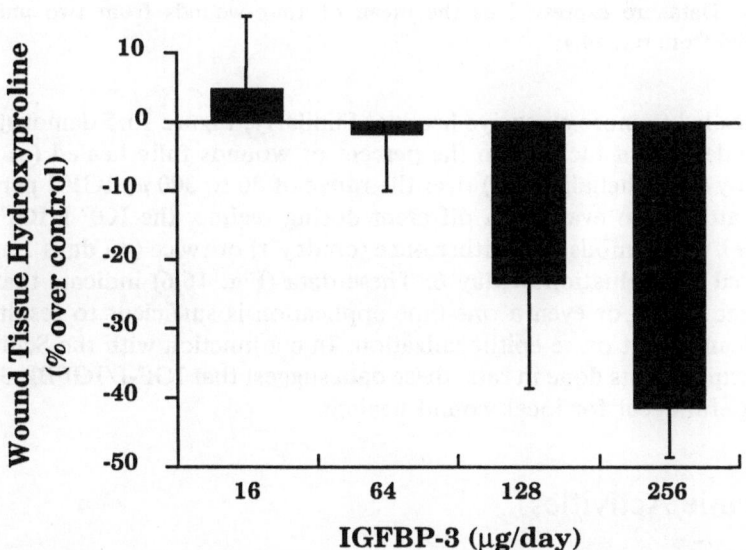

FIGURE 16.3. Effect of exogenous IGFBP-3 on collagen accumulation in the Schilling-Hunt chambers. Chambers were implanted in rats as above and injected daily with the indicated doses of IGFBP-3 for 17 days. Tissue was collected and hydroxyproline was measured as previously described. Data are expressed relative to placebo and are mean $\pm$ SEM for $n = 5$. (Adapted from ref. 24.)

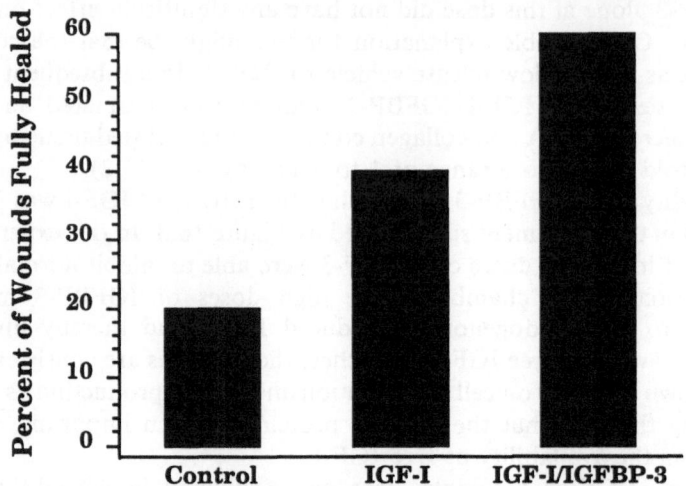

FIGURE 16.4. Comparison of equimolar doses of IGFBP-3 (373 μg), IGF-I (100 μg), and the IGF-I/IGFBP-3 complex (475 μg) in split-thickness wounds in pigs. Dermal wounds (1200 μm deep; 2.5 cm × 2.5 cm in area) were made in domestic pigs. Wounds were either treated with vehicle (3% methylcellulose in PBS, 0.1% BSA), or the indicated drug formulated in above formulation in a final volume of 1 ml. Wounds were treated daily and analyzed on day 6. Wounds were analyzed histologically for the percentage of the wound resurfaced by epithelium. Wounds covered by a layer of epithelium were considered "fully healed" for the purposes of scoring. Data are expressed as the mean of four wounds from two animals. (Adapted from ref. 24.)

complex led to more extensive healing. Similarly, Figure 16.5 demonstrates a dose-dependent increase in the percent of wounds fully healed (as measured by re-epithelialization) over the range of 30 to 300 μg IGF-I per day. In an attempt to evaluate a different dosing regime, the IGF-I/IGFBP-3 complex was administered either once (on day 1) or twice (on days 1 and 2) followed by evaluation at day 6. These data (Fig. 16.6) indicate that less frequent dosing or even a one-time application is sufficient to result in a significant effect on re-epithelialization. In conjunction with the Schilling-Hunt experiments done in rats, these data suggest that IGF-I/IGFBP-3 may be a useful agent for local wound healing.

Systemic Activities

Unlike most other growth factors being evaluated for enhancement of wound healing, the IGF-I/IGFBP-3 complex has the potential advantage of also being useful for systemic wound healing applications. IGF-I/IGFBP-3

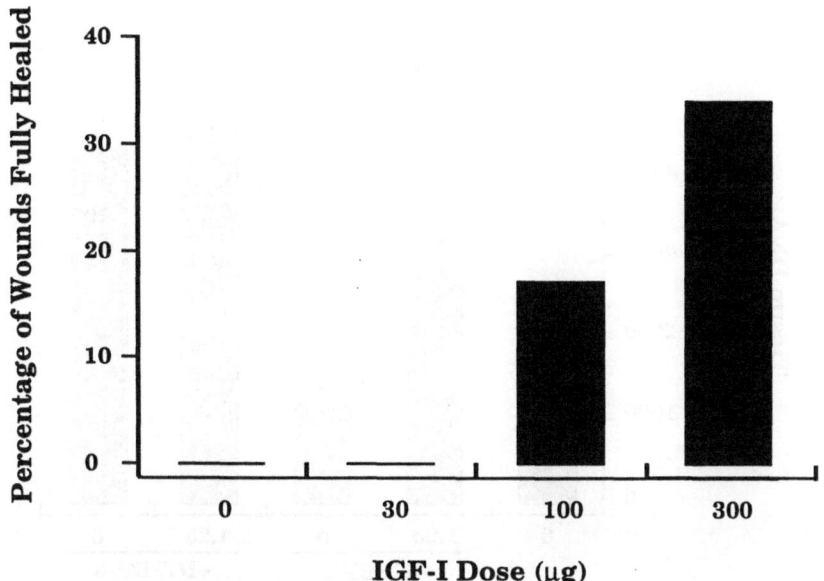

FIGURE 16.5. Effect of the IGF-I/IGFBP-3 complex (SomatoKine) on dermal wound healing in domestic pigs. Wounds were prepared and analyzed as described in Figure 16.4. Wounds were treated daily with the indicated doses of SomatoKine for 6 days. Doses are expressed as IGF-I equivalents (indicated doses of IGF-I complexed to an equimolar amount of IGFBP-3). Data are expressed as the % of wounds fully healed (as described for Figure 16.4) and are the mean of four wounds from two animals.

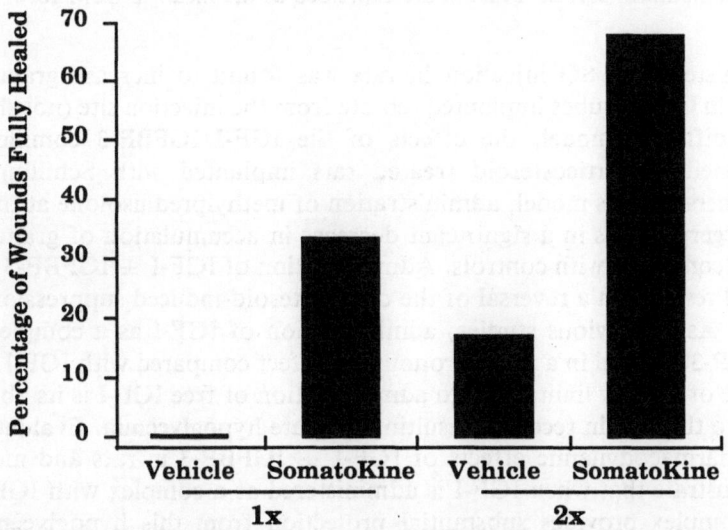

FIGURE 16.6. Effect of limited dosing with SomatoKine on wound healing. Wounds were created in pigs as described previously. SomatoKine (300 μg IGF-I + 1130 μg IGFBP-3) was applied to wounds either on day 1 (1x) or twice 2x; on days 1 and 2), and then analyzed on day 6. Data are expressed as percentage of wounds fully healed (as described for Figure 16.4) and are the mean of four wounds from two animals.

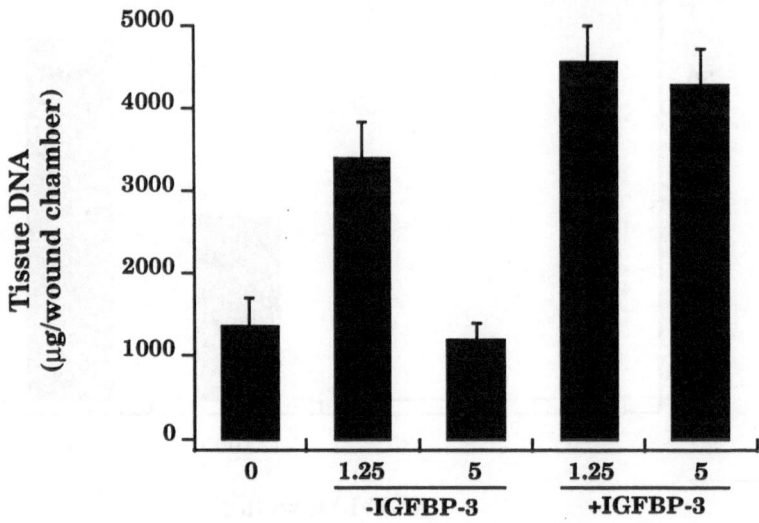

FIGURE 16.7. Effect of systemic administration of SomatoKine on corticosteroid suppressed wound healing. Rats were implanted with Schilling-Hunt chambers as described for Figure 16.1 and were given methylprednisolone (8 mg/rat) at the time of surgery to suppress the healing response. Chambers were injected daily for 17 days with the indicated doses of IGF-I either alone (– IGFBP-3) or complexed to an equal molar amount of IGFBP-3. Data are expressed as the mean ± SEM for $n = 5$.

administered by SQ injection in rats was found to increase granulation tissue in Gortex tubes implanted remote from the injection site (not shown). In a different model, the effects of the IGF-I/IGFBP-3 complex was evaluated in corticosteroid treated rats implanted with Schilling-Hunt chambers. In this model, administration of methylprednisolone at the time of surgery results in a significant decrease in accumulation of granulation tissue compared with controls. Administration of IGF-I ± IGFBP-3 in this model resulted in a reversal of the corticosteroid-induced suppression (Fig. 16.7). As in previous studies, administration of IGF-I as a complex with IGFBP-3 resulted in a more pronounced effect compared with IGF-I alone.

One of the key limitations to administration of free IGF-I is its ability to bind to the insulin receptor resulting in acute hypoglycemia. Evaluation of the pharmacodynamic effects of IGF-I ± IGFBP-3 in rats and monkeys demonstrate that when IGF-I is administered as a complex with IGFBP-3, the complex provides substantial protection from this hypoglycemic response. Figure 16.8 portrays an experiment where IGF-I is given as an IV bolus injection at a dose of 2 mg/kg (± IGFBP-3). At this dose, the monkeys become severely hypoglycemic with the free IGF-I, but exhibit no

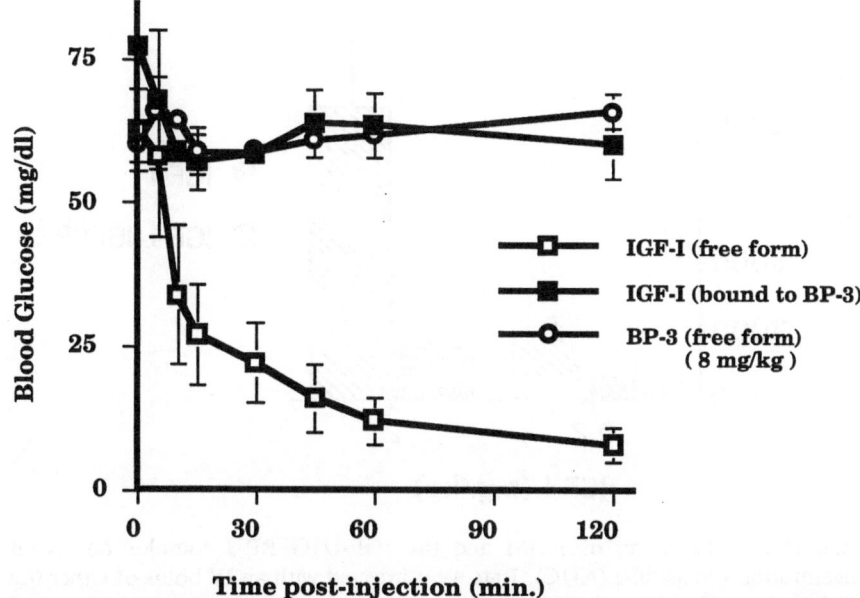

FIGURE 16.8. Comparison of equimolar doses of IGF-I (2 mg/kg), IGFBP-3 (8 mg/kg), and the IGF-I/IGFBP-3 complex (10 mg/kg) on blood glucose levels in cynamologous monkeys. IGF-I (open squares), IGFBP-3 (open circles), or IGF-I/IGFBP-3 (solid squares) were formulated in 105 mM NaCl, 20 mM sodium acetate, pH 5.5, and injected by IV administration into cynamologous monkeys. Blood was drawn at the indicated times and analyzed for glucose. Data are the mean ± SEM for $n = 3$.

significant change in blood glucose when IGF-I is administered as a complex with IGFBP-3. Similarly, equivalent doses of IGFBP-3 alone had no significant effect on blood glucose levels. In other studies, we have been able to demonstrate that administration of IGF-I as a complex with IGFBP-3 also prevented acute side effects, such as hypoglycemia, with doses as much as 20-fold higher (on an equal molar basis).

Recent pharmacokinetic studies have shown that there is a substantial difference in the systemic exposure of free IGF-I compared with Somato-Kine as determined by the area under the serum concentration versus time curve (AUC) values. In both rats (Fig. 16.9) and monkeys (not shown), the AUC for SomatoKine is significantly greater than it is for an equimolar concentration of free IGF-I, indicating an enhanced systemic exposure for SomatoKine compared with an equivalent dose of IGF-I. Together these data suggest that SomatoKine represents a potentially safer and more efficacious method of administering IGF-I.

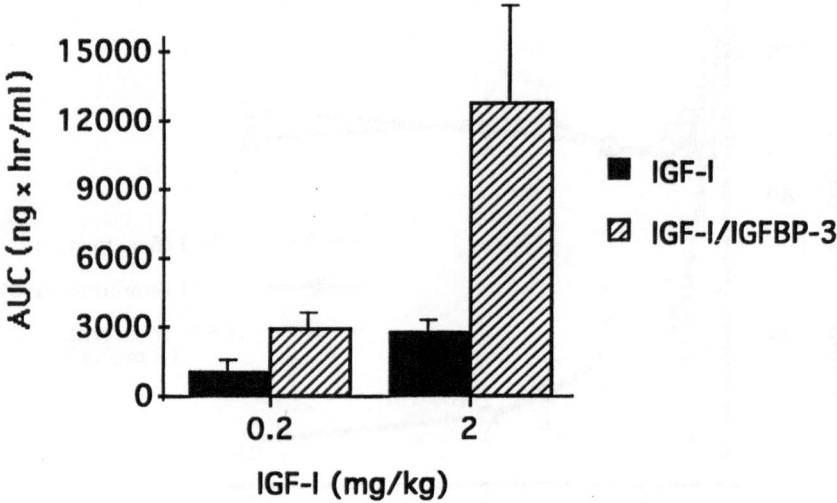

FIGURE 16.9. Comparison of IGF-I and the IGF-I/IGFBP-3 complex on serum concentration versus time (AUC). Rats were injected with an IV bolus of either 0.2 or 2.0 mg/kg of free IGF-I (solid bars) or the IGF-I complexed to IGFBP-3 (hatched bars). Blood was collected at various times over a 24-hour period and analyzed for the presence of human IGF-I using an immunoradiometric assay (IRMA) (DSL laboratories). Data are expressed as ng-hr/ml and are presented as the mean ± SEM for $n = 3$.

Potential Clinical Utility

Published reports by several investigators have demonstrated that circulating levels of IGF-I and IGFBP-3 are significantly reduced after severe trauma, such as burns (13–16) or major surgery (17, 18). These patients also exhibit an impaired ability to heal. Growth hormone therapy has been shown to successfully stimulate or enhance wound healing in children with burns (19, 20). However, it has also been reported that critically ill patients have near-normal levels of growth hormone, but significantly reduced levels of circulating IGF-I (21). In addition, septic patients who have been given growth hormone have also been reported to have a significantly attenuated response in terms of IGF-I production (22). Thus, in critically ill or traumatized patients, the normal growth hormone–IGF-I axis may be altered and growth hormone treatment may not result in the expected or desired increase in circulating levels of IGF-I (23). Therefore, these patient populations might be particularly well suited to IGF-I/IGFBP3 therapy. These findings, along with the well-documented anabolic activity of IGF-I, suggest that the IGF-I/IGFBP-3 complex may be an attractive therapeutic or hormone replacement therapy for patients who have experienced severe trauma, such as those with severe burns.

Acknowledgments. The authors would like to thank Drs. T.K. Hunt and E.M. Spencer (University of California–San Francisco) and Drs. L. Nanney and J. Davidson (Vanderbilt University) for their contributions to the wound healing studies in rats and pigs. We would also like to acknowledge the contributions of Drs. Henryk Cudney, Robert Chang, and Yasushi Ogawa and their groups for supplying and analyzing the IGF-I and IGFBP-3 required for these studies. Finally, we thank Dr. Cedo Bagi, Shirley Chu, Estalita DeLeon, and Conan Liu for their help with the pharmacokinetic studies.

References

1. Baxter RC. Insulin-like growth factor binding proteins in the human circulation: a review. Horm Res 1994;42:140–4.
2. Baxter RC. Circulating binding proteins for the insulin-like growth factors. Trends Endocrinol Metab 1993;4:91–6.
3. Cohen P, Rosenfeld RG. Physiological and clinical relevance of the insulin-like binding proteins. Curr Opin Pediatr 1994;6:462–7.
4. Drop SL, Schuller AG, Lindenbergh-Kortleve DJ, Groffen C, Brinkman A, Zwarthoff EC. Structural aspects of the IGFBP family. Growth Regul 1992; 2:69–79.
5. Clemmons DR, Jones JI, Busby WH, Wright G. Role of insulin-like growth factor binding proteins in modifying IGF actions. Ann NY Acad Sci 1993; 692:10–21.
6. Clemmons DR. IGF binding proteins and their functions. Mol Reprod Dev 1993;35:368–74.
7. Schuller AGP, Zwarthoff EC, Drop SLS. Gene expression of the six insulin-like growth factor binding proteins in the mouse conceptus during mid- and late gestation. Endocrinology 1993;132:2544–50.
8. Martin JL, Baxter RC. Insulin-like growth factor binding protein-3: biochemistry and physiology. Growth Regul 1992;2:88–99.
9. Lewitt MS, Saunders H, Phuyal JL, Baxter RC. Complex formation by human insulin-like growth factor-binding protein-3 and human acid-labile subunit in growth hormone-deficient rats. Endocrinology 1994;134:2402–09.
10. Mueller RV, Spencer M, Sommer A, Maack CA, Suh D, Hunt TK. The role of IGF-I and IGFBP-3 in wound healing. In: Spencer EM, ed. Modern concepts of insulin-like growth factors. New York: Elsevier, 1991:185–92.
11. Karey KP, Sirbasku DA. Human platelet-derived mitogens II. Subcellular localization of insulin-like growth factor I to the alpha granules and release in response to thrombin. Blood 1989;74:1093–100.
12. Cohick WS, Clemmons DR. The insulin-like growth factors. Annu Rev Physiol 1993;55:131–53.
13. Moller S, Jensen M, Svenson P, Skakkebaek NE. Insulin-like growth factor I (IGF-I) in burn patients. Burns 1991;17:279–81.
14. Abribat T, Brazeau O, Davignon I, Garrel DR. Insulin-like growth factor-I blood levels in severely burned patients: effects of time post injury, age of patient, and severity of burn. Clin Endocrinol 1993;39:583–9.

15. Huang KF, Chung DH, Herdon DN. Insulin-like growth factor-I (IGF-I) reduces gut atrophy and bacterial translocation after severe burn injury. Arch Surg 1993;128:47–53.
16. Ghahary A, Fu S, Shen YJ, Shankowski HA, Tredget EE. Differential effects of thermal injury on circulating levels of insulin-like growth factor binding proteins in burn patients. Mol Cell Biochem 1994;135:171–80.
17. Hughs SCC, Cotterill AM, Malloy AR, et al. The induction of specific proteases for insulin-like growth factor binding proteins following major heart surgery. J Endocrinol 1992;135:135–45.
18. Tacke J, Bolder U, Löhlein D. Improved nitrogen balance after administration of recombinant growth hormone in patients undergoing gastrointestinal surgery. Infusionsther Transfusionsmed 1994;21:24–9.
19. Gilpin DA, Barrow RE, Rutan RL, Broemeling L, Herndon DN. Recombinant human growth hormone accelerates wound healing with large cutaneous burns. Ann Surg 1994;220:19–24.
20. Herndon DN, Barrow RE, Kunkel KR, Broemeling L, Rutan RL. Effects of human recombinant growth hormone on donor site healing in severely burned children. Ann Surg 1990;211:424–31.
21. Ross RJM, Freeman E, Jones J, Mathews DR, Preece MA, Buchanan C. Critically ill patients have high basal growth hormone levels with attenuated oscillatory activity associated with low levels of insulin-like growth factor-1. Clin Endocrinol 1991;35:47–54.
22. Dahn MS, Lange MP, Jacobs LA. Insulin-like growth factor I production is inhibited in human sepsis. Arch Surg 1988;123:1409–14.
23. Cotterill AM. The therapeutic potential of recombinant human insulin-like growth factor-I. Clin Endocrinol 1992;37:11–6.
24. Sommer A, Maack CA, Spratt SK, et al. Molecular genetics and action of recombinant insulin-like growth factor binding protein-3. In: Spencer EM, ed. Modern concepts of insulin-like growth factors. New York: Elsevier, 1991: 715–32.

Part V

Clinical Application of Peptide Growth Factors

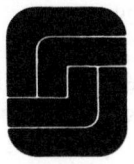

17

Roles of Keratinocyte Growth Factor in Epithelial Growth and Regeneration

Sharon Lea Aukerman, Jeffrey S. Rubin, and Glenn F. Pierce

Keratinocyte growth factor (KGF) is a cytokine that was first identified in 1989 as a mesenchymally derived paracrine mediator of epithelial cell growth (1-3). Upon sequencing, approximately 35% to 40% homology was found with other members of the fibroblast growth factor (FGF) family; hence, KGF is designated as FGF7. In contrast to many other members of the FGF family, cells responsive to KGF appear to be confined to epithelial lineages (4). The KGF receptor (KGFR) is an alternatively spliced tyrosine kinase product of the FGF receptor 2 gene (FGFR2, bek) (5, 6). KGF and acidic FGF (FGF1) bind with high affinity to KGFR, while basic FGF (FGF2) binds with lower affinity (7, 8). The basis for a more KGF selective binding to the KGFR is found in a 49 amino acid stretch beginning in the C-terminal half of the third immunoglobulin loop in FGFR2 (9). A synthetic peptide from this region can block KGF interaction with the KGFR, demonstrating the specificity for KGF conferred by the alternative splicing event (10). Further work suggests elements of the second 1 g loop are also important for high-affinity binding to KGF (11). In contrast to acidic and basic FGF, KGF has a signal sequence and is secreted from mesenchymal cells in a conventional manner.

Target Tissues of KGF

Finch, Rubin, and coworkers (1) first identified KGF in a human lung fibroblast line, and purified the activity using the BALB/MK keratinocyte line as a target. Early work demonstrated that KGF messenger RNA (mRNA) was present in the dermis, while KGFR mRNA was present in the epidermis, implying a paracrine role for KGF. Subsequent work from several laboratories has supported and extended this hypothesis.

KGF and the KGF receptor have frequently been detected within the same organs by ribonuclease (RNase) protection assay analyses (12). In general, epithelial organs having mesenchymal components contain high levels of ligand and receptor mRNA (e.g., lung, skin, gastrointestinal tract). In situ hybridization studies have supported the hypothesis that the ligand is usually synthesized in underlying mesenchyme while the KGF receptor is present in overlying epithelia (3, 13, 14; reviewed in 15). This relationship is not absolute, however, since ligand mRNA has been detected in the developing heart and both ligand and receptor mRNAs have been found in developing cartilage and bone (14).

KGF can stimulate proliferation, and in some cases, differentiation of a number of specific epithelial lineages contained within many organs. Collectively, these observations indicate KGF may function in normal tissue homeostasis, and in epithelial regeneration following injury. An autocrine role for KGF in malignancies has not been established, although a paracrine role in tumor growth and benign cellular proliferations (e.g., psoriasis) has not been ruled out.

KGF and the Skin

Werner and colleagues (16) first demonstrated an enormous upregulation of KGF expression in the surrounding dermis of full-thickness skin excisions made in rats, suggesting elevated KGF levels were a response to injury. Subsequent work using porcine excisions and rabbit ear excisions that were treated with topical recombinant KGF (rKGF) demonstrated enhanced reepithelialization, but also accelerated maturation of the neoepidermis (17, 18). These observations were supported by finding increased differentiation of cultured keratinocytes in response to KGF (19). In addition, increased proliferation of hair follicle keratinocytes and sebocytes and increased size (i.e., differentiation) of the corresponding hair follicles and sebaceous glands were detected within dermis adjacent to wounds treated with topical rKGF. These observations prompted further analysis of KGF's therapeutic potential in a chemotherapy-induced alopecia model, a nude mouse model, and a porcine partial-thickness burn model (20, 21).

In all three models, increased proliferation of hair follicle keratinocytes was detected following systemic treatment with rKGF. In the chemotherapy-induced alopecia model in newborn rats, pretreatment with rKGF was required prior to administration of cytosine arabinoside. Approximately 50% of the hair remained on animals pretreated with rKGF, versus complete hair loss in placebo-treated animals. Hair regrowth was not accelerated in rKGF treated animals, suggesting KGF has a cytoprotective mechanism of action for existing follicles subjected to the toxic insult.

The precise genetic defect in the nu/nu mouse responsible for lack of hair is unknown, but is probably unrelated to the immune deficiency, since a partial chromosomal deletion is present in these animals. Minoxidil, a drug used to treat male-pattern baldness, is ineffective in stimulating hair follicles in the nude mouse. In contrast, systemic delivery of rKGF resulted in abundant but variable hair growth in the nude mouse (20). These results suggest the hair follicles in the nude mouse are capable of synthesizing hair, but may either lack sufficient stimulus or be unresponsive to a stimulatory signal, for which pharmacologic doses of rKGF can partially compensate.

KGF is induced by proinflammatory cytokines such as interleukin (IL)-1 and IL-6 (22, 23), which presumably contributes to the increase in KGF expression following injury. The large induction of KGF seen in mouse skin following full-thickness lesion is reduced and delayed during wound healing in the skin of genetically diabetic mice (24). Similarly, the inhibitory effect of glucocorticoids on healing may be due in part to its inhibitory effects on KGF expression (25, 26). A role for the KGF signaling pathway in skin healing was inferred from a transgenic study in which a dominant negative KGFR was expressed in the epidermis (via keratin 14 promoter) (27). Knockout of KGF itself did not appear to impair wound healing in a couple of models, nor did the concomitant knockout of transforming growth factor-α (TGF-α) (28), implying there is indeed redundancy of growth factors involved in wound healing.

A growth factor capable of stimulating adnexal elements within the dermis may be of use in partial-thickness skin injuries, which heal via the sprouting of keratinocytes from remaining viable adnexa. Previous findings in the partial-thickness rabbit ear model supported the development of a porcine burn model to evaluate the ability of topically applied rKGF to stimulate reepithelialization (18). The porcine burn model is considered a more relevant wound than the acute partial-thickness skin wound for predicting therapeutic utility of a candidate drug (29). Despite detecting KGFR and marked stimulation by topical KGF of hair follicles and wound border keratinocytes, clinically insignificant effects on wound closure and time to full healing were observed (21). Combination therapy with epidermal growth factor or platelet-derived growth factor-BB (PDGF-BB) failed to accelerate closure, although PDGF-BB markedly enhanced underlying granulation tissue formation. These results were surprising, in light of the expected synergy one might expect in using either two epithelial cell growth factors [KGF and epidermal growth factor (EGF)] signaling via different signal transaction pathways, or the combination of an epithelial and fibroblast/vascular stimulator (KGF and PDGF-BB) and the recognized contribution of a healthy granulation tissue bed toward promoting re-epithelialization. However, in light of no detectable synergism between these growth factors, perhaps the limiting variables within healing wounds require reevaluation (29).

KGF and the GI Tract

In situ hybridization and RNase protection studies in the embryonic and adult mouse and rat demonstrate the genes for KGF and the KGF receptor are expressed throughout the gastrointestinal system to varying degrees (12–14). This information as well as the data obtained from molecular and cellular studies in vitro demonstrate that KGF is synthesized mainly in stroma or mesenchyme and may function primarily as a paracrine growth factor for epithelial tissues of the gut. Thus, it was of interest to characterize KGF's activity when administered in vivo to adult animals.

Systemic treatment with rKGF produced striking changes in the gastrointestinal tract of rodents. Epithelial hyperplasia was induced in the pancreatic ductal system of adult rats (30). The first change observed after rKGF administration was the appearance of proliferating cells throughout the entire pancreatic ductal system within 24 hours after rKGF administration. This increase in proliferation was followed by histologic evidence of ductal epithelial cell proliferation mainly within the intralobular ducts adjacent to or within the islets of Langerhans. Of importance is the fact that these intralobular ducts, along with intercalated ducts, are thought to be the site of stem cells required both for regeneration of islet and acinar cell populations. rKGF is one of the first purified proteins known to induce pancreatic ductal epithelial proliferation in normal adult rats that have not undergone a preceding injury to the pancreas. The role of rKGF in regenerating islet cells postinjury is currently under investigation.

Recombinant KGF also has been demonstrated to elicit potent mitogenic and differentiative effects on specific epithelial tissues of the gastrointestinal system following in vivo administration of pharmacologic doses of rKGF to adult rats (12). The liver demonstrates a marked increase in hepatocyte proliferation peaking at one day post-rKGF administration. The proliferative index 24 hours post-rKGF is six- to eightfold higher than proliferation in the normal, quiescent, liver. This increase in proliferation is accompanied by an increase in liver weight as well. These results are consistent with findings obtained in cultured hepatocytes, which showed KGF could induce proliferation (31, 32).

Besides a stimulatory effect on hepatocyte mitogenesis, numerous serum parameters of liver function such as albumin, cholesterol, and triglycerides were significantly elevated in sera obtained from rKGF-treated animals (1 and 5 mg/kg/day, qd $\times$ 4) compared with control animals (12). In rats treated with 5 mg/kg/day rKGF, serum albumin and total protein were increased at 4 days and remained elevated through day 7, suggesting KGF accelerates hepatocyte differentiation following proliferation. A rapid increase of serum triglycerides and cholesterol beginning after 1 day of rKGF treatment indicated an influence on fat metabolism. The increased cholesterol levels were due to increased high- and low-density lipoprotein

(HDL and LDL) fractions (33). The serum transaminases, aspartate aminotransferase, and alanine aminotransferase were minimally elevated.

Because hepatocyte cell size did not change in treated animals, the increased liver weight was due primarily to a transient increase in the number of hepatocytes. However, because rKGF did not induce all hepatocytes to enter the cell cycle, the target cells could be a subpopulation that retains relatively more proliferative capacity, such as oval cells derived from a hepatic stem cell compartment (34). At day 7, mild biliary duct hyperplasia was present in animals treated with rKGF daily for 4 days. Finding bile duct hyperplasia and pancreatic ductal hyperplasia also in rKGF-treated rats is consistent with their shared lineage with hepatocyte precursors.

One day after a single intraperitoneal injection of rKGF, proliferation of epithelial cells was detected in the stomach, small intestine, and large intestine as well as the liver and pancreas. Daily treatment resulted in the marked selective induction of mucin-producing cell lineages throughout the GI tract in a dose-dependent fashion. Other cell lineages were either unaffected (e.g., Paneth cells), or relatively decreased (e.g., parietal cells) in rKGF-treated rats.

In the stomach, 1, 4, and 7 days of rKGF treatment induced a widening of the isthmus above the mucus neck cell layer, and numerous bromodeoxyuridine (BrdU) positive proliferating cells were visible. The isthmus above the mucus neck layer of the glandular stomach is the location of progenitor cells within the stomach. Following cell division, cells from this layer migrate upward, toward the gut lumen, to form mucin surface cells or downward, toward the serosal surface, to generate other differentiated cell types that occupy the gastric glands. By 4 and 7 days of rKGF treatment, increased numbers of gastric pit mucin-producing cells were detected throughout the glandular gastric mucosa. While rKGF promotes selective proliferation of mucus neck cells that move toward the lumen, it appears to induce a depletion of parietal cells, suggesting both cell types arise from the same multipotential lineage that responds to rKGF selectively. Animals treated with rKGF for 4 and 7 days had mildly elongated gastric glands and the depth of the mucous layer from the luminal surface of the gastric mucosa was also markedly increased after 4 and 7 days of rKGF treatment.

The small intestine of adult mice and rats treated with rKGF demonstrated markedly increased numbers of mucus-producing goblet cells within the proliferative crypt region and along the length of the villi after treatment. The duodenum, jejunum, and ileum regions were all affected by rKGF administration. Because the size or length of the villi within the small intestine were not increased in rKGF-treated rodents, this suggests that the transit time of mucin-positive cells in the villi may be accelerated by KGF treatment.

A dramatic increase in mucus-producing goblet cells throughout the proximal and distal colon was detected in rKGF-treated rats and mice. In control animals, the number of goblet cells decreased toward the luminal surface of colonic crypts, leaving only an occasional positive cell in the upper one-third of the crypt. In contrast, treated animals as early as 4 days showed marked increases in goblet cells in the upper one-half of the colonic crypts. By 7 days of treatment, the crypt lumen was obscured and appeared packed throughout the entire length of the crypt. Alcian blue and periodic acid-Schiff (PAS) staining yielded similar results, indicating that mucins induced by rKGF were qualitatively normal although markedly increased. Concomitant with these changes in cellular content, the net weight of the colon was increased in rKGF-treated rats. As with the effects on other organs, all the effects observed in the GI tract were entirely reversible by discontinuing KGF administration (12, 30, 35, 36).

Thus, rKGF is a uniquely potent inducer of proliferation and differentiation in specific lineages throughout the GI tract and suggests a role for KGF in normal maintenance of the gut. As has been observed in the lung, skin, pancreas, and male genital tract, selective stimulation of cell lineages by rKGF may yield new insights on stem cells, and differentiation processes within the gastrointestinal tract and liver as well.

Specific diseases where mucosal proliferation and/or mucin production in the gastrointestinal tract are limited, or states of liver hepatocyte or endocrine pancreas injury may be candidates for pharmacologic intervention with rKGF. In that regard, rKGF has been administered in several models of epithelial cell injury. In a model of acetic-acid–induced gastric mucosal injury in the rat, KGF demonstrated a modest effect on the area of the ulcer when measured at 10 to 24 days postinjury (37). In this model, therapy was begun on day 4 after injury when the ulcer size is at its maximum size and was continued until day 10. By delaying the initiation of therapy until injury is at its maximum, rKGF elicited its effects through accelerating epithelial repair. Other investigators have demonstrated KGF mRNA expression in the normal rat gastric submucosal and muscular layers that was not increased after an acute gastric mucosal injury induced with indomethecin (38). rKGF has also been tested for efficacy in a trinitrobenzene-induced experimental colitis model in rats (39). In this model, rKGF induced a 40% to 50% decrease in the macroscopic and microscopic ulceration induced in the colon when it was administered systematically for 1 week beginning 24 hours after colitis induction. KGF mRNA has also been demonstrated to be elevated in colonic tissue from patients with inflammatory bowel disease (40). Recently, rKGF has been found to prolong survival of mice if administered prior to chemotherapy and radiation (Farrell et al., personal communication). Taken together, these results suggest KGF may be therapeutically useful in treating diseases of the gut requiring epithelial regeneration.

KGF and the Lung

Because KGF was initially purified from a lung fibroblast line, lung epithelia was considered a potential paracrine target of the cytokine. Ulich and coworkers (35) administered KGF to normal rats via intratracheal administration, and saw a highly specific, transient burst of type II pneumocyte proliferation. The micropapillary epithelial proliferation within alveoli was shown by surfactant protein B immunohistochemistry and electron microscopy to consist of proliferating and differentiated type II pneumocytes. The effect of exogenous KGF treatment, as in the GI tract, was entirely reversible. Simultaneously, Panos and colleagues (41) demonstrated that KGF directly stimulates cultured type II pneumocytes, providing further support for the in vivo observations. Small brochiolar epithelium was also transiently stimulated by KGF treatment, while large airways were unaffected, consistent with the pattern of KGF receptor expression. In contrast to the GI tract, mucus-producing goblet cells of the lung were unaffected by KGF. Further studies have shown that KGF can ameliorate oxygen-induced injury to rat lungs (42), suggesting a potential clinical role in treating alveolar injury in premature infants and adults.

KGF and Other Epithelial Targets

Many normal tissues can respond to exogenous KGF, extending the hypothesis that endogenous KGF may play a role in normal epithelial tissue homeostasis. Systemic administration of KGF to normal adult rats results in a profound stimulation of ductal epithelium in the mammary glands of both male and nulliparous female animals (36). Ductal epithelium became stratified and markedly increased ductal arborization was detected. No lactational differentiation was found. In contrast, in mice KGF administration caused marked dilation of mammary ducts in addition to the focal ductal epithelial hyperplasia seen in rats (43). In mice, estrogen appeared to potentiate the effects of KGF. The cystic dilation of ducts seen in mice in response to KGF resembles fibrocystic disease in humans, and is fully reversible upon cessation of KGF treatment.

KGF is also a candidate andromedin. Cunha and coworkers (44, 45) have found that testosterone stimulates differentiation of fetal prostate and seminal vesicles via KGF synthesis by stromal cells in these organs. Thus KGF appears to be a major endogenous modulator of male sex organ differentiation in the newborn period (3, 45; reviewed in 46). KGF also appears to be a progestomedin in primate endometrium (47). KGF is induced by progesterone within stromal cells and vascular smooth muscle cells, suggesting it may stimulate adjacent endometrial glandular cells.

Recently, systemic KGF was found to stimulate proliferation of urothelium in the bladder, as well as the epithelial lining of the ureters and collecting tubules of the kidney by Yi and coworkers (48). High levels of KGF message were found in the underlying mesenchyme of the bladder wall, while KGF receptor expression was found in the epithelium of all three responsive tissues. These results suggest that a KGF antagonist might be of use in treating bladder cancer.

In the thymus, high levels of KGF receptor were localized by in situ hybridization to thymic nurse cells (49). These cells are epithelial in origin, and are thought to participate in the differentiation of T lymphocytes within the thymic milieu. Administration of KGF increases the number of nurse cells, and decreases cellularity of the thymic medulla. The functional significance of these changes has not yet been established. Activated $\gamma\delta$-T cells from skin and intestine express KGF in contrast to lymphoid $\gamma\delta$-T cells, which do not express this mitogen. This observation suggests a role for $\gamma\delta$-T cells in surveillance and/or repair of damaged epithelium (50).

Summary

Since its discovery in 1989, KGF has been found to have remarkable proliferative, differentiative, and cytoprotective effects on epithelial tissues in numerous organs. The widespread distribution of the ligand and its specific receptor, coupled with the response of many tissues in normal adult animals, suggests KGF has a role in normal homeostasis and epithelial cell turnover, in addition to its likely roles in embryonic development and specific disease states. While the mechanisms of action of KGF in each organ system are not fully understood, preclinical models have suggested several relevant clinical targets that may benefit from KGF treatment. In addition, the results suggest that specific antagonists of KGF may be of benefit in diseases of excess epithelial proliferation. For instance, psoriasis, which is caused by excess keratinocyte proliferation possibly due to growth factors released from infiltrating T lymphocytes, may respond to a KGF antagonist. Likewise, specific epithelial tumors bearing KGF receptors, such as breast, stomach, colon, kidney, and bladder, might be candidates for therapy that targeted KGF receptor bearing cells.

References

1. Rubin JS, Osada H, Finch PW, Taylor WG, Rudikoff S, Aaronson SA. Purification and characterization of a newly identified growth factor specific for epithelial cells. Proc Natl Acad Sci USA 1989;86:802–6.
2. Finch PW, Rubin JS, Miki T, Ron D, Aaronson SA. Human KGF is FGF-related with properties of a paracrine effector of epithelial cell growth. Science 1989;245:752–5.
3. Rubin JS, Bottaro DP, Chedid M, et al. Keratinocyte growth factor as a cytokine that mediates mesenchymal-epithelial interaction. In: Goldberg I,

Rosen E, eds. Epithelial-mesenchymal interactions in cancer. Basel/ Switzerland: Birkhauser Verlag: 1995.

4. Aaronson SA, Bottaro DP, Miki T, et al. Keratinocyte growth factor: a fibroblast growth factor family member with unusual target cell specificity. Ann NY Acad Sci 1991;638:62–77.

5. Miki T, Fleming TP, Bottaro DP, Rubin JS, Ron D, Aaronson SA. Expression cDNA cloning of the KGF receptor by creation of a transforming autocrine loop. Science 1991;251:72–5.

6. Hattori Y, Odagiri H, Nakatani H, et al. K-sam, an amplified gene in stomach cancer, is a member of the heparin-binding growth factor receptor genes. Proc Natl Acad Sci USA 1990;87:5983–7.

7. Bottaro DP, Rubin JS, Ron D, Finch PW, Florio C, Aaronson SA. Characterization of the receptor for keratinocyte growth factor: evidence for multiple fibroblast growth factor receptors. J Biol Chem 1990;265:126767–70.

8. Dell KR, Williams LT. A novel form of fibroblast growth factor receptor 2: alternative splicing of the third immunoglobulin-like domain confers ligand binding specificity. J Biol Chem 1992;267:21225–9.

9. Miki T, Bottaro DP, Fleming TP, et al. Determination of ligand-binding specificity by alternative splicing: two distinct growth factor receptors encoded by a single gene. Proc Natl Acad Sci USA 1992;89:246–50.

10. Bottaro DP, Fortney E. A keratinocyte growth factor receptor-derived peptide antagonist identifies part of the ligand binding site. J Biol Chem 1993; 268:9180–3.

11. Cheon HG, LaRochelle WJ, Bottaro DP, Burgess WH, Aaronson SA. High-affinity binding sites for related fibroblast growth factor ligands reside within different receptor immunoglobulin-like domains. Proc Natl Acad Sci USA 1994;91:989–93.

12. Housley RM, Morris CF, Boyle W, et al. Keratinocyte growth factor induces proliferation of hepatocytes and epithelial cells throughout the rat gastrointestinal tract. J Clin Invest 1994;94:1764–77.

13. Mason IJ, Fuller-Pace F, Smith R, Dickson C. FGF-7 (keratinocyte growth factor) expression during mouse development suggests roles in myogenesis, forebrain regionalisation and epithelial-mesenchymal interactions. Mech Dev 1994;45:15–30.

14. Finch PW, Cunha GR, Rubin JS, Wong J, Ron D. Pattern of keratinocyte growth factor and keratinocyte growth factor receptor expression during mouse fetal development suggests a role in mediating morphogenetic mesenchymal-epithelial interactions. Dev Dynamics 1995;203:223–40.

15. Orr-Urtreger A, Bedford MT, Burakova T, et al. Developmental localization of the splicing alternatives of fibroblast growth factor receptor-2 (FGFR2). Dev Biol 1993;158:475–86.

16. Werner S, Peters KG, Longaker MT, Fuller-Pace F, Banda MJ, Williams LT. Large induction of keratinocyte growth factor expression in the dermis during wound healing. Proc Natl Acad Sci USA 1992;89:6896–900.

17. Staiano-Coico L, Krueger JG, Rubin JS, et al. Human keratinocyte growth factor effects in a porcine model of epidermal wound healing. J Exp Med 1993;178:865–78.

18. Pierce GF, Yanagihara D, Klopchin K, et al. Stimulation of all epithelial elements during skin regeneration by keratinocyte growth factor. J Exp Med 1994;179:831–40.

19. Marchese C, Rubin J, Ron D, et al. Human keratinocyte growth factor activity on proliferation and differentiation of human keratinocytes: differentiation response distinguishes KGF from EGF family. J Cell Physiol 1990;144: 326–32.

20. Danilenko DM, Ring BD, Yanagihara D, et al. Keratinocyte growth factor is an important endogenous mediator and hair follicle growth, development and differentiation: influence in the nu/nu defect and chemotherapy-induced alopecia. Am J Pathol 1995;147:145–54.

21. Danilenko DM, Ring BD, Tarpley JE, et al. Growth factors in porcine full and partial thickness burn repair: differing targets and effects of keratinocyte growth factor, platelet-derived growth factor-BB, epidermal growth factor, and neu differentiation factor. Am J Pathol 1995;147:1261–77.

22. Chedid M, Rubin JS, Csaky KG, Aaronson SA. Regulation of keratinocyte growth factor gene expression by interleukin 1. J Biol Chem 1994;269:10752–67.

23. Brauchle M, Angermeyer K, Hübner G, Werner S. Large induction of keratinocyte growth factor expression by serum growth factors and pro-inflammatory cytokines in cultured fibroblasts. Oncogene 1994;9:3199–204.

24. Werner S, Breeden M, Hübner G, Greenhalgh DG, Longaker MT. Induction of keratinocyte growth factor expression is reduced and delayed during wound healing in the genetically diabetic mouse. J Invest Dermatol 1994;103:469–73.

25. Brauchle M, Fässler R, Werner S. Suppression of keratinocyte growth factor expression by glucocorticoids in vitro and during wound healing. J Invest Dermatol 1995;105:579–84.

26. Chedid M, Hoyle JR, Csaky KG, Rubin JS. Glucocorticoids inhibit keratinocyte growth factor production in primary dermal fibroblasts. Endocrinology 1996; 137:2232–7.

27. Werner S, Smola H, Liao X, et al. The function of KGF in morphogenesis of epithelium and reepithelialization of wounds. Science 1994;266:819–21.

28. Guo L, Degenstein L, Fuchs E. Keratinocyte growth factor is required for hair development but not for wound healing. Gene Dev 1996;10:165–75.

29. Mustoe TA, Pierce GF. Pharmacologic treatment of wounds. Annu Rev Med 1995;46:449–63.

30. Yi ES, Yin S, Harclerode DL, et al. Keratinocyte growth factor induces pancreatic ductal epithelial proliferation. Am J Pathol 1994;145:80–5.

31. Itoh T, Suzuki M, Mitsui Y. Keratinocyte growth factor as a mitogen for primary culture of rat hepatocytes. Biochem Biophys Res Commun 1993; 192:1011–15.

32. Strain AJ, McGuinnes G, Rubin JS, Aaronson SA. Keratinocyte growth factor and fibroblast growth factor action on DNA synthesis in rat and human hepatocytes: modulation by heparin. Exp Cell Res 1994;210:253–9.

33. Nonogaki K, Pan X-M, Moser AH, Staprans I, Feingold KR, Grunfeld C. Keratinocyte growth factor increases fatty acid mobilization and hepatic triglyceride secretion in rats. Endocrinology 1995;136:4278–84.

34. Thorgeirsson SS. Commentary: hepatic stem cells. Am J Pathol 1993; 142:1331–3.

35. Ulich TR, Yi ES, Longmuir K, et al. Keratinocyte growth factor is a growth factor for type II pneumocytes in vivo. J Clin Invest 1994;93:1298–306.

36. Ulich TR, Yi ES, Cardiff R, et al. Keratinocyte growth factor is a growth factor for mammary epithelium in vivo: the mammary epithelium of lactating rats are resistant to the proliferative action of KGF. Am J Pathol 1994;144:862–8.

37. Ohning GV, Guth PH. Keratinocyte growth factor promotes healing and acetic acid-induced gastric ulcers in rats. Gastroenterology 1994;106:A624(abstr).
38. Kinoshita Y, Nakata H, Hassan S, et al. Gene expression of keratinocyte and hepatocyte growth factors during the healing of rat gastric mucosal lesions. Gastroenterology 1995;109:1068–77.
39. Zeeh JM, Procaccino F, Hoffmann P, et al. Keratinocyte growth factor ameliorates mucosal injury in an experimental model of colitis in rats. Gastroenterology 1996;110:1077–83.
40. Finch PW, Pricolo V, Wu A, Finkelstein SD. Increased expression of keratinocyte growth factor messenger RNA associated with inflammatory bowel disease. Gastroenterology 1996;110:441–51.
41. Panos RJ, Rubin JS, Csaky KG, Aaronson SA, Mason RJ. Keratinocyte growth factor and hepatocyte growth factor/scatter factor are heparin-binding growth factors for alveolar type II cells in fibroblast-conditioned medium. J Clin Invest 1993;92:969–77.
42. Panos RJ, Bak PM, Simonet WS, Rubin JS, Smith LJ. Intratracheal instillation of keratinocyte growth factor decreases hyperoxia-induced mortality in rats. J Clin Invest 1995;96:2026–33.
43. Yi ES, Bedoya AA, Lee H, et al. Keratinocyte growth factor causes cystic dilation of the mammary glands of mice: interactions of keratinocyte growth factor, estrogen, and progesterone in vivo. Am J Pathol 1994;145:1015–22.
44. Cunha GR, Sugimura Y, Foster BA, Rubin JS, Aaronson SA. The role of growth factors in the development and growth of the prostrate and seminal vesicle. Biomed Pharmacother 1996;48(suppl 1):(in press).
45. Alarid ET, Rubin JS, Young P, et al. Keratinocyte growth factor functions in epithelial induction during seminal vesicle development. Proc Natl Acad Sci USA 1994;91:1074–8.
46. Yan G, Fukabori Y, Nikolaropoulos S, Wang F, McKeehan WL. Heparin-binding keratinocyte growth factor is a candidate stromal-to-epithelial-cell andromedin. Mol Endocrinol 1992;6:2123–8.
47. Koji T, Chedid M, Rubin JS, et al. Progesterone-dependent expression of keratinocyte growth factor mRNA in stromal cells of the primate endometrium: keratinocyte growth factor as a progestomedin. J Cell Biol 1994;125:393–401.
48. Yi ES, Shabaik AS, Lacey DL, et al. Keratinocyte growth factor causes proliferation of urothelium in vivo. J Urol 1995;154:1566–70.
49. Danilenko DM, Ring BD, Trebasky LD, et al. Keratinocyte growth factor alters thymocyte development via stimulation of thymic epithelial cells. FASEB J 1996;10:A1148(abstr).
50. Boismenu R, Havran WL. Modulation of epithelial cell growth by intraepithelial γδ T cells. Science 1994;266:1253–6.

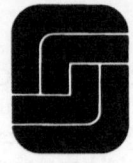

18

Hepatocyte Growth Factor

DONALD P. BOTTARO, VITTORIA CIOCE, ANDREW M.-L. CHAN,
DAVID H. ADAMS, AND JEFFREY S. RUBIN

Hepatocyte growth factor (HGF) was originally detected in the circulation
of hepatectomized animals on the basis of its ability to stimulate hepatocyte
proliferation in another animal with an intact liver (1–3). It was purified
from serum, plasma, or blood platelets in the form of a disulfide-linked
heterodimer of ~60-kd heavy (alpha) and ~32-kd light (beta) polypeptide
chains (1–3). HGF was independently isolated from the conditioned medium of cultured fibroblasts based on its mitogenic activity on a variety of
cellular targets (4), or its ability to stimulate the dispersion of epithelial and
vascular endothelial cells (5–7). These sources yielded a ~90-kd monomeric
polypeptide that copurified with the aforementioned heterodimer (4–6).
Analysis of these polypeptides and subsequent molecular cloning and
recombinant expression of HGF revealed that it was synthesized and
secreted in the monomeric ~90-kd form (4), and proteolytically converted
to the disulfide-linked heterodimer. Several laboratories have shown that
proteolytic conversion of the monomeric precursor to the heterodimer,
which can occur in situ, is required for biologic activity (8–10). The strong
affinity of HGF for heparin was exploited as a major enrichment step in
many of the purification schemes (1–6, 11), and the interaction between
HGF and this ubiquitous extracellular matrix component may play an
important role in HGF sequestration and signaling, as has been demonstrated for members of the fibroblast growth factor family (reviewed in 12).

Structural and Biologic Properties

Oligonucleotide probes based on HGF amino acid sequence were used to
obtain cDNA clones from placental (13), liver (14), and fibroblast libraries
(4, 15). Analysis of these clones revealed a single open reading frame
encoding a 728 amino acid molecule with a striking sequence similarity to
plasminogen: 38% overall amino acid identity, conservation of repeated

kringle motifs (~80 amino acids containing a characteristic set of three internal disulfide bonds), and a serine protease-like domain (4, 13, 14). HGF has four kringle domains, while plasminogen has five; all of these kringles are roughly 40% to 50% identical to each other. The serine protease-like region of HGF differs from that of plasminogen at two of the three amino acids required for catalysis (14), and HGF appears to lack proteolytic activity.

HGF stimulates DNA synthesis and/or the proliferation of hepatocytes (1-3), biliary epithelial cells (16), mammary epithelial cells (4), kerati-nocytes (4), renal tubular epithelial cells (4, 17), melanocytes and melanoma cells (4, 18), and vascular endothelial cells (4). HGF also supports the proliferation and differentiation of myeloid progenitor cells from bone marrow (19), and the differentiation of the promyelocyte leukemia cell, HL-60, into granulocyte-like cells (20). "Scatter activity" was first charac-terized using Madin-Darby canine kidney (MDCK) cells, which do not proliferate in response to HGF treatment (21). These polygonal epithelial cells normally form tightly adherent colonies in culture, but are dispersed as single cells in the presence of HGF and acquire a spiky, fibroblastoid phenotype. Primary mammary epithelial cells (21), several carcinoma cell lines (6), as well as vascular endothelial cells (7) also respond to HGF by changes in cell shape and motility, in some cases in addition to a proliferative response.

When grown in collagen gels, MDCK cells form organized tubular structures in response to HGF (22). HGF stimulates the formation of similar structures by epithelial carcinoma cells, and activated HGF recep-tors have been observed on the luminal surface of cells forming these structures both in vitro and in sections of whole breast tissue (23). HGF also has been reported to induce angiogenesis in vivo (24, 25). The pleiotropic effects of HGF, and the temporal and spatial distribution of its expression, suggest that it may be an important mediator of both mesenchymal-epithelial interaction and interconversion (reviewed in 26). The morpho-logic changes that accompany cell scattering and tubular morphogenesis in vitro have been compared to epithelial-mesenchymal transitions that occur during development when cell migration is required (27). Alternatively, fibroblasts overexpressing HGF and its receptor appear to undergo me-senchymal to epithelial conversion when injected into nude mice (23). Other studies, examining the coexpression of HGF and its receptor during development and/or testing the effects of added HGF or antibodies against HGF in model systems, implicate this pathway in the development of several organs including kidney, liver, and spleen (26).

The fundamental role of HGF in early development has been evaluated by studying the effects of targeted disruption of the HGF gene (28, 29). Mice lacking the HGF gene were smaller than normal, showed abnormal development of several organs, and died in utero. Two organs affected most noticeably were liver and placenta. Reduction in liver mass was noted between embryonic days 12 and 15; he liver structure appeared to be disrupted by enlarged sinusoidal spaces and dissociation of the parenchymal cells, which showed obvious signs of apoptosis (28). The most striking placental abnormality was a marked reduction in the number of labyrinthine trophoblast cells (29). The growth of trophoblast cells was stimulated by HGF in vitro, and HGF activity was produced by primary cultures of allantoic fibroblasts from normal but not mutant embryos. These observations suggest that HGF mediates interactions between allantoic mesenchyme and trophoblastic epithelia that are required for placental organogenesis (29).

In the adult, HGF may participate in differentiation associated with tissue renewal, in cell growth associated with wound healing, and possibly in the onset and progression of cancer. Coexpression of HGF and its receptor in fibroblasts can confer tumorigenicity when these cells are injected into mice (30), and HGF stimulates the motility and invasiveness of carcinoma cells (31). HGF is angiogenic, and thus may contribute to the growth and metastasis of solid tumors (25). Overexpression of HGF and/or its receptor occurs in a variety of tumors, and a high level of HGF in primary breast tumors is a strong, independent predictor of relapse and death (32). HGF produced by normal stromal cells can stimulate adjacent tumor tissue in a paracrine manner, and tumor factors may enhance this mesenchymal-epithelial interaction abnormally (31, 33). It is by no means clear, however, that HGF expression inevitably leads to tumor progression; HGF also has cytotoxic or growth-inhibitory properties in some situations (20, 34). Cytotoxic effects were potent on certain mouse sarcoma cell lines, but more modest on a few human carcinoma cell lines (20). HGF inhibits the proliferation of several gastric and hepatocellular carcinomas in culture, although there are other examples of these tumor cell types that respond positively to the factor (35, 36). While the mechanisms underlying these divergent effects are not understood, similar phenomena have been reported for other growth regulators such as transforming growth factor-β (35).

Although HGF is generally considered as a mesenchymally derived factor with epithelial targets, it also has mesenchymal targets, including lymphocytes (37), chondrocytes (38), and peripheral blood T-cells (39). HGF is released from cells involved in inflammation and wound repair, including platelets, monocytes, and fibroblasts (1, 4, 40). HGF can enhance both neutrophil and B-lymphocyte functions (37, 41), and can stimulate motility in cultured monocytes (34). HGF has also been detected on the surface of vascular endothelial cells in vivo (42), presumably immobilized by heparin-like proteoglycans in the extracellular matrix. HGF was found to stimulate the chemokinetic migration of resting human T-cells through polycarbonate membranes when present in solution or when immobilized by heparan sulfate proteoglycan (39). HGF acted within seconds, and with equal or greater potency than other T-cell chemokines such as interleukin-6 (IL-6),

IL-8 and macrophage inflammatory protein-1β (39). Concomitantly, HGF triggered integrin-mediated adhesion to fibronectin, dramatic cytoskeletal rearrangement and actin polymerization, and the tyrosyl-phosphorylation of intracellular proteins (39). Thus HGF, released at a wound site by infiltrating inflammatory cells and immobilized by heparin-like proteoglycan present on the endothelial surface, might in turn recruit passing lymphocytes by activating T-cell integrins and initiating T-cell adhesion and subsequent migration into tissue.

HGF Receptors

The binding of HGF to immobilized heparin proteoglycan (HPG) is likely to profoundly influence the deposition, availability, and biological signaling of HGF (21, 43, 44). Although initially exploited as a means of affinity purification, the affinity of growth factors for HPG has become increasingly important in understanding how, when, and where heparin-binding growth factors will act; the fibroblast growth factors (FGFs) serve as a model in this regard. HPG serves as a reservoir of FGF storage; FGF bound to HPG in the extracellular matrix is protected from proteolytic cleavage and thermal breakdown (reviewed in 12). FGF delivery is thus controlled at several levels: protein synthesis, secretion, or by enzymatic turnover of the extracellular matrix. Finally, the interaction of FGFs with tyrosine-kinase cell surface receptors, and subsequent FGF signaling, is modulated by (or may even require) simultaneous interaction with HPG (12). Several parallels between the FGFs and HGF can already be made: HGF can be retained in the extracellular matrix in a biologically active form (39). The mitogenic effects of HGF on epithelial and endothelial cells can be blocked by the addition of soluble heparin in vitro (4), while in primary hepatocytes enhanced HGF potency has been reported (43, 45). HPG has not been shown to be required for HGF signaling, but all known biologically active forms of HGF bind HPG, and research aimed at identifying the structural determinants of HGF/HPG interactions may be the first step toward an accurate assessment of the biologic significance of HPG and HGF signaling.

HGF binds with high affinity to the c-Met proto-oncogene product (46, 47). The *met* oncogene was originally identified in a chemical carcinogen-treated human osteogenic sarcoma cell line by NIH 3T3 transfection analysis (48). Its cloning revealed that the oncogene encoded a truncated tyrosine kinase activated by chromosomal rearrangement (49). While the oncogene product is predominantly a cytosolic kinase, the proto-oncogene product is a transmembrane receptor-like protein composed of disulfide-linked 50-kd α- and 145-kd β-subunits (50). In the fully processed Met product, the α-subunit is extracellular, and the β-subunit has extracellular, transmembrane and tyrosine kinase domains as well as sites of tyrosine phosphorylation (51, 52). HGF binding results in the rapid autophosphorylation and activation of the intracellular catalytic domain of this enzyme. Several subsequent intracellular events have been characterized that are likely to constitute portions of intracellular HGF signaling pathways (reviewed in 53). Several studies have demonstrated that Met is required for most known HGF biological effects (47). Thus, the variety of HGF responses may reflect cell-specific differences in the expression of signal transduction pathway components downstream of the receptor itself.

In at least one case, however, HGF effects may be mediated by another, yet undiscovered receptor: evidence of Met expression in biologically responsive T-cells could not be demonstrated by immunoblotting, Northern blotting, or polymerase chain reaction (PCR) analysis (39). A Met-related receptor-like molecule, the c-Sea proto-oncogene product, is expressed by circulating lymphocytes in chickens (54, 55), and this molecule is strikingly similar to the receptor for human macrophage-stimulating protein (MSP), an HGF-related cytokine (see below; 56). Evidence presented in the latter study, however, suggests that HGF does not interact with the MSP receptor. Clearly more research is needed to clarify the ligand-binding characteristics of known Met receptor-like molecules and/or identify other, yet uncharacterized molecules that might mediate the potent biologic effects of HGF on T cells.

Isoforms and Related Molecules

Northern blot analysis and comparison of different HGF cDNA clones demonstrated the existence of multiple mRNA transcripts with lengths of 6, 3, 2, and 1.3 kd (4). The 6- and 3-kb transcripts each specify transcripts that either contain or lack a 15-bp stretch encoding the 5 amino acids FLPSS in the first HGF kringle domain (4). The resulting variant HGF isoforms of 728 and 723 amino acids exhibit comparable mitogenic, scattering, and cytotoxic activities, although quantitative differences have been reported (57). Whether these variants have any unique biologic functions remains to be elucidated.

The presence of the 1.3-kb transcript was associated with the expression of a smaller molecule that was immunologically cross-reactive with HGF (58). This transcript was recognized by oligonucleotide probes derived from HGF heavy chain, but not light chain, sequences. Based on this pattern of hybridization, cDNA clones corresponding to the 1.3-kb transcript were isolated and nucleotide sequencing revealed that it encoded a protein extending from the HGF signal peptide sequence to the end of the second kringle domain, followed by an additional three amino acids, a termination codon, and a distinct 3'-untranslated sequence (58). The 1.3-kb transcript is produced by the alternative splicing of a kringle 2 exon with an exon having an in-frame termination signal, rather than a portion of the kringle 3 sequence (13, 58).

This truncated HGF isoform, designated HGF/NK2, was purified from conditioned medium of a human tumor cell line that expressed relatively high levels of the 1.3-kb transcript (58). HGF/NK2 lacked mitogenic activity on either a normal cultured mammary epithelial cells or melanocytes, but it specifically blocked HGF mitogenic activity when present at a tenfold molar excess (58). It has been reported to have scattering activity, although with only ~3% the potency of full-length HGF (59). Covalent affinity cross-linking experiments with [125I]-HGF/NK2 demonstrated that it and HGF bound specifically to the same high-affinity cell surface receptor, the c-Met protein (58, 59). A survey of several different cell lines suggests that the physiologic impact of HGF in vivo may be transcriptionally regulated by varying the expression of full-length HGF, and by alternative splicing to generate its own competitive antagonist (58). A similar hypothesis has been proposed to explain alternative splicing of transcripts from the acidic fibroblast growth factor gene (60).

The 2-kb HGF transcript also encodes a truncated form of HGF (61). The cDNA clone was isolated by the same strategy used to isolate the HGF/NK2 transcript, and encoded 210 amino acids consisting of the HGF signal peptide, amino-terminal, and first kringle domains (61). This isoform, designated HGF/NK1, terminated immediately downstream of kringle 1 and included two additional amino acids and a stop codon not found in the corresponding region of HGF. Recombinantly expressed HGF/NK1 protein bound to immobilized heparin similar to full-length HGF, but exhibited unique biological properties (61). Unlike HGF/NK2, HGF/NK1 showed mitogenic activity on cultured mammary epithelial cells, although it was less potent than HGF itself. Interestingly, the maximal mitogenic activity of HGF could not be attained with HGF/NK1 at any dose, and HGF/NK1 partially blocked HGF-stimulated DNA synthesis when present in 40-fold molar excess. HGF/NK1 could also stimulate cell scattering, although with ~50-fold lower potency than HGF (61). All of the known HGF isoforms appear to bind and induce the autophosphorylation of the c-Met receptor-kinase. Subtle differences in receptor phosphorylation, and in downstream events relevant to biologic signaling, may account for the distinct biologic responses elicited by these different ligands.

Another molecule related to HGF, but encoded by a different gene, was cloned from a genomic library by hybridization with a cDNA probe encoding the kringle domains of prothrombin under reduced stringency conditions (62). The predicted protein sequence of 711 amino acids included a signal peptide and an internal proteolytic processing site that would yield a disulfide-linked heterodimer. Like HGF, the amino-terminal chain contained four kringle domains while the carboxy-terminal portion had serine protease structure but lacked an intact catalytic triad. The complete amino acid sequence is approximately 50% identical to that of HGF (62). Similar to the convergence of research that led to the identity of HGF and scatter factor, this HGF-like protein was found to be identical to MSP (56). MSP was purified from human plasma and makes resident peritoneal macrophages capable of responding to the chemoattractant complement component C5a, and it causes marked macrophage spreading and morphologic changes in vitro (56). These observations link MSP to activation of the C3b receptor (CR1) of peritoneal macrophages and cultured human blood monocytes, which has been implicated in host defense against microbial pathogens, cellular injury in immune complex disease, and the destruction of neoplastic cells (56).

Interestingly enough, MSP binds and activates a cell surface molecule that closely resembles the c-Met proto-oncogene product (63, 64). The cDNA encoding the MSP receptor, designated Ron, was obtained by screening several libraries with oligonucleotide probes coding for highly conserved sequences of protein tyrosine kinase genes (65). Among known tyrosine kinases, Ron is most closely related to Met an a chicken proto-oncogene product known as c-Sea (55, 65). Despite the sequence similarity between Ron and Sea, it remains uncertain as to whether Ron represents the human homologue of the chicken Sea protein (65).

The v-*sea* oncogene was isolated from the S13 avian erythroblastosis retrovirus, which produces a syndrome characterized by sarcomas, erythroblastosis, and anemias, and encoded a tyrosine kinase fused in frame with the viral envelope gene, resulting in the expression of a cell surface tyrosine kinase molecule resembling an unregulated growth factor receptor (54, 55). The c-*sea* counterpart encodes a membrane spanning, tyrosine kinase receptor expressed in peripheral white blood cell populations and in the intestine, with ~34% overall amino acid identity to human Met, and ~46% overall identity to human Ron (54–66). In addition to conserved sequence in their intracellular tyrosine kinase domains, both Ron and Sea share similarities with Met in the structural organization and processing of their extracellular domains, including conserved cysteine residues and proteolytic cleavage of the nascent monomer into mature α- and β-subunits (55, 63, 64). Identification of the Sea ligand and further investigation of the possible interactions between HGF-related and Met-related molecules should broaden our perspective of the overall importance of these molecular families in normal development, homeostasis, and disease.

Potential Clinical Relevance

The expression of HGF and its receptor (reviewed in 53) in a variety of organs both during development and in the adult suggests a wide range of effects and possible applications. Serum HGF levels appear to have prognostic value in monitoring fulminant hepatic failure (67). In view of HGF induction in models of liver injury (68, 69) and elevated circulating levels in conditions characterized by active liver regeneration (70), systemic administration of HGF may augment the rate of hepatocyte proliferation and reduce liver damage in some instances of liver injury (71). Similarly, the correlation of HGF induction with the compensatory hypertrophic response to unilateral nephrectomy suggests that HGF may contribute to repair in the kidney (72). In addition to stimulating the proliferation of parenchymal cells, HGF may foster wound healing by promoting angiogenesis (24, 25). The ability of HGF to stimulate endothelial cell migration, proliferation, and tubular morphogenesis might be particularly useful when angiogenesis is compromised by an underlying disease. Alternatively, the potential contribution of HGF to neovascularization associated with pathologic conditions like diabetic retinopathy might be selectively blocked by the administration of antagonists, such as HGF/NK2.

Blocking the HGF signaling pathway may also be a useful adjunct to conventional cancer therapy. HGF receptor overexpression has been documented in carcinomas of the lung, pancreas, thyroid, colon, and stomach (53). Half of all thyroid follicular carcinomas examined exhibited as much as a 100-fold increase in c-Met protein, and were associated with a poor prognosis (73). A high frequency of c-*met* gene amplification was observed in scirrhous-type stomach cancer (74), and the oncogenic *tpr-met* rearrangement was identified in cell lines derived from other gastric carcinomas and in premalignant gastric lesions (75). Based on its ability to stimulate certain epithelial cells to invade collagen gels (6) or grow in soft agar (76), HGF is suspected of promoting tumor expansion and metastasis in certain settings. Autocrine expression of HGF and Met has been observed in some sarcomas, and appears to confer an enhanced metastatic potential (77, 78). The detection of HGF in malignant pleural effusions associated with primary lung, mesothelial, and breast malignancies is consistent with a role for this molecule neoplasia (79). Paradoxically, the cytotoxic effects of HGF for certain tumor cells in vitro suggest the possibility that some tumors might regress following HGF treatment.

The widespread and pleiotropic effects of HGF that occur throughout development and adulthood underscore the fundamental importance of HGF signaling pathways. In light of this it is not surprising that the expression, availability, and cellular responses to HGF are regulated at several levels. As a consequence of this complexity, the contribution of HGF in various systems, and the outcome of artificially modulating HGF pathways therapeutically, are not easily predicted. Gaining a better understanding of the regulatory mechanisms, signal transduction events, and the structure-function relationships that govern HGF actions are important goals that may lead ultimately to the successful application of this knowledge to complex clinical problems.

References

1. Nakamura T, Nawa K, Ichihara A, Kaise N, Nishino T. Purification and subunit structure of hepatocyte growth factor from rat platelets. FEBS Lett 1987;224:311–6.

2. Gohda E, Tsubouchi H, Nakayama H, et al. Purification and partial characterization of hepatocyte growth factor from plasma of a patient with fulminant hepatic failure. J Clin Invest 1988;81:414–9.
3. Zarnegar R, Michalopoulos G. Purification and biological characterization of human hepatopoietin A, a polypeptide growth factor for hepatocytes. Cancer Res 1989;49:3314–20.
4. Rubin JS, Chan AM, Bottaro DP, et al. A broad-spectrum human lung fibroblast-derived mitogen is a variant of hepatocyte growth factor. Proc Natl Acad Sci USA 1991;88:415–9.
5. Gherardi E, Gray J, Stoker M, Perryman M, Furlong R. Purification of scatter factor, a fibroblast-derived basic protein that modulates epithelial interactions and movement. Proc Natl Acad Sci USA 1989;86:5844–8.
6. Weidner KM, Behrens J, Vandekerckhove J, Birchmeier W. Scatter factor: molecular characteristics and effect on the invasiveness of epithelial cells. J Cell Biol 1990;111:2097–108.
7. Rosen EM, Meromsky L, Goldberg I, Bhargava M, Setter E. Studies on the mechanism of scatter factor. Effects of agents that modulate intracellular signal transduction, macromolecular synthesis and cytoskeleton assembly. J Cell Sci 1990;96:639–49.
8. Naka D, Ishii T, Yoshiyama Y, et al. Activation of hepatocyte growth factor by proteolytic conversion of a single chain form to a heterodimer. J Biol Chem 1992;267:20114–9.
9. Gak E, Taylor WG, Chan AM, Rubin JS. Processing of hepatocyte growth factor to the heterodimeric form is required for biological activity. FEBS Lett 1992;311:17–21.
10. Naldini L, Tamagnone L, Vigna E, et al. Extracellular proteolytic cleavage by urokinase is required for activation of hepatocyte growth factor/scatter factor. EMBO J 1992;11:4825–33.
11. Rosen EM, Goldberg ID, Kacinski BM, Buckholz T, Vinter DM. Smooth muscle releases an epithelial cell scatter factor which binds to heparin. In Vitro Cell Dev Biol 1989;25:163–73.
12. Rapraeger AC, Giumond S, Krufka A, Olwin BB. Regulation by heparan sulfate in fibroblast growth factor signaling. Methods Enzymol 1994;245:219–40.
13. Miyazawa K, Tsubouchi H, Naka D, et al. Molecular cloning and sequence analysis of cDNA for human hepatocyte growth factor. Biochem Biophys Res Commun 1989;163:967–73.
14. Nakamura T, Nishizawa T, Hagiya M, et al. Molecular cloning and expression of human hepatocyte growth factor. Nature 1989;342:440–3.
15. Weidner KM, Arakaki N, Hartmann G, et al. Evidence for the identity of human scatter factor and human hepatocyte growth factor. Proc Natl Acad Sci USA 1991;88:7001–5.
16. Joplin R, Hishida T, Tsubouchi H, et al. Human intrahepatic biliary epithelial cells proliferate in vitro in response to human hepatocyte growth factor. J Clin Invest 1992;90:1284–9.
17. Igawa T, Kanda S, Kanetake H, et al. Hepatocyte growth factor is a potent mitogen for cultured rabbit renal tubular epithelial cells. Biochem Biophys Res Commun 1991;174:831–8.
18. Halaban R, Rubin JS, Funasaka Y, et al. Met and hepatocyte growth factor/scatter factor signal transduction in normal melanocytes and melanoma cells. Oncogene 1992;7:2195–206.

19. Kmiecik TE, Keller JR, Rosen E, Vande Woude GF. Hepatocyte growth factor is a synergistic factor for the growth of hematopoietic progenitor cells. Blood 1992;80:2454–7.
20. Shima N, Itagaki Y, Nagao M, Yasuda H, Morinaga T, Higashio K. A fibroblast-derived tumor cytotoxic factor/F-TCF (hepatocyte growth factor/HGF) has multiple functions in vitro. Cell Biol Int Rep 1991;15:397–408.
21. Stoker M, Perryman M. An epithelial scatter factor released by embryo fibroblasts. J Cell Sci 1985;77:209–23.
22. Montesano R, Schaller G, Orci L. Induction of epithelial tubular morphogenesis in vitro by fibroblast-derived soluble factors. Cell 1991;66:697–711.
23. Tsarfaty I, Resau JH, Rulong S, Keydar I, Faletto DL, Vande Woude GF. The met proto-oncogene receptor and lumen formation. Science 1992;257:1258–61.
24. Bussolino F, Di Renzo MF, Ziche M, et al. Hepatocyte growth factor is a potent angiogenic factor which stimulates endothelial cell motility and growth. J Cell Biol 1992;119:629–41.
25. Grant DS, Kleinman HK, Goldberg ID, et al. Scatter factor induces blood vessel formation in vivo. Proc Natl Acad Sci USA 1993;90:1937–41.
26. Rosen EM, Nigam SK, Goldberg ID. Scatter Factor and the c-Met receptor: a paradigm for mesenchymal/epithelial interaction. J Cell Biol 1994;127:1783–7.
27. Thiery JP, Duband JL, Tucker GC. Cell migration in the vertebrate embryo: role of cell adhesion and tissue environment in pattern formation. Annu Rev Cell Biol 1985;1:91–113.
28. Schmidt C, Bladt F, Goedecke S, et al. Scatter factor/hepatocyte growth factor is essential for liver development. Nature 1995;373:699–702.
29. Uehara Y, Minowa O, Mori C, et al. Placental defect and embryonic lethality in mice lacking hepatocyte growth factor/scatter factor. Nature 1995;373:702–5.
30. Rong S, Bodescot M, Blair D, et al. Tumorigenicity of themet proto-oncogene and the gene for hepatocyte growth factor. Mol Cell Biol 1992;12:5152–8.
31. Rosen EM, Knesel J, Goldberg ID, et al. Scatter factor modulates the metastatic phenotype of the EMT6 mouse mammary tumor. Int J Cancer 1994;57:706–14.
32. Yamashita J, Ogawa M, Yamashita S, et al. Immunoreactive hepatocyte growth factor is a strong and independent predictor of recurrence and survival in human breast cancer. Cancer Res 1994;54:1630–3.
33. Seslar MA, Nakamura T, Byers SW. Regulation of fibroblast hepatocyte growth factor/scatter factor expression by human breast carcinoma cell lines and peptide growth factors. Cancer Res 1993;53:1233–8.
34. Tajima H, Matsumoto K, Nakamura T. Regulation of cell growth and motility by hepatocyte growth factor and receptor expression in various cell species. Exp Cell Res 1992;202:423–31.
35. Shibamoto S, Hayakawa M, Hori T, et al. Hepatocyte growth factor and transforming growth factor-beta stimulate both cell growth and migration of human gastric adenocarcinoma cells. Cell Struct Funct 1992;17:185–90.
36. Shiota G, Rhoads DB, Wang TC, Nakamura T, Schmidt EV. Hepatocyte growth factor inhibits growth of hepatocellular carcinoma cells. Proc Natl Acad Sci USA 1992;89:373–7.
37. Delaney B, Koh WS, Yang KH, Strom SC, Kaminski NE. Hepatocyte growth factor enhances B-cell activity. Life Sci 1993;53:PL89–93.
38. Takebayashi T, Iwamoto M, Jikko A, et al. Hepatocyte growth factor/scatter factor modulates cell motility, proliferation, and proteoglycan synthesis of chondrocytes. J Cell Biol 1995;129:1411–9.

39. Adams DH, Harvath L, Bottaro DP, et al. Hepatocyte growth factor and macrophage inflammatory protein 1B: structurally distinct cytokines that induce rapid cytoskeletal changes and subset-perferential migration in T-cells. Proc Natl Acad Sci USA 1994;91:7144-8.
40. Seki T, Ihara I, Sugimura A, et al. Isolation and expression of cDNA for different forms of hepatocyte growth factor from human leukocyte. Biochem Biophys Res Commun 1990;172:321-7.
41. Jiang W, Puntis MC, Nakamura T, Hallett MB. Neutrophil priming by hepatocyte growth factor, a novel cytokine. Immunology 1992;77:147-9.
42. Wolf HK, Zarnegar R, Michalopoulos GK. Localization of hepatocyte growth factor in human and rat tissues: an immunohistochemical study. Hepatology 1991;14:488-94.
43. Naka D, Ishii T, Shimomura T, Hishida T, Hara H. Heparin modulates the receptor-binding and mitogenic activity of hepatocyte growth factor on hepatocytes. Exp Cell Res 1993;209:317-24.
44. Arakaki N, Hirono S, Ishii T, et al. Identification and partial characterization of two classes of receptors for human hepatocyte growth factor on adult rat hepatocytes in primary culture. J Biol Chem 1992;267:7101-7.
45. Zioncheck TF, Richardson L, Liu J, et al. Sulfated oligosaccharides promote hepatocyte growth factor association and govern its mitogenic activity. J Biol Chem 1995;270:16871-8.
46. Bottaro DP, Rubin JS, Faletto DL, et al. Identification of the hepatocyte growth factor receptor as the c-met proto-oncogene product. Science 1991; 251:802-4.
47. Weidner KM, Sachs M, Birchmeier W. The Met receptor tyrosine kinase transduces motility, proliferation, and morphogenic signals of scatter factor/ hepatocyte growth factor in epithelial cells. J Cell Biol 1993;121:145-54.
48. Cooper CS, Park M, Blair DG, et al. Molecular cloning of a new transforming gene from a chemically transformed human cell line. Nature 1984;311:29-33.
49. Park M, Dean M, Cooper CS, et al. Mechanism of met oncogene activation. Cell 1986;45:895-904.
50. Park M, Dean M, Kaul K, Braun MJ, Gonda MA, Vande Woude G. Sequence of MET protooooncogene cDNA has features characteristic of the tyrosine kinase family of growth-factor receptors. Proc Natl Acad Sci USA 1987;84:6379-83.
51. Giordano S, Di Renzo MF, Narsimhan RP, Cooper CS, Rosa C, Comoglio PM. Biosynthesis of the protein encoded by the c-met proto-oncogene. Oncogene 1989;4:1383-8.
52. Ferracini R, Longati P, Naldini L, Vigna E, Comoglio PM. Identification of the major autophosphorylation site of the Met/hepatocyte growth factor receptor tyrosine kianse. J Biol Chem 1991;266:19558-64.
53. Rubin JS, Bottaro DP, Aaronson SA. Hepatocyte growth factor/scatter factor and its receptor, the c-met proto-oncogene product. Biochim Biophys Acta 1993;1155:357-71.
54. Hayman MJ, Kitchener G, Vogt PK, Beug H. The putative transforming protein of S13 avian erythroblastosis virus is a transmembrane glycoprotein with an associated protein kinase activity. Proc Natl Acad Sci USA 1985;82:8237-41.
55. Huff JL, Jelinek MA, Borgman CA, Lansing TJ, Parsons JT. The protoooncogene c-sea encodes a transmembrane protein-tyrosine kinase related to the Met/hepatocyte growth factor/scatter factor receptor. Proc Natl Acad Sci USA 1993;90:6140-4.

56. Skeel A, Yoshimura T, Showalter SD, Tanaka S, Appella E, Leonard EJ. Macrophage stimulating protein: purification, partial amino acid sequence, and cellular activity. J Exp Med 1991;173:1227–34.
57. Furlong RA, Takehara T, Taylor WG, Nakamura T, Rubin JS. Comparison of biological and immunochemical properties indicates that scatter factor and hepatocyte growth factor are indistinguishable. J Cell Sci 1991;100:173–7.
58. Chan AM, Rubin JS, Bottaro DP, Hirschfield DW, Chedid M, Aaronson SA. Identification of a competitive HGF antagonist encoded by an alternative transcript. Science 1991;254:1382–5.
59. Hartmann G, Naldini L, Weidner KM, et al. A functional domain in the heavy chain of scatter factor/hepatocyte growth factor binds the c-Met receptor and induces cell dissociation but not mitogenesis. Proc Natl Acad Sci USA 1992;89:11574–8.
60. Yu YL, Kha H, Golden JA, Migchielsen AA, Goetzl EJ, Turck CW. An acidic fibroblast growth factor protein generated by alternate splicing acts like an anatogonist. J Exp Med 1992;175:1073–80.
61. Cioce V, Casky KG, Chan AM-L, et al. HGF/NK1 is a naturally occurring HGF/SF variant with partial agonist/antagonist activity. J Biol Chem 1996; in press.
62. Han S, Stuart LA, Degen SJ. Characterization of the DNF15S2 locus on human chromosome 3: identification of a gene coding for four kringle domains with homology to hepatocyte growth factor. Biochemistry 1991;30:9768–80.
63. Gaudino G, Follenzi A, Naldini L, et al. Ron is a heterodimeric tyrosine kinase receptor activated by the HGF homologue MSP. EMBO J 1994;13:3524–32.
64. Wang M-H, Skeel A, Leonard EJ, et al. Identification of the Ron gene product as the receptor for the human macrophage stimulating protein. Science 1994; 266:117–9.
65. Ronsin C, Muscatelli F, Mattei MG, Breathnach R. A novel putative receptor protein tyrosine kinase of the met family. Oncogene 1993;8:1195–202.
66. Smith DR, Vogt PK, Hayman MJ. The v-sea oncogene of avian erythroblastosis retrovirus S13: another member of the protein-tyrosine kinase gene family. Proc Natl Acad Sci USA 1989;86:5291–5.
67. Tsubouchi H, Kawakami S, Hirono S, et al. Prediction of outcome in fulminant hepatic failure by serum human hepatocyte growth factor [letter]. Lancet 1992;340:307.
68. Okajima A, Miyazawa K, Kitamura N. Primary structure of rat hepatocyte growth factor and induction of its mRNA during liver regeneration following hepatic injury. Eur J Biochem 1990;193:375–81.
69. Zarnegar R, Defrances MC, Kost DP, Lindroos P, Michalopoulos GK. Expression of hepatocyte growth factor mRNA in regenerating rat liver after partial hepatectomy. Biochem Biophys Res Commun 1991;177:559–65.
70. Tsubouchi H, Niitani Y, Hirono S, et al. Levels of the human hepatocyte growth factor in serum of patients with various liver diseases determined by an enzyme-linked immunosorbent assay. Hepatology 1991;13:1–5.
71. Ishiki Y, Ohnishi H, Muto Y, Matsumoto K, Nakamura T. Direct evidence that hepatocyte growth factor is a hepatotrophic factor for liver regeneration and has a potent antihepatitis effect in vivo. Hepatology 1992;16:1227–35.
72. Nagaike M, Hirao S, Tajima H, et al. Renotropic functions of hepatocyte growth factor in renal regeneration after unilateral nephrectomy. J Biol Chem 1991;266:22781–4.

73. Di Renzo MF, Olivero M, Ferro S, et al. Overexpression of the c-MET/HGF receptor gene in human thyroid carcinomas. Oncogene 1992;7:2549–53.
74. Kuniyasu H, Yasui W, Kitadai Y, Yokozaki H, Ito H, Tahara E. Frequent amplification of the c-met gene in scirrhous type stomach cancer. Biochem Biophys Res Commun 1992;189:227–32.
75. Soman NR, Correa P, Ruiz BA, Wogan GN. The TPR-MET oncogenic rearrangement is present and expressed in human gastric carcinoma and precursor lesions. Proc Natl Acad Sci USA 1991;88:4892–6.
76. Uehara Y, Kitamura N. Expression of a human hepatocyte growth factor/ scatter factor cDNA in MDCK epithelial cells influences cell morphology, motility, and anchorage-independent growth. J Cell Biol 1992;117:889–94.
77. Tsarfaty I, Rong S, Resau JH, et al. Met mediated signaling in mesenchymal to epithelial cell conversion. Science 1994;263:98–101.
78. Jeffers M, Rong S, Vande Woude GF. Enhanced tumorigenicity and invasion-metastasis by hepatocyte growth factor/scatter factor-Met signalling in human cells concomitant with induction of the urokinase proteolysis network. Mol Cell Biol 1996;16:1115–25.
79. Kenworthy P, Dowrick P, Baillie-Johnson H, et al. The presence of scatter factor in patients with metastatic spread to the pleura. Br J Cancer 1992; 66:243–47.

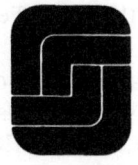

19

The Biology of Vascular Endothelial Growth Factor, a Specific Regulator of Angiogenesis

NAPOLEONE FERRARA

The establishment of a vascular supply is required for organ development and differentiation as well as for tissue repair and reproductive functions in the adult (1–3). Neovascularization (angiogenesis) is also implicated in the pathogenesis of a number of disorders: proliferative retinopathies, age-related macular degeneration, tumors, rheumatoid arthritis, and psoriasis. In the case of proliferative retinopathies and age-related macular degeneration, the new blood vessels are responsible for many of the destructive events characteristic of these conditions, as leakage and bleeding may ultimately lead to retinal detachment or irreversible damage to the macula (4). Conversely, in neoplasms neovascularization provides nourishment to the growing tumor, thus allowing tumor cells to express their critical growth advantage (2, 3). Accordingly, a strong correlation has been noted between density of microvessels in primary breast cancers and their nodal metastases and patient survival (5, 6). Similarly, a correlation has been reported between vascularity and invasive behavior in several other tumors (7–11).

A variety of factors have been previously identified as potential positive regulators of angiogenesis (1–3). This chapter reviews the molecular properties of vascular endothelial growth factor (VEGF), an endothelial cell mitogen and angiogenesis inducer, and discusses its role in normal and pathologic angiogenesis (12–15). VEGF and its receptors appear to play a major role in the regulation of physiologic angiogenesis, such as embryonic and reproductive angiogenesis (16–18). Also, VEGF administration is sufficient to achieve therapeutic end points in animal models of coronary or limb ischemia (19–22). Furthermore, recent studies point to VEGF as a key mediator of neovascularization associated with a variety of disorders (23–25).

Biologic Activities of VEGF

VEGF is a potent mitogen [median effective dose (ED_{50}) 2 to 10 pM] for vascular endothelial cells derived from small or large vessels but is apparently devoid of appreciable mitogenic activity for other cell types. VEGF is also able to induce angiogenesis in a variety of in vivo models (26–28). VEGF has been shown to promote angiogenesis in a tridimensional in vitro model (29). Also, VEGF induces sprouting from rat aortic rings embedded in a collagen gel (30). This model emphasizes the specificity of the growth factor for endothelial cells, as the proliferation induced by VEGF consisted almost exclusively of vascular endothelial cells (30).

Furthermore, VEGF induces expression of the serine proteases urokinase-type and tissue-type plasminogen activators (PA) and of PA inhibitor-1 (PAI-1) in cultured bovine microvascular endothelial cells (31). Also, VEGF induces expression of the metalloproteinase interstitial collagenase in human umbilical vein endothelial cells but not in dermal fibroblasts (32). Recent studies have shown that VEGF induces expression of urokinase receptor in vascular endothelial cells (33).

VEGF has been independently purified and cloned as a vascular permeability factor (VPF) based on its ability to induce vascular leakage in guinea pig skin (34, 35). It has been proposed that an increase in microvascular permeability is a crucial step in angiogenesis associated with tumors and wounds (36, 37). According to this hypothesis, a major function of VEGF in angiogenesis is to induce plasma protein leakage. This would result in the formation of an extravascular fibrin gel, a substrate for endothelial and tumor cell growth.

Additional effects of VEGF on the vascular endothelium are the stimulation of hexose transport (38) and the induction of tissue factor expression (39).

Interestingly, VEGF has also been shown to induce vasodilatation in vitro in a dose-dependent fashion (40). This results in a transient hypotension in vivo (unpublished observations). Such effects appear to be mediated primarily by endothelial cell-derived nitrous oxide (NO), as assessed by the requirement for an intact endothelium and the prevention of the effect by N-methyl-arginine (41).

It has been recently shown (42) that the mitogenic and the permeability-enhancing activity of VEGF can be potentiated by placenta growth factor (PlGF), a molecule having significant structural homology with VEGF (43). While PlGF has little or no direct mitogenic or permeability-enhancing activity, it significantly potentiates the activity of low, marginally efficacious, concentrations of VEGF (42).

The VEGF Proteins

By alternative messenger RNA (mRNA) splicing of a single gene, VEGF may exist as one of four different molecular species, having respectively 121, 165, 189, and 206 amino acids (VEGF$_{121}$, VEGF$_{165}$, VEGF$_{189}$, VEGF$_{206}$) (26, 43, 44). VEGF purified from a variety of species and sources is a basic, heparin-binding, homodimeric glycoprotein of 45,000 daltons (13). These properties correspond to those of $VEGF_{165}$, the predominant isoform. $VEGF_{121}$ is a weakly acidic polypeptide that fails to bind to heparin (48). $VEGF_{189}$ and $VEGF_{206}$ are more basic and bind to heparin with greater affinity than $VEGF_{165}$ (45). $VEGF_{121}$ is secreted as a freely soluble protein in the conditioned medium of transfected cells. $VEGF_{165}$ is also secreted but a significant fraction remains bound to the cell surface or the extracellular matrix (ECM). In contrast, $VEGF_{189}$ and $VEGF_{206}$ are almost completely sequestered in the ECM (46). However, they may be released from the bound state by suramin, heparin or heparinase. Furthermore, these longer forms may be released in a biologically active form by plasmin cleavage (45, 46). Recent studies have shown that the bioactive product of plasmin action is composed of the 110 NH_2 terminal amino acids of VEGF (unpublished observations). Plasminogen activation and generation of plasmin have been shown to play an important role in the angiogenesis cascade (47). However, loss of heparin binding, whether due to alternative splicing or plasmin cleavage, results in a substantial loss of mitogenic activity for vascular endothelial cells (unpublished observations).

Interestingly, evidence has been provided for the existence in the conditioned medium of a rat glioma cell line of heterodimers between VEGF and PlGF (48). The VEGF.PlGF heterodimer was ~7-fold less potent than the VEGF homodimer in promoting endothelial cell growth.

Regulation of VEGF Expression

Oxygen tension has been shown to play a major role in the regulation of VEGF gene expression, both in vitro and in vivo. VEGF messenger RNA (mRNA) expression is rapidly and reversibly induced by exposure to low pO_2 in a variety of cultured cells (49–51). Occlusion of the left anterior descending coronary artery results in a dramatic increase in VEGF RNA levels in the pig myocardium, suggesting that VEGF is a mediator of the spontaneous revascularization that follows myocardial ischemia (52).

Goldberg and Schneider (53) have shown that similarities exist between the mechanisms leading to hypoxic regulation of VEGF and erythropoietin (Epo). Also, hypoxia-inducibility appears to be conferred to both genes by homologous sequences. A 28-base sequence has been identified in the 5' promoter of the rat VEGF gene, which mediated hypoxia-induced transcription in transient assays (54). Such sequence reveals a high degree of homology and similar protein binding characteristics as the hypoxia-inducible factor-1 (HIF-1) binding site within the Epo gene, which behaves like a classic 3' transcriptional enhancer (55). HIF-1 has been identified as a mediator of transcriptional responses to hypoxia (56). Also, activation of c-Src has been shown to participate in the hypoxic upregulation of VEGF gene expression (57).

Several cytokines of growth factors upregulate VEGF mRNA expression and/or induce release of VEGF protein. Exposure of quiescent human keratinocytes to serum, epidermal growth factor (EGF), transforming growth factor-β (TNF-β) or keratinocyte growth factor (KGF) resulted in a marked induction of VEGF mRNA expression (58). In addition, treatment of quiescent cultures of several epithelial and fibroblastic cell lines with TGF-β resulted in induction of VEGF mRNA and release of VEGF protein into the medium (59). Furthermore, interleukin-1β (IL-1β) induces VEGF expression in aortic smooth muscle cells (60).

Differentiation appears to play a pivotal role in the regulation of VEGF gene expression, at least in some models of cellular differentiation (61). The VEGF mRNA was markedly upregulated during the conversion of 3T3 preadipocytes into adipocytes. Conversely, VEGF gene expression was dramatically suppressed during the differentiation of the pheochromocytoma cell line PC12 into nonmalignant, neuron-like, cells. These studies also indicate that induction of VEGF mRNA expression requires pathways mediated by both protein kinase C and protein kinase A activation (61).

Specific transforming events also result in induction of VEGF gene expression. For example, a mutated form of the murine p53 tumor suppressor gene (ala135 > val) has been shown to induce VEGF mRNA expression and potentiate phorbol ester stimulated VEGF mRNA expression in NIH 3T3 cells in transient transfection assays (62). Likewise, oncogenic mutation or amplification of H*ras* led to VEGF upregulation in rat-1 cells (unpublished observations). It is tempting to speculate that VEGF-induced angiogenesis is a final common pathway for multiple and apparently unrelated alterations in cell growth regulatory pathways, leading to uncontrolled in vivo proliferation and tumorigenesis.

The VEGF Receptors

Two classes of high-affinity VEGF binding sites have been identified on the cell surface of cultured bovine endothelial cells (63, 64). The K_d values are 10 pM and 100 pM, respectively (63, 64). Thieme et al. (65) have recently shown that hypoxia increases VEGF receptor number by 50%, without changing the affinity, in cultured bovine retinal capillary endothelial cells.

In agreement with the hypothesis that VEGF is an endothelial cell-specific factor, ligand autoradiography studies on fetal and adult rat tissue sections have demonstrated that high-affinity VEGF binding sites are localized to the vascular endothelium of large or small vessels, but not to other cell types (66, 67).

Two tyrosine kinases have been identified as VEGF receptors (68–71). The fms-like tyrosine kinase (Flt-1) and kinase domain region (KDR) proteins have been shown to bind VEGF with high affinity (68, 69). Fetal liver kinase-1 (Flk-1), the murine homologue of KDR, also binds VEGF (70,

71). Both Flt-1 and KDR/Flk-1 have seen immunoglobulin (Ig)-like domains in the extracellular domain (ECD), a single transmembrane region
and a tyrosine kinase sequence that is interrupted by a kinase-insert domain
(68–71). In addition, a soluble form of Flt-1, consisting of the six
NH_2-terminal domains in the ECD, has been identified in human umbilical
vein endothelial cells (72).

The Flt-1 and KDR proteins have been shown to have different signal
transduction properties (73). Porcine aortic endothelial cells lacking endogenous VEGF receptors display chemotaxis and mitogenesis in response to
VEGF when transfected with an expression vector coding for KDR. In
contrast, transfected cells expressing Flt-1 lack such responses (73, 74).
While KDR/Flk-1 undergoes strong ligand-dependent tyrosine phosphorylation in intact cells (70, 71), Flt-1 reveals a very weak or undetectable
response (68, 73, 74). Transfection of Flt-1 cNDA in NIH 3T3 led to a weak
VEGF-dependent tyrosine phosphorylation that did not generate any
mitogenic signal (74). Accordingly, PlGF, which binds with high affinity to
Flt-1 but not to KDR/Flk-1, lacks direct mitogenic or permeability-
enhancing properties or the ability to effectively stimulate tyrosine phosphorylation in endothelial cells (41). These findings indicate that interaction
with KDR/Flk-1 is a critical requirement to elicit the full spectrum of VEGF
biologic responses.

Recent studies have demonstrated that both Flt-1 and KDR/Flk-1 are
essential for normal development of embryonic vasculature, although their
respective roles appear to be distinct (75, 76). Mouse embryos homozygous
for a targeted mutation in the Flt-1 locus died in utero at day 8.5 (75).
Endothelial cells developed in both embryonic and extraembryonic sites but
failed to organize in normal vascular channels. Mice in which the Flk-1 gene
had been inactivated revealed a more profound deficit, as they not only
lacked vasculogenesis but also failed to develop blood islands (76). Hematopoietic precursors were severely disrupted and organized blood vessels
failed to develop throughout the embryo or the yolk sac, resulting in death
in utero between day 8.5 and 9.5.

Expression of VEGF During Physiologic Circumstances

VEGF mRNA is expressed within the first few days following implantation
in the giant cells of the trophoblast (16, 67). At later developmental stages
in mouse and rat embryos, the VEGF mRNA is expressed in a variety of
organs, including heart, vertebral column, kidney, and along the surface of
the spinal cord and brain. In the developing mouse brain, the highest levels
of mRNA expression are associated with the choroid plexus and the
ventricular epithelium (16, 67).

In the human fetus (16 to 22 weeks), VEGF mRNA expression is
detectable in virtually all tissues and is most abundant in lung, kidney, and

spleen. VEGF protein, as assessed by immunocytochemistry, is expressed in epithelial cells and myocytes, but not vascular endothelial cells (77). Interestingly, VEGF expression is also detectable, both in the fetus and in the adult, around microvessels in areas where endothelial cells are quiescent, such as kidney glomerulus, pituitary, heart, lung, and brain (13, 77, 78). These findings raise the possibility that VEGF is required not only to induce active vascular proliferation but also for the maintenance of the differentiated state of blood vessels, at least in some circumstances (13).

In situ hybridization studies on the rat and primate ovary (17, 79) have shown that VEGF mRNA expression is temporally and spatially related to the proliferation of microvessels. Minimal hybridization was detected in avascular granulosa cells of preovulatory follicles while a strong hybridization signal was present in the corpus luteum, where 50% to 60% of the total cell population is represented by capillary endothelial cells and pericytes. These findings suggest that VEGF is involved in a major physiologic event such as corpus luteum angiogenesis.

Cultured human keratinocytes express VEGF mRNA, suggesting that VEGF may be important in processes such as wound healing (58). Interestingly, decreased expression of VEGF mRNA has been observed in the skin of genetically diabetic db/db mice (58). Therefore, an altered regulation of VEGF gene expression could contribute to the defective angiogenesis and impaired wound healing characteristic of this genetic disorder.

The Role of VEGF in Pathologic Angiogenesis

Angiogenesis Associated with Tumors

In situ hybridization studies have shown that the VEGF mRNA is markedly upregulated in most human tumors examined. These include renal, bladder, breast, ovarian, and gastrointestinal tract carcinomas (80), and several intracranial tumors including glioblastoma multiforme (50, 81, 82) and sporadic as well as von Hippel-Lindau syndrome–associated capillary hemangioblastoma (83, 84). Only sections of lobular carcinoma of the breast and papillary carcinoma of the bladder failed to reveal significant VEGF mRNA expression (80). In all of these circumstances, VEGF mRNA is expressed by tumor cells but not by endothelial cells. Interestingly, the VEGF protein is detectable by immunohistochemistry not only in the tumor cells but also in the vasculature (50, 80). This discrepancy indicates that tumor-secreted VEGF accumulates in the target cells. A strong correlation exists between degree of vascularization of the malignancy and VEGF mRNA expression (83). In addition, the mRNA for the VEGF receptors, Flt-1 and KDR, is upregulated in the tumor vasculature (80, 81, 85). These findings are consistent with the hypothesis that VEGF-expressing tumor cells may have a growth advantage in vivo due to stimulation of angiogenesis (86).

More direct evidence for a role of VEGF in tumorigenesis has been made possible by the availability of specific monoclonal antibodies capable of inhibiting VEGF-induced angiogenesis in vivo and in vitro (87). Such antibodies exert a dramatic inhibitory effect on the growth of a variety of human tumor cell lines injected subcutaneously in nude mice, including glioblastoma multiforme, rhabdomyosarcoma, leiomyosarcoma, and colon and ovarian carcinoma (23, 85). Neither the antibodies nor VEGF itself had any effect on the in vitro growth of the tumor cells. In agreement with the hypothesis that inhibition of angiogenesis is the mechanism of tumor suppression, the density of microvessels was significantly lower in sections of tumors from antibody-treated animals as compared with controls (23, 85).

It has been shown that VEGF is a major mediator of the in vivo growth of human colon carcinoma cells in a nude mouse model of liver metastasis (85). Treatment with anti-VEGF monoclonal antibodies resulted in a dramatic decrease in the number and size of metastases. Most of the tumors in the treated group were under 1 mm in diameter and all were under 3 mm. Also, neither blood vessels nor Flk-1 mRNA expression could be demonstrated in such metastases.

An independent verification of the hypothesis that VEGF action is necessary for tumorigenesis has been provided by the finding that retrovirus-mediated expression of a negative dominant Flk-1 mutant suppresses growth of glioblastoma cells in vivo (88).

Angiogenesis Associated with Other Conditions

Diabetes mellitus, occlusion of the central retinal vein, and prematurity with subsequent exposure to oxygen can all be associated with intraocular vascular proliferation (89). The new blood vessels may lead to vitreous hemorrhage, retinal detachment, neovascular glaucoma, and eventual blindness (4). Diabetic retinopathy is the leading cause of blindness in the working population (90). All of these conditions are known to be associated with retinal ischemia (91). As early as 1948, Michaelson (92) proposed that the key event in pathogenesis of such disorders is the release, by the ischemic retina, of diffusible angiogenic factor(s). Until now, the identity of such factor(s) has been unknown. VEGF, by virtue of its diffusible nature and hypoxia inducibility, is an attractive candidate. Recently, elevations of VEGF levels in the aqueous and vitreous of eyes with proliferative retinopathy have been reported (24, 93, 94). In a large series in which 164 patients and 210 samples of ocular fluid were examined, a strong correlation was found between levels of immunoreactive VEGF in the aqueous and vitreous humors and active proliferative retinopathy (24). In agreement with these findings, in situ hybridization studies demonstrated upregulation of VEGF mRNA in the retina of patients with proliferative retinopathies secondary to diabetes, central retinal vein occlusion, retinal detachment, or intraocular tumors (95).

More direct evidence for the hypothesis that VEGF is a mediator of intraocular neovascularization has been provided in a primate model of iris neovascularization that closely mimics human disease and in a mouse model of retinopathy of prematurity. In the former model, intraocular administration of anti-VEGF antibodies dramatically inhibited the neovascularization that follows occlusion of central retinal veins (96). Likewise, soluble Flt-1 or Flk-1 fused to an IgG suppressed retinal angiogenesis in the mouse model (97). Therefore, treatment with inhibitors of VEGF may prevent the consequences of neovascularization secondary to ischemic retinal disorders.

It has been proposed that VEGF is involved in the angiogenesis associated with rheumatoid arthritis (98, 99). Levels of immunoreactive VEGF were high in the rheumatoid synovial fluid while they were very low or undetectable in the synovial fluid of patients affected by other forms of arthritis or by degenerative joint disease.

It has been also shown that VEGF mRNA expression is increased in psoriatic skin (80). Increased vascularity and permeability are characteristic of psoriasis. Also, elevations in VEGF expression in the skin have been recently described in three bullous disorders: bullous pemphigoid, erythema multiforme, and dermatitis herpetiformis (100).

Interestingly, Lyttle et al. (101) have identified at least two sequences having a significant homology to VEGF in the genome of *orf* virus, a parapoxvirus that affects goats, sheeps, and occasionally humans. Intriguingly, the lesions of goats and humans following *orf* virus infection are characterized by extensive microvascular proliferation in the skin, raising the possibility that the product of the viral VEGF-like gene is responsible for such lesions.

VEGF as a Therapeutic Agent

Growth factors able to promote the growth of new collateral vessels would be potentially of major therapeutic value for the treatment of disorders characterized by inadequate tissue perfusion. For example, chronic limb ischemia, most frequently secondary to obstructive atherosclerosis affecting the superficial femoral artery, is associated with a high rate of morbidity and mortality and treatment is currently limited to surgical revascularization or endovascular interventional therapy (102). No pharmacological therapy has been shown to be effective for this condition. Intraarterial or intramuscular administration of rhVEGF$_{165}$ significantly augments perfusion and development of collateral vessels in a rabbit model where chronic hindlimb ischemia was created by surgical removal of the femoral artery (21, 103). Arterial gene transfer with a cDNA encoding VEGF$_{165}$ also led to revascularization of rabbit ischemic limbs (22). In addition, the angiogenesis initiated by the administration of VEGF results in improved muscle function as well as increased exercise-induced hyperemia (104). Similarly, it has been shown that both maximal flow velocity and maximal blood flow, as assessed by Doppler, are significantly increased in ischemic limbs following VEGF administration (91). Thus, the neovascularization seen in response to rhVEGF$_{165}$ results in improvements of clinically relevant physiologic parameters. Recent studies have shown that VEGF administration also leads to a recovery of normal endothelial reactivity in dysfunctional endothelium (105).

Furthermore, intraluminal VEGF administration promotes increase in coronary blood flow in a dog model of coronary insufficiency (19). In addition, Harada et al. (20) have recently demonstrated that extraluminal administration of as little as 2 μg of rhVEGF results in a significant increase in coronary blood flow in a pig model of chronic myocardial ischemia created by ameroid occlusion of the proximal circumflex artery. In this model, VEGF treatment led to 2.6-fold decrease in the size of left ventricular infarct (20).

An additional potential therapeutic application of VEGF is the prevention of restenosis following percutaneous transluminal angioplasty (PTA). It has been proposed that damage to the endothelium is the crucial event triggering fibrocellular intimal proliferation (106). Interestingly, VEGF administration accelerates re-endothelialization and attenuates intimal hyperplasia in balloon-injured rat carotid artery (107) or rabbit aorta (108). Therefore, it is tempting to speculate that rapid re-endothelialization promoted by VEGF may prove effective at preventing the cascade of events leading to neointima formation and restenosis in patients.

Conclusion

The recent finding that targeted mutations inactivating the VEGF receptors genes result in a profound deficit in vasculogenesis and blood island formation, leading to early intrauterine death, emphasizes the pivotal role played by the VEGF/VEGF-receptor system in the development of the vascular system.

An intriguing possibility is that the VEGF protein or gene therapy with a VEGF cDNA may be used in the future to promote endothelial cell growth and collateral vessel formation. This would represent a novel therapeutic modality for conditions that frequently are refractory to conservative measures and unresponsive to pharmacologic therapy.

The high expression of VEGF mRNA in the vast majority of human tumors, and the presence of the VEGF protein in ocular fluids of individuals with proliferative retinopathies and in the synovial fluid of RA patients support the hypothesis that VEGF is a key mediator of angiogenesis associated with various pathologic conditions. The ability of anti-

VEGF antibodies or soluble VEGF receptors to block tumor growth or neovascularization associated with ischemic retinal disorders provide more compelling evidence for such hypothesis. Therefore, VEGF antagonists have the potential to be of therapeutic value for a variety of highly vascularized and aggressive malignancies as well as for other angiogenic disorders.

References

1. Folkman J, Shing Y. Angiogenesis. J Biol Chem 1992;267:10931–4.
2. Klagsbrun M, D'Amore PA. Regulators of angiogenesis. Annu Rev Physiol 1991;53:217–39.
3. Folkman J. What is the evidence that tumors are angiogenesis-dependent? J Natl Cancer Inst 1991;82:4–6.
4. Garner A. Vascular diseases. In: Garner A, Klintworth GK, eds. Pathobiology of ocular disease. A dynamic approach, 2nd ed. New York: Marcel Dekker, 1994:1625–710.
5. Weidner N, Semple P, Welch W, Folkman J. Tumor angiogenesis and metastasis. Correlation in invasive breast carcinoma. N Engl J Med 1991; 324:1–6.
6. Weidner N, Folkman J, Pozza F, et al. Tumor angiogenesis: a new significant and independent prognostic indicator in early-stage breast carcinoma. J Natl Cancer Inst 1992;84:1875–88.
7. Wakui S, Furusato M, Sasaki H, et al. Tumor angiogenesis in prostatic carcinoma with and without bone metastasis: a morphometric study. J Pathol 1992;168:257–62.
8. Chodak GW, Haudenschild C, Gittes RF, Folkman J. Angiogenic activity as a marker of neoplastic and preneoplastic lesions of the human bladder. Ann Surg 1980;192:762–71.
9. Macchiarini P, Fontanini G, Hardin MJ, Squartini F, Angeletti CA. Relation of neovascularization to metastasis of non-small cell lung carcinoma. Lancet 1992;340:145–6.
10. Sillman F, Boyce J, Fruchter R. The significance of atypical vessels and neovascularization in cervical neoplasias. Am J Obstet Gynecol 1981; 139:154–7.
11. Smith-McCune KS, Weidner N. Demonstration and characterization of the angiogenic properties of cervical dysplasia. Cancer Res 1994;54:804–8.
12. Ferrara N, Henzel WJ. Pituitary follicular cells secrete a novel heparin-binding growth factor specific for vascular endothelial cells. Biochem Biophys Res Commun 1989;161:851–9.
13. Ferrara N, Houck K, Jakeman L, Leung DW. Molecular and biological properties of the vascular endothelial growth factor family of proteins. Endocr Rev 1992;13:18–32.
14. Plöuet J, Schilling J, Gospodarowicz D. Isolation and characterization of a newly identified endothelial cell mitogen produced by AtT20 cells. EMBO J 1989;8:3801–7.
15. Conn G, Bayne M, Soderman L, et al. Amino acid and cDNA sequence of a vascular endothelial cell mitogen homologous to platelet-derived growth factor. Proc Natl Acad Sci USA 1990;87:2628–32.

16. Breier G, Albrecht U, Sterrer S, Risau W. Expression of vascular endothelial growth factor during embryonic angiogenesis and endothelial cell differentiation. Development 1992;114:521-32.
17. Phillips HS, Hains J, Leung DW, Ferrara N. Vascular endothelial growth factor is expressed in rat corpus luteum. Endocrinology 1990;127:965-68.
18. Shweiki D, Itin A, Neufeld G, Gitay-Goren H, Keshet E. Patterns of expression of vascular endothelial growth factor (VEGF) and VEGF receptors in mice suggest a role in hormonally regulated angiogenesis. J Clin Invest 1993;91:2235-43.
19. Banai S, Jaktlish MT, Shou M, et al. Angiogenic-induced enhancement of collateral blood flow to ischemic myocardium by vascular endothelial growth factor in dogs. Circulation 1994;89:2183-9.
20. Harada K, Friedman M, Lopez J, et al. Vascular endothelial growth factor improves coronary flow and myocardial function in chronically ischemic porcine hearts. Am J Physiol 1996;270:H1791-802.
21. Takeshita S, Zhung L, Brogi E, et al. Therapeutic angiogenesis: a single intra-arterial bolus of vascular endothelial growth factor augments collateral vessel formation in a rabbit ischemic hindlimb model. J Clin Invest 1994;93:662-70.
22. Takeshita S, Zheng LP, Cheng D, et al. Therapeutic angiogenesis following arterial gene transfer of vascular endothelial in a rabbit model of hindlimb ischemia. Biochem Biophys Res Commun 1996;227:628-35.
23. Kim KJ, Li B, Winer J, et al. Inhibition of vascular endothelial growth factor-induced angiogenesis suppresses tumour growth in vivo. Nature 1993;362:841-4.
24. Aiello LP, Avery R, Arrigg R, et al. Vascular endothelial growth factor in ocular fluid of patients with diabetic retinopathy and other retinal disorders. N Engl J Med 1994;331:1480-7.
25. Ferrara N. Vascular endothelial growth factor—the trigger for neovascularization in the eye. Lab Invest 1995;72:615-18.
26. Leung DW, Cachianes G, Kuang W-J, Goeddel DV, Ferrara N. Vascular endothelial growth factor is a secreted angiogenic mitogen. Science 1989; 246:1306-9.
27. Phillips GD, Stone AM, Jones BD, Schultz JC, Whitehead RA, Knighton DR. Vascular endothelial growth factor (rhVEGF165) stimulates direct angiogenesis in the rabbit cornea. In Vivo 1995;8:961-5.
28. Connolly DT, Heuvelman DM, Nelson R, et al. Tumor vascular permeability factor stimulates endothelial cell growth and angiogenesis. J Clin Invest 1989;84:1470-8.
29. Pepper MS, Ferrara N, Orci L, Montesano R. Potent synergism between vascular endothelial growth factor and basic fibroblast growth factor in the induction of angiogenesis in vitro. Biochem Biophys Res Commun 1992; 189:824-31.
30. Nicosia RF, Nicosia SV, Smith M. Vascular endothelial growth factor, platelet-derived growth factor and insulin-like growth factor-1 promote rat aortic angiogenesis in vitro. Am J Pathol 1995;145:1023-29.
31. Pepper MS, Ferrara N, Orci L, Montesano R. Vascular endothelial growth factor (VEGF) induces plasminogen activators and plasminogen activator inhibitor type 1 in microvascular endothelial cells. Biochem Biophys Res Commun 1991;181:902-8.

32. Unemori E, Ferrara N, Bauer EA, Amento EP. Vascular endothelial growth factor induces interstitial collagenase expression in human endothelial cells. J Cell Physiol 1992;153:557–62.

33. Mandriota S, Montesano R, Orci L, et al. Vascular endothelial growth factor increses urokinase receptor expression in vascular endothelial cells. J Biol Chem 1995;270:9709–16.

34. Connolly DT, Olander JV, Heuvelman D, et al. Human vascular permeability factor. Isolation from U937 cells. J Biol Chem 1989;254:20017–24.

35. Keck PJ, Hauser SD, Krivi G, et al. Vascular permeability factor, an endothelial cell mitogen related to platelet derived growth factor. Science 1989;246:1309–12.

36. Senger DR, Galli SJ, Dvorak AM, Perruzzi CA, Harvey VS, Dvorak HF. Tumor cells secrete a vascular permeability factor that promotes accumulation of ascites fluid. Science 1983;219:983–5.

37. Dvorak HF, Harvey VS, Estrella P, Brown LF, McDonagh J, Dvorak AM. Fibrin containing gels induce angiogenesis: implications for tumor stroma generation and wound healing. Lab Invest 1987;57:673–86.

38. Pekala P, Marlow M, Heuvelman D, Connolly D. Regulation of hexose transportin aortic endothelial cells by vascular permeability factor and tumor necrosis factor-alpha, but not by insulin. J Biol Chem 1990;265:18051–4.

39. Clauss M, Gerlach M, Gerlach H, et al. Vascular permeability factor: a tumor-derived polypeptide that induces endothelial cell and monocyte procoagulant activity, and promotes monocyte migration. J Exp Med 1990;172:1535–45.

40. Ku DD, Zaleski JK, Liu S, Brock T. Vascular endothelial growth factor induces EDRF-dependent relaxation of coronary arteries. Am J Physiol 1993;265:H586–92.

41. Park JE, Chen H, Winer J, Houck K, Ferrara N. Placenta growth factor. Potentiation of vascular endothelial growth factor bioactivity, in vitro and in vivo, and high affinity binding to Flt-1 but not to Flk-1/KDR. J Biol Chem 1994;269:25646–54.

42. Maglione D, Guerriero V, Viglietto G, Delli-Bovi P, Persico MG. Isolation of a human placenta cDNA coding for a protein related to the vascular permeability factor. Proc Natl Acad Sci USA 1991;88:9267–71.

43. Tisher E, Mitchell R, Hartmann T, et al. The human gene for vascular endothelial growth factor. J Biol Chem 1991;266:11947–54.

44. Houck KA, Ferrara N, Winer J, Cachianes G, Li B, Leung DW. The vascular endothelial growth factor family: identification of a fourth molecular species and characterization of alternative splicing of RNA. Mol Endocrinol 1991;5:1806–14.

45. Houck KA, Leung DW, Rowland AM, Winer J, Ferrara N. Dual regulation of vascular endothelial growth factor bioavailability by genetic and proteolytic mechanisms. J Biol Chem 1992;267:26031–7.

46. Park JE, Keller G-A, Ferrara N. The vascular endothelial growth factor (VEGF) isoforms: differential deposition into the subepithelial extracellular matrix and bioactivity of ECM-bound VEGF. Mol Biol Cell 1993;4:1317–26.

47. Mignatti P, Tsuboi R, Robbins E, Rifkin DB. In vitro angiogenesis on the human amniotic membrane: requirement for basic fibroblast growth factor-induced proteinases. J Cell Biol 1989;108:671–82.

48. DiSalvo J, Bayne ML, Conn G, et al. Purification and characterization of a

naturally occurring vascular endothelial growth factor placenta growth factor heterodimer. J Biol Chem 1995;270:7717–23.

49. Minchenko A, Bauer T, Salceda S, Caro J. Hypoxic stimulation of vascular endothelial growth factor expression in vivo and in vitro. Lab Invest 1994;71:374–9.

50. Shweiki D, Itin A, Soffer D, Keshet E. Vascular endothelial growth factor induced by hypoxia may mediate hypoxia-initiated angiogenesis. Nature 1992;359:843–5.

51. Shima DT, Adamis AP, Ferrara N, et al. Hypoxic induction of vascular endothelial cell growth factors in the retina: Identification and characterization of vascular endothelial growth factor (VEGF) as the sole mitogen. Mol Med 1995;2:64–71.

52. Banai S, Shweiki D, Pinson A, Chandra M, Lazarovici G, Keshet E. Upregulation of vascular endothelial growth factor expression induced by myocardial ischemia: implications for coronary angiogenesis. Cardiovasc Res 1994;28:1176–9.

53. Goldberg MA, Schneider TJ. Similarities between the oxygen-sensing mechanisms regulating the expression of vascular endothelial growth factor and erythropoietin. J Biol Chem 1994;269:4355–61.

54. Levy AP, Levy NS, Wegner S, Goldberg MA. Transcriptional regulation of the rat vascular endothelial growth factor gene by hypoxia. J Biol Chem 1995;270:13333–40.

55. Madan A, Curtin PT. A 24-base pair sequence 3′ to the human erythropoietin contains a hypoxia-responsive transcriptional enhancer. Proc Natl Acad Sci USA 1993;90:3928–32.

56. Wang GL, Jiang BH, Rue EA, Semenza GL. Hypoxia-inducible factor-1 is a basic helix-loop helix-PAS heterodimer regulated by cellular O_2 tension. Proc Natl Acad Sci USA 1995;92:5510–4.

57. Mukhopadhyay D, Tsilokas L, Zhou X-M, Foster D, Brugge JS, Sukhatme VP. Hypoxic induction of human vascular endothelial growth factor expression through c-Src activation. Nature 1995;375:577–81.

58. Frank S, Hubner G, Breier G, Longaker MT, Greenhalgh DG, Werner S. Regulation of VEGF expression in cultured keratinocytes. Implications for normal and impaired wound healing. J Biol Chem 1995;270:12607–13.

59. Pertovaara L, Kaipainen A, Mustonen T, et al. Vascular endothelial growth factor is induced in response to transforming growth factor-β in fibroblastic and epithelial cells. J Biol Chem 1994;269:6271–4.

60. Li J, Perrella MA, Tsai JC, et al. Induction of vascular endothelial growth factor gene expression by interleukin-1 beta in rat aortic smooth muscle cells. J Biol Chem 1995;270:308–12.

61. Claffey KP, Wilkinson WO, Spiegelman BM. Vascular endothelial growth factor. Regulation by cell differentiation and activated second messenger pathways. J Biol Chem 1992;267:16317–22.

62. Kieser A, Weich H, Brandner G, Marme D, Kolch W. Mutant p53 potentiates protein kinase C induction of vascular endothelial growth factor expression. Oncogene 1994;9:963–9.

63. Vaisman N, Gospodarowicz D, Neufeld G. Characterization of the receptors for vascular endothelial growth factor. J Biol Chem 1990;265:19461–9.

64. Ploüet J, Moukadiri HJ. Characterization of the receptors to vasculotropin on

bovine adrenal cortex-derived capillary endothelial cell. J Biol Chem 1990; 265:22071-5.

65. Thieme H, Aiello LP, Ferrara N, King GL. Comparative analysis of VEGF receptors on retinal and aortic endothelial cells. Diabetes 1995;44:98-103.

66. Jakeman LB, Winer J, Bennett GL, Altar CA, Ferrara N. Binding sites for vascular endothelial growth factor are localized on endothelial cells in adult rat tissues. J Clin Invest 1992;89:244-53.

67. Jakeman LB, Armanini M, Phillips HS, Ferrara N. Developmental expression of binding sites and mRNA for vascular endothelial growth factor suggests a role or this protein in vasculogenesis and angiogenesis. Endocriniology 1993;133:848-59.

68. deVries C, Escobedo JA, Ueno H, Houck KA, Ferrara N, Williams LT. The fms-like tyrosine kinase, a receptor for vascular endothelial growth factor. Science 1992;255:989-91.

69. Terman BI, Vermazen MD, Carrion ME, et al. Identification of the KDR tyrosine kinase as a receptor for vascular endothelial growth factor. Biochem Biophys Res Commun 1992;34:1578-86.

70. Quinn T, Peters KG, de Vries C, Ferrara N, Williams LT. Fetal liver kinase 1 is a receptor for vascular endothelial growth factor and is selectively expressed in vascular endothelium. Proc Natl Acad Sci USA 1993;90:7533-7.

71. Millauer B, Wizigmann-Voos S, Schnurch H, et al. High affinity binding and developmental expression suggest Flk-1 as a major regulator of vasculogenesis and angiogenesis. Cell 1993;72:835-46.

72. Kendell RL, Thomas KA. Inhibition of vascular endothelial growth factor by an endogenously encoded soluble receptor. Proc Natl Acad Sci USA 1993; 90:10705-9.

73. Waltenberger J, Claesson-Welsh L, Siegbahn A, Shibuya M, Heldin C-H. Different signal transduction properties of KDR and Flt1, two receptors for vascular endothelial growth factor. J Biol Chem 1994;269:26988-95.

74. Seetharam L, Gotoh N, Maru Y, Neufeld G, Yamaguchi S, Shibuya M. A unique signal transduction pathway for the FLT tyrosine kinase, a receptor for vascular endothelial growth factor. Oncogene 1995;10:135-47.

75. Fong G-H, Rassant J, Gertenstein M, Breitman M. Role of Flt-1 receptor tyrosine kinase in regulation of assembly of vascular endothelium. Nature 1995;376:66-70.

76. Shalabi F, Rossant J, Yamaguchi TP, et al. Failure of blood island formation and vasculogenesis in Flk-1 deficient mice. Nature 1995;376:62-6.

77. Shifren JL, Doldi N, Ferrara N, Mesiano S, Jaffe RB. In the human fetus, vascular endothelial growth factor (VEGF) is expressed in epithelial cells and myocytes, but not vascular endothelium: implications for mode of action. J Clin Endocrinol Metab 1994;79:316-22.

78. Monacci W, Merrill M, Oldfield E. Expression of vascular permeability factor/vascular endothelial growth factor in normal rat tissues. Am J Physiol 1993;264:C995-1002.

79. Ravindranath N, Little-Ihrig L, Phillips HS, Ferrara N, Zeleznick AJ. Vascular endothelial growth factor mRNA expression in the primate ovary. Endocrinology 1992;131:254-60.

80. Dvorak HF, Brown LF, Detmar M, Dvorak AM. Vascular permeability factor/vascular endothelial growth factor, microvascular permeability and angiogenesis. Am J Pathol 1995;146:1029-39.

81. Plate KH, Breier G, Weich HA, Risau W. Vascular endothelial growth is a potential tumour angiogenesis factor in vivo. Nature 1992;359:845–7.
82. Phillips HS, Armanini M, Stavrou D, Ferrara N, Westphal M. Intense focal expression of vascular endothelial growth factor mRNA in human intracranial neoplasms: association with regions of necrosis. Int J Oncol 1993;2:913–9.
83. Berkman RA, Merrill MJ, Reinhold WC, et al. Expression of the vascular permeability/vascular endothelial growth factor gene in central nervous system neoplasms. J Clin Invest 1993;91:153–9.
84. Wizigmann-Voss S, Breier G, Risau W, Plate K. Up-regulation of vascular endothelial growth factor and its receptors in von Hippel-Lindau disease-associated and sporadic hemangioblastoma. Cancer Res 1994;55:1358–64.
85. Warren RS, Yuan H, Matli MR, Gillett NA, Ferrara N. Regulation by vascular endothelial growth factor of human colon cancer tumorigenesis in a mouse model of experimental liver metastasis. J Clin Invest 1995;95:1789–97.
86. Ferrara N, Winer J, Burton T, et al. Expression of vascular endothelial growth factor does not promote transformation but confers a growth advantage in vivo to chinese hamster ovary cells. J Clin Invest 1993;91:160–70.
87. Kim KJ, Li B, Houck K, Winer J, Ferrara N. The vascular endothelial growth factor proteins: identification of biologically relevant regions by neutralizing monoclonal antibodies. Growth Factors 1992;7:53–64.
88. Millauer B, Shawver LK, Plate KH, Risau W, Ullrich A. Glioblastoma growth is inhibited in vivo by a negative dominant Flk-1 mutant. Nature 1994; 367:576–9.
89. Patz A. Studies on retinal neovascularization. Invest Ophthalmol Vis Sci 1980;19:1133–8.
90. Olk RJ, Lee CM. Diabetic retinopathy: practical management. Philadelphia: Lippincott, 1993.
91. Bauters C, Asahara T, Zheng LP, et al. Physiologic assessment of augmented vascularity induced by VEGF in a rabbit ischemic hindlimb model. Am J Physiol 1994;267:H1263–71.
92. Michaelson IC. The mode of development of the vascular system of the retina with some observations on its significance for certain retinal disorders. Trans Ophthalmol Sci UK 1948;68:137–80.
93. Adamis AP, Miller JW, Bernal M-T, et al. Increased vascular endothelial growth factor in the vitreous of eyes with proliferative diabetic retinopathy. Am J Ophthalmol 1994;118:445–50.
94. Malecaze F, Clemens S, Simorer-Pinotel V, et al. Detection of vascular endothelial growth factor mRNA and vascular endothelial growth factor-like activity in proliferative diabetic retinopathy. Arch Ophthalmol 1994;112:1476–82.
95. Pe'er J, Shweiki D, Itin A, Hemo I, Gnessin H, Keshet E. Hypoxia-induced expression of vascular endothelial growth factor (VEGF) by retinal cells is a common factor in neovascularization. Lab Invest 1995;72:638–45.
96. Adamis AP, Shima DT, Tolentino M, et al. Inhibition of VEGF prevents ocular neovascularization in a primate. Arch Ophthalmol 1996;144:66–71.
97. Aiello LP, Pierce EA, Foley ED, et al. Suppression of retinal neovascularization in vivo by inhibition of vascular endothelial growth factor (VEGF) using soluble VEGF-receptor chimeric proteins. Proc Natl Acad Sci USA. In press.
98. Koch E, Harlow L, Haines GK, et al. Vascular endothelial growth factor: a cytokine modulating endothelial function in rheumatoid arthritis. J Immunol 1994;152:4149–5.

99. Fava RA, Olsen NJ, Spencer-Green G, et al. Vascular permeability factor/ vascular endothelial growth factor (VPF/VEGF): accumulation and expression in human synovial fluids and rheumatoid arthritis. J Exp Med 1994;180:340-6.

100. Brown LF, Harris TJ, Yeo KT, et al. Increased expression of vascular permeability factor (vascular endothelial growth factor) in bullous pemphigoid, dermatitis herpetiformis and erythema multiforme. J Invest Dermatol 1995;104:744-9.

101. Lyttle DJ, Fraser KM, Flemings SB, Mercer AA, Robinson AJ. Homologs of vascular endothelial growth factor are encoded by the poxvirus orf virus. J Virol 1994;68:84-92.

102. Graor RA, Gray BH. Interventional treatment of peripheral vascular disease. In: Young JR, Graor RA, Olin JW, Bartholomew JR, eds. Peripheral vascular diseases. St. Louis: Mosby, 1991:111-33.

103. Takeshita S, Pu L-Q, Stein LA, et al. Intramuscular administration of vascular endothelial growth factor induces dose-dependent collateral artery augmentation in a rabbit model of chronic limb ischemia. Circulation 1994;90:II228-34.

104. Waler CE, Errett CJ, Ogez J, et al. Vascular endothelial growth factor (VEGF) improves blood flow and function in a chronic ischemic hind-limb model. J Cardiovasc Pharmacol 1966;27:91-8.

105. Bauters C, Asahara T, Zheng LP, et al. Recovery of disturbed endothelium-dependent flow in collateral-perfused rabbit ischemic hindlimb following administration of VEGF. Circulation 1995;91:2793-01.

106. Essed CD, Brand MVD, Becker AE. Transluminal coronary angioplasty and early restenosis. Br Heart J 1983;49:93-02.

107. Asahara T, Bauters C, Pastore C, et al. Local delivery of vascular endothelial growth factor accelerates re-endothelialization and attenuates intimal hyperplasia in balloon-injured rat carotid artery. Circulation 1995;91:2802-09.

108. Callow AD, Choi ET, Trachtenberg JD, et al. Vascular permeability factor accelerates endothelial regrowth following balloon angioplasty. Growth Factors 1994;10:223-8.

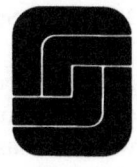

20

FDA Regulatory Concerns for Wound Healing Biologics

Kurt Stromberg

Major recent changes within the Food and Drug Administration (FDA) include the Prescription Drug User Fee Act of 1992 with its associated managed review process, and substantial involvement of the FDA with the International Conference on Harmonization (ICH). Within the Center for Biologics Evaluation and Review (CBER) the effect of the former has been (1) to expand the number of clinical reviewers, (2) to enhance the staff training and computer capabilities, and (3) to facilitate a reorganization of CBER that has streamlined the biologics approval process. The global regulatory activity of the ICH is expected to also result in greater consistency and promptness in regulatory review. Specifically in respect to wound healing, a new development has been the formation of a tricenter Wound Healing Clinical Focus Group in which reviewers from the Centers for Drugs, Devices, and Biologics meet monthly to exchange information and promote consistency. In addition, many FDA documents are now available by FAX: CDER, 301-827-0577; CBER, 301-594-1939; and CDRH, 301-827-0111. These will assist a sponsor in preparing for product submission.

The basic biology of the healing process is unclear and clinical trials of wound healing agents are difficult and expensive to carry out due to the length of treatment, level of compliance, etc. To reduce complexity, several common sense suggestions are offered: (1) focus the clinical indication and enroll a homogeneous patient population; (2) include a standardized care arm at the phase 2 stage to evaluate the effect of the vehicle alone on healing; (3) establish an effective clinical dosage, formulation, and administrative regime prior to phase 3 pivotal trials; and (4) enroll an adequate number of patients to overcome individual patient variability and to obtain adequate statistical power to support the primary end point.

Particular issues in wound healing regulation include (1) product sterility; (2) combinations of wound healing products, in which increasing flexibility is developing on regulation of multiple agent therapy, in part because synergistic interaction and safety concerns for the individual components often can be established in preclinical studies; (3) standard of clinical care, or optimum basic wound care in clinical trials; and (4) product jurisdiction, which is based upon the primary mode of action of the proposed product. These first three topics, among many other issues, are discussed in an article in *Wound Repair and Regeneration* (1994;2:155–64); the last, product jurisdiction, is discussed in a forthcoming article in *Tissue Engineering*.

In summary, changes are under way at the FDA to speed the regulatory process, and to increase the consistency of review. However, the most expeditious path of a sponsor to product approval remains solid basic, preclinical, and clinical science.

FDA Regulation of Growth Factors

As a background for clinical and laboratory investigators, my first aim is to briefly provide an overview of the FDA regulatory process for biologics. What is an IND application and what are the steps in the review process? Second, I address several recent developments at FDA: the ICH and the Prescription Drug User Fee Act of 1992 with its associated managed review process. I then describe how the three FDA centers (CBER, CDER, and CDRH) meet to deal in common with wound healing products. Collectively, these efforts illustrate the increasing integration, consistency, and accessibility of these three FDA centers. Third, I make suggestions for clinical trials of wound healing agents and address FDA concerns particular to wound healing such as topical product sterility, combination products, product jurisdiction among the three centers, and the design and performance of clinical trials.

Recent Clinical Trials

A press release (September 18, 1995) announced the results of a phase 3 trial done under an IND of rhPDGF-BB in nonhealing diabetic foot ulcers. The company (Johnson and Johnson/Chiron) plan is to continue to develop this product. If this PDGF-BB were to go successfully through the subsequent product license application process, it would be the first recombinant biologic or drug approved for a chronic wound indication. On the other hand, in 1994 alone there were 74 new noninteractive products cleared for marketing through the 510k (i.e., premarket notification) process. These dressing-type products are hydrogels, hydrocolloids, occlusive tapes, and porcine products for which there is much experience relating to safety and effectiveness. Only one interactive wound dressing (Biobrain II for third-degree burns) has been approved via the premarket approval (PMA) process. Overall, the biotech INDs received in CBER increased in a linear manner during the 1980s to essentially plateau thus far in the early 1990s. I suspect this was true for wound healing products in particular as well.

Brief Review of the IND Process

Because recombinant growth factors are overwhelmingly regulated as biologics, a brief overview of their regulation by the CBER is appropriate. The statutes that regulate biologic products are section 351 of the PHS Act and the Food, Drug, and Cosmetic Act (FDCA). The former defines biologics and prohibits their interstate transport unless approved and manufactured in a licensed facility. Sections 201 and 301 of the FDCA note that biologics may be drugs or devices according to their intended use. It prohibits interstate commerce of a drug or a device that is misbranded or adulterated. It is important to realize that the definition of interstate commerce also includes shipment of any of a product's components across state lines, as well as the finished product itself. Exemptions to this prohibition are biologics approved as safe and effective for a given indication, i.e., licensed for a defined indication. To permit movement across state lines for products under clinical investigation for determination of their safety and efficacy, an investigational new drug (IND) application is made (Section 505 (i), FDCA). This exempts investigational drugs from the new drug approval requirements, and thus permits their interstate commerce. Section 21 of the Code of Federal Regulations (CFR) Part 601.21 states that investigational biologics also fall within this exemption from new drug regulations. The manufacturing aspects of drug regulation of product purity, potency, consistency, and stability are not considered in this chapter.

The use of an investigational drug in a clinical investigation begins with filing an IND for review. An IND is effective 30 days after filing unless notified by the FDA. The IND review team consists of at least three reviewers: primary product or manufacturing, pharmacology/toxicology, and clinical. In addition, consultant reviewers with special knowledge may be brought into the process. Basically, the questions asked are: What is the product? Can it be consistently made? Does it work in animal models? What is the risk of using it in humans? How would it work in the human body (biological rationale)? How will efficacy be shown? Have good science, statistics, and medicine been employed? In summary, is it safe and effective?

Besides manufacturing deficiencies, grounds for withholding permission for a product to enter clinical trials can be patient risk, unqualified clinical investigators, an inadequate investigator brochure or informed consent form, or lack of information to assess risk. Avoiding these problems comes about by seeking early interaction with FDA in the development process, usually in the form of a pre-IND meeting. These can occur within 4 to 6 weeks after a request is made, and meeting packages should contain information on manufacturing, preclinical work completed, prior experience in humans, the clinical protocol, and most importantly, a list of what issues the sponsor wishes to discuss.

The traditional three phases of clinical investigation are well known. The objectives of phase 1 are primarily devoted to safety considerations, i.e., determining side effects with increasing doses, and the pharmacology of the product. Trials of biologics for dermal ulcers have generally enrolled 15 to 20 patients per arm. Phase 2 objectives are controlled studies designed to identify some measure of patient benefit, to define an active dose and manner of administration, and to learn the common short-term side effects and risks. About 50 to 75 patients per arm have generally been included in phase 2 wound healing trials. Phase 3 generally represents expanded (usually 120 to 150 patients per arm), adequate and well-controlled, statistically powered, studies that determine overall risk-benefit information on safety and efficacy, and provide the basis for product labeling.

FDA Developments

Wound Healing Clinical Focus Group

Changes within the FDA affect the regulation of wound healing products. The regulation of recombinant wound healing biologics is not unique; they are regulated like other recombinant biologics. Overall, I think the FDA is moving toward greater integration, consistency, and more accessibility. In respect to wound healing, an example of this is a tricenter Wound Healing Clinical Focus Group in which reviewers from the Centers for Drugs, Devices, and Biologics meet monthly to exchange information. The aim is to educate one another on the various disciplines within wound healing and to achieve greater regulatory consistency within the three centers. We sponsor conferences, develop FDA response positions vis-à-vis industry, organizational, or academic groups, and invite academic experts to speak on topics such as wound healing animal models, instrumentation to provide quantitative assessments of efficacy of wound closure, and burn wound biology and clinical care.

International Conference on Harmonization

Two major developments within the FDA during the last several years are the International Conference on Harmonization (ICH) and the Prescription Drug User Fee Act of 1992. Changes brought by the ICH will benefit sponsors and regulators alike, a process that began several years ago and is now issuing position statements in nearly final form in the areas of product quality, safety, and efficacy. The impact of these changes will be to smooth and codify the regulatory process of an international basis. Briefly, drug regulatory bodies of the three regions and their respective pharmaceutical trade organizations have been meeting periodically since 1991 to harmonize the drug approval process, and in the process bring new drugs to the market sooner. The objectives are to remove the need for duplicate studies, thus avoiding repetitious clinical studies, reducing animal usage, and making research more economical. In the United States, the ICH/FDA procedures are integrated, and are presented in the Federal Register in proposal form for public comment and then in final form. For example, the Federal Register issues of July 9, 1993, and August 2 and 9, September 22, and November 28, 1994, presented notices about various stages of the ICH process. In summary, this global regulatory activity should expedite the development of wound healing products, which are often sponsored by multinational pharmaceutical corporations.

Prescription Drug User Fee Act of 1992

Within CBER, I believe the effect of the Prescription Drug User Fee Act of 1992 has been to expand the number of clinical reviewers, to enhance the staff training and development programs and computer capabilities, and to facilitate a reorganization of CBER that is intended to streamline the biologics approval process by what is termed the "managed review process." Briefly, this process sets a regulatory framework and timetable for reviewing products. For CBER, a joint PLA/ELA filing will be accepted or rejected with explanations within 45 days, and a decision made within 6 or 12 months depending on whether it receives a priority or standard review. Consequently, if a novel and clearly safe and effective wound healing product is received today, its PLA could be processed to approval within 6 months. CBER's 5-year goal is to have 80% of submissions processed within these time frames by 1996, and 100% by 1998.

In respect to accessibility of information, a wide array of FDA information is now available by fax (Table 20.1). The CBER Fax Information System, or "Fax On DEMAND" number is 301-594-1938, which provides a voice-prompt menu that includes guidelines and Points to Consider documents, Federal Register notices, memoranda, letter to manufacturers, to sponsors, to health professionals, draft background information, etc. In all, 96 documents are listed for CBER alone. The Center for Drug Evaluation and Research (fax 301-827-0577) has a list of guidelines that runs 17 pages. The Center for Devices and Radiological Health's fax on demand number is 301-827-0111, and its list of publications is also extensive. Consequently, the range of information and speed of response of this system are impressive.

Another change for CBER is found in the July 11, 1995, Federal Register announcement that states that pilot manufacturing facilities of recombinant

TABLE 20.1. Points to consider and related documents.

Available without costs for Biologics from the Congressional and Consumer Affairs Branch, HFM-11, Woodmont Office Center, Suite 200 North, 1401 Rockville Pike, Rockville, MD 20852-1448, 301-594-2000 (phone), 301-594-1939 (fax on demand); for Medical Devices from Division of Small Manufacturers Assistance, HFZ-220, 1350 Piccard Drive, Rockville, MD 20850-4307, 800-638-2041 (phone), 800-899-0381 or 301-827-0111 (fax on demand); and for Drug Products from Executive Secretariat Staff, CDER, HFG-8 Room 151, 7520 Standish Place, Rockville, MD 20855, 301-594-1012 (phone), 800-342-2722 or 310-827-0577 (fax on demand). A list of documents and corresponding codes on each facsimile system can be obtained by dialing either "1" (DCER and CDRH) or follow voice-prompts (CBER).

Points to Consider in the Manufacture of In Vitro Monoclonal Antibody Products Subject to Licensure (1983).

Points to Consider in the Manufacture and Testing of Monoclonal Antibody Products for Human Use (1987). Updated 1994.

Points to Consider in the Production and Testing of Interferon Intended for Investigational Use in Humans (1983).

Points to Consider in the Manufacture of In Vitro Monoclonal Antibody Products for Further Manufacture into Blood Grouping Reagent and Anti-Human Globulin (1992).

Points to Consider in the Manufacture and Clinical Evaluation of In Vitro Tests to Detect Antibodies to the Human Immunodeficiency Virus, Type 1 (1989) (draft).

Points to Consider in the Production and Testing of New Drugs and Biologicals Produced by Recombinant DNA Technology (1985).

Supplement to the Points to Consider in the Production and Testing of New Drugs and Biologicals Produced by Recombinant DNA Technology: Nucleic Acid Characterization and Genetic Stability (1992). Update 1995.

Guidelines for Research Involving Recombinant DNA Molecules (1986).

Points to Consider in the Characterization of Cell Lines Used to Produce Biologicals (1993).

Points to Consider in the Collection, Processing, and Testing of Ex Vivo–Activated Mononuclear Leukocytes for Administration to Humans (1989).

FDA, CDER: Guideline for the Format and Content of the Clinical and Statistical Sections of New Drug Applications. July 1988.

Points to Consider in Computer Assisted Submissions for License Applications (1990).

FDA's Policy Statement Concerning Cooperative Manufacturing Arrangements for Licensed Biologicals (1992).

OELPS Advertising and Promotional Labeling Staff Procedural Guide (1993).

Cytokine and Growth Factor Prepivotal Trial Package: With a Special Emphasis on Products Identified for Consideration Under 21 CFR 312 Subpart E. "Drugs Intended to Treat Life-Threatening and Severely Debilitating Illnesses" (1990) (Draft).

Points to Consider in Human Somatic Cell Therapy and Gene Therapy (1991).

Points to Consider in the Safety Evaluation of Hemglobin-Based Oxygen Carriers (1990).

Guildelines on Validation of the Limulus Amebocyte Lysate Test as an End Product Endotoxin Test for Human and Animal Parenteral Drugs, Biological Products, and Medical Devices (1987).

Guideline for Submitting Documentation for the Stability of Human Drugs and Biologics (1987).

Submitting Documentation for Packaging for Human Drugs and Biologicals (1987).

Sterile Drug Products Produced by Aseptic Processing (1987).

Guideline on General Principles of Process Validation (1987).

Test for Residual Moisture for Biological Products (1990).

Draft Guideline for Adverse Experience Reporting for Licensed Biological Products (1995).

TABLE 20.1. (*Continued*)

Draft Guidance for the Preparation of an IDE Submission for an Interactive Wound and
Burn Dressing (CDRH, revised 1995).

Draft Guidance for the Preparation of a Premarket Notification for a Non-Interactive
Wound and Burn Dressing (CDRH, revised 1995).

Three Intercenter Agreements of 1991 Regarding Product Jurisdiction Among the Centers
for Biologics Evaluation and Research, Drug Evaluation and Research, and Devices and
Radiological Health.

CFR, Federal Register Notices, and Articles Relevant to Wound Healing:

56 F.R. 58756 of November 21, 1991 and 21 CFR 3.2 define "Combination Products."

58 F.R. 65514 of December 14, 1993 for regulatory jurisdiction of "minially processed
human tissue."

21 CFR 600.3 (h), Federal Register announcement of October 14, 1993 (58 F.R. 53248)
for definition if somatic cell therapy.

Institutional Review Board approval is described in 21 CFR 56, and that for informed
patient consent is in 21 CFR 50.

60 F.R. 36808 of July 18, 1995, regarding "Public Hearing: Products Comprised of
Living Autologous Cells Manipulated Ex Vivo and Intended for Implantation for
Structural Repair or Reconstruction."

60 F.R. document of July 11, 1995 concerning "Use of Pilot Manufacturing Facilities for
the Development and Manufacture of Biological Products."

Regulatory Concerns in the Development of Topical Recombinant Ophthalmic and
Cutaneous Wound Healing Biologics. *Wound Repair and Regeneration* 1994;2:155–164.

Responses from the Wound Healing Clinical Focus Group at the FDA to the
Government Relations Committee of the Wound Healing Society. *Scars and Stripes*
Autumn 1994;4:5–12.

Product Jurisdiction Considerations for Tissue-Engineered Products. *Tissue Engineering*,
in press.

---

biologics are eligible for licensure if they are qualified, validated, and
operate in accordance with GMPs. This might be thought of as part of a
more general move toward uncoupling of the PLA and ELA approval
process. Thus, the Center for Biologics is considering allowing biotech
products that are well characterized to be regulated under a single application. One would think that many recombinant growth factors for wound
healing would qualify for consideration under these procedures.

Wound Healing Regulatory Concerns

Overall, the only modest success thus far of single growth factors in wound
healing may be related to several issues. The basic biology of the healing
process and its essentials in content and sequence are only emerging and are
very complicated, as this book has demonstrated. Within this context of
relative ignorance and absolute complexity, a number of single biologics
have been evaluated in clinical trials that were themselves full of variables.

To reduce this complexity, and in the process to clarify the results of
clinical trials, several "common sense" suggestions seem appropriate.

1. Narrow the clinical indication and make the patient population as homogeneous as possible. For example, inclusion criteria for a diabetic foot ulcer trial might include (a) assurance that the diabetes is under control via hemoglobin A1c determination; (b) one nonhealing stage III chronic ulcer present for a minimum of about 8 weeks; (c) a narrow size range of approximately 2 to 10 cm^2 in area after sharp surgical debridement; (d) a transcutaneous oxygen tension measurement of, for example, at least 30 mm Hg; (e) infection under control as defined by a wound infection score, or by quantitative bacteriology of less that 100,000 colonies per gram of tissue; (f) as a measure of adequate nutrition, a serum albumin level greater than 3 g/dl; and, most importantly; (g) assurance that pressure off-loading can be maintained. This would require that all principal investigators agree on a uniform definition and manner of debridement and non–weight bearing.

2. Include a standardized care arm at the phase 2 stage to evaluate the effect of the vehicle itself on healing, and to judge the quality of the wound care the patients are receiving.

3. Establish an optimized clinical dosage and treatment method prior to phase 3 "pivotal" trials. This implies that a sponsor has completed dose-ranging in phase 2, and the manner of use and formulation are set. Issues such as whether to use single or multiuse dispensing, whether the product is to be sterile, whether or not a preservative will be included, and other such manufacturing questions should be resolved early in development.

4. Enroll an adequate number of patients to overcome individual patient variability, and to obtain adequate statistical power to support the primary end point.

Beyond these suggestions to clarify clinical trials, I think other relevant issues include product sterility, combinations of wound healing products, standard of clinical care or optimum basic wound care in clinical trials, and product jurisdiction.

As noted in an article in *Wound Repair and Regeneration* (1994; 2:155–64), there currently are insufficient data to support a scientifically based decision concerning a requirement for the sterility of the final formulation of all topical wound healing products. However, the safest approach for a topical product is to make it sterile with a preservative or in a single-use container, and therefore this is strongly recommended. While this recommendation is clearly true for ocular products, it is also probably appropriate for burn wounds. Chronic cutaneous ulcers are microbially contaminated at the outset, and so the issue is one of avoiding an additional microbial load in a product that might further delay healing. This becomes particularly true if a nonsterile product contains particularly invasive pathogenic flora, such as *Staphylococcus aureus* and *Bacteroides fagilis*. In addition, the presence of bacteria can reduce product stability. Consequently, sterility for both recombinant protein(s) and vehicle is recommended also in the case of topical biologics for chronic ulcers. Appropriate preservatives, single-use containers, and a very low bioburden (e.g., less than 10 colony-forming units per gram or milliliter with both aerobic and anaerobic species are examined) are required in topical products that are not manufactured to be sterile. The specific expectations in the nonsterile product, including microbial identity and preservative effectiveness tests, are detailed in the article in Fall, 1994 issue of *Wound Repair and Regeneration* cited above. In addition, there is an FDA Guideline on Sterile Drug Products Produced by Aseptic Processing (Table 20.1), and the USP Preservative Effectiveness Test and the Microbial Limits and Identity Tests, which are also available to guide manufacturers.

With regard to wound healing combination products, it is clear that the topical healing process is mediated by a cascade of multiple endogenous growth factors. The preclinical research of many investigators has documented the additive or synergistic benefit of using multiple growth factors. Consequently, intuition and animal model research provide a rationale for use of more than one biologic, or perhaps their use in a sequential manner, to enhance healing in humans. Traditionally, the constituent biologics of combination products have been examined for their individual contribution to safety and efficacy. I think there is a move toward increasing flexibility on multiple-agent therapy for chronic wound indications. The experimental basis for additive and synergistic interaction among growth factors can be established in preclinical studies, and by increasing dosing to toxic levels in animal models; it is hoped that major safety in humans can be anticipated. The aim should be to reduce, by phase 2–level clinical studies, the number of therapeutic compartments or trial arms so that the phase 3 trials will be sufficiently powered for a robust statistical evaluation.

There is a widely acknowledged need for consensus on standardized wound care for any given type of chronic ulcer or burn wound indication. Good clinical trial science, managed care considerations, and reimbursement concerns drive this need to establish clinical care guidelines. By agreement of all investigative sites to use identical wound care, the contribution of vehicle or formulation, as well as actual product, to the healing process can be determined. In addition, until "optimum" clinical care of a particular type of chronic wound is established, this approach permits a comparison among studies as to what, in fact, is the best care. Having a standardized care arm, over time and in the aggregate, will help establish better guidelines for clinical care. I think the FDA's view is that the standardized care arm should be incorporated into a phase 2–level study, at the same stage when a sponsor is trying to determine the optimal dosage and treatment method.

An aspect of disagreement in wound management is how to debride the chronic wound. Should it be sharp surgical? Done under sterile conditions in the operating room? Done with the assistance of enzymatic products? In fact, these questions lend themselves to analysis by clinical trials, and research is needed to address these issues. Touching upon this is the impact of containment of wound infection, and bacterial "balance" (less than 100,000 colonies per gram of tissue). The treatment impact of debridement and infection are subjects that may be clarified by inclusion of a standardized care arm in wound healing trials.

Wound healing product jurisdiction is important because it governs which of the three FDA centers will review the proposed vulnerary product, and under which regulatory authority, either an IND, NDA, or IDE depending on the product's primary mode of action. For example, if the product is a device that is not a significant risk, a sponsor need not even file an IDE prior to beginning clinical studies. Only permission of the institutional review board of an investigative site is required. Also, the designation of product jurisdiction influences the nature and extent of the regulatory process. For instance, a Premarket Notification Application, i.e., 510(k), for a device that is substantially equivalent to an already legally marketed device will entail less review.

Formal determination of product jurisdiction for a product that is not obvious is obtained through a Request For Designation (from Amanda Peterson, HF-7, Room 14-84, FDA, 5600 Fisher's Lane, Rockville, MD 20857, phone 301-443-1306, and fax 301-594-6807). Each center has a coordinator for product jurisdiction: Eugene Berk for devices (301-594-1190), Janet Jones for drugs (301-594-6758), and Joy Cavagnaro for biologics (301-827-0372). There are intercenter agreements among CDER, CBER, and CDRH that clarify which center will regulate which products. These agreements can be obtained from the Dockets Management Branch, HFA-305, FDA, Room 1-23, 12420 Parklawn Dr., Rockville, MD 20857. In brief, for wound healing products, the Center for Biologics handles recombinant products, and products derived from living tissues and fluids; the Center for Drugs regulates low molecular weight molecules that can be manufactured through organic synthesis; the Center for Devices has traditionally overseen dressings, burn, and bone products.

An area of some controversy is the FDA's regulation of autologous products that have been manipulated, particularly products derived from a patient's own cells or fluids, because these can often merge into the practice of medicine, which is outside of the FDA's purview. To address some of these issues, a public FDA hearing was held on November 16–17, 1995 in Gaithersburg, Maryland, on "Products Comprised of Living Autologous Cells Manipulated Ex Vivo and Intended for Repair or Reconstruction." In respect to wound healing, these waters can become merky as the following hypothetical composite skin product illustrates: a releasate from a patient's platelets, added to a bovine collagen gel matrix that has been impregnated with several protease inhibitors and infiltrated with the patient's ex vivo amplified dermal fibroblasts and then overlaid with allogenic keratinocytes transfected with plasmids expressing relevant human growth factor genes. This obviously extreme example serves to illustrate the profound potential complexity of wound healing regulation and product jurisdiction, and the inevitable shared involvement in the regulatory process of the Centers for Drugs, Biologics, and Devices. I want to emphasize that, despite the complexity of wound healing products, real progress has been made in coordinating tricenter activities to make the regulation of wound healing products more consistent and expeditious.

In summary, wound healing biologic products are not regulated differently than other recombinant biologics. However, as the complexity of the product increases, involving potentially a drug, biologic, and a device component, new regulatory arrangements among the three centers are required, and they are developing. Today's FDA aims to be increasingly fast and responsive, as well as consistent, while remaining science based. Ultimately, the basic requirement for regulatory success with any proposed product is good science in its manufacture and preclinical studies, and good science in clinical trials supporting the product's safety and efficacy.

Acknowledgments. I wish to thank my FDA colleagues Drs. Earl S. Dye, Charles N. Durfor, Angel S. Torres-Cabassa, Gail G. Gantt, Bette A. Goldman, and Louis L. Marzella for their assistance in preparation of this manuscript.

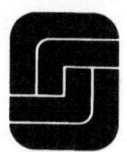

Author Index

345

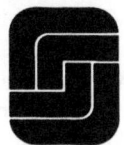

Subject Index